ABC of
Orthopaedics and Trauma

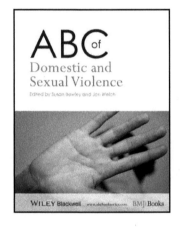
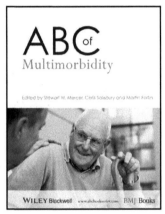
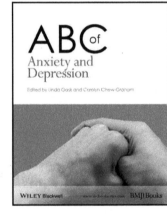
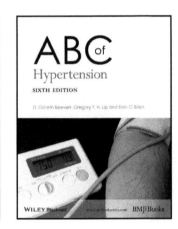
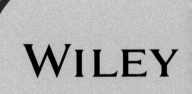

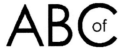

Orthopaedics and Trauma

EDITED BY

Kapil Sugand

MSk Lab, Charing Cross Hospital
Imperial College London
London
UK
and
North West London Rotation
London
UK

Chinmay M. Gupte

MSk Lab, Charing Cross Hospital
Imperial College London
London
UK
and
Imperial College Healthcare NHS Trust
London
UK

WILEY Blackwell

Registered Office(s)
John Wiley & Sons, Inc., 111 River Street, Hoboken, NJ 07030, USA
John Wiley & Sons Ltd, The Atrium, Southern Gate, Chichester, West Sussex, PO19 8SQ, UK

Editorial Office
9600 Garsington Road, Oxford, OX4 2DQ, UK

For details of our global editorial offices, customer services, and more information about Wiley products, visit us at www.wiley.com.

Wiley also publishes its books in a variety of electronic formats and by print-on-demand. Some content that appears in standard print versions of this book may not be available in other formats.

Library of Congress Cataloging-in-Publication Data

Names: Sugand, Kapil, editor. | Gupte, Chinmay M., editor.
Title: ABC of orthopaedics and trauma / edited by Kapil Sugand, Chinmay M. Gupte.
Description: Hoboken, NJ : Wiley 2018. | Series: ABC series | Includes bibliographical references and index. |
Identifiers: LCCN 2018016196 (print) | LCCN 2018016893 (ebook) | ISBN 9781118561218 (epdf) |
    ISBN 9781118561201 (epub) | ISBN 9781118561225 (pbk.)
Subjects: | MESH: Orthopedic Procedures–methods | Musculoskeletal System–injuries | Physical Examination–methods
Classification: LCC RD731 (ebook) | LCC RD731 (print) | NLM WE 168 | DDC 616.7–dc23
LC record available at https://lccn.loc.gov/2018016196

Cover Design: Wiley
Cover Image: Courtesy of Kapil Sugand

Set in 9.25/12pt Minion by SPi Global, Pondicherry, India
Printed and bound by CPI Group (UK) Ltd, Croydon, CR0 4YY

C9781118561225_200224

KS: To my support network: my mother Poonam, family, colleagues and friends for their constant support and faith in me. I thank Mr. Gupte, my supervisor and mentor, for his guidance, motivation, and help.

CMG: To my wife, Thia, and my two wonderful children, India and Adi, for their unbridled support, encouragement and forebearance.

Contents

Foreword

ABC of Orthopaedics and Trauma

Students of medicine have a tough life in many ways: the body of knowledge continues to grow at a pace, so any supposed 'core of knowledge' has a definite date stamp. For this reason, the ABC of Orthopaedics and Trauma, in its first edition, is a useful snapshot of the state of our understanding in 2018 – a world of 3D printing and holograms, as well as the ancient arts of fracture reduction. Chinmay Gupte and Kapil Sugand have assembled a bright group of co-authors who have scoped out each field, and condensed it to be comprehensible and readable introduction to our world. Key to this project has been an editorial style that allows the reader to survey the whole field at a similar level – quite a feat across so many areas.

For every anatomic site, and in both the fields of trauma and orthopaedics, the reader will find the principles of the diseases we treat, and the foundations on which our management strategies are based. So the common approaches and operations for common conditions, are easily accessible, and basic sciences and mechanics are also explained, with illustrations of the important points, and a few key references.

In 2018, a physical library is no longer an essential key to student life, but the core text books continue to have an important place for the successful student – chapter layout and illustrations help us understand and retain information in a structured way. So this book will have a place on the shelves of students around the world, and its physical layout will be part of the memories that will serve its readers for their working life. Congratulations to all the contributors, and happy reading to this new generation of students and clinicians – it is an exciting world. Come and join us!

Prof. Justin P Cobb
Chair, Section of Orthopaedics
MSk Lab, Advancing musculoskeletal research and treatment
Imperial College London

Contributors

Ali Abbasian

Consultant Orthopaedic Surgeon, Guy's & St. Thomas' Hospital, London, UK

Hani B Abdul-Jabar

Consultant Orthopaedic Surgeon, Imperial College Healthcare NHS Trust, London, UK

Sonya Abraham

Consultant in Rheumatology and General Internal Medicine, Imperial College Healthcare NHS Trust, London, UK

Syed Aftab

Royal National Orthopaedic Hospital, Stanmore, UK

Issaq Ahmed

Consultant Orthopaedic Surgeon, Royal Infirmary of Edinburgh, Edinburgh, UK

Adil Ajuied

Consultant Orthopaedic Surgeon, Guy's & St. Thomas' Hospitals, London, UK

Nawfal Al-Hadithy

Orthopaedic Specialist Trainee, Imperial College Healthcare NHS Trust, London, UK

Rajarshi Bhattacharya

Consultant Orthopaedic Surgeon, Imperial College Healthcare NHS Trust, London, UK

Rej Bhumbra

Consultant Orthopaedic Surgeon, Barts Health Orthopaedic Centre, London, UK

Jasvinder Daurka

Imperial College Healthcare NHS Trust, London, UK

Rishi Dhir

Orthopaedic Specialist Trainee, Royal National Orthopaedic Hospital, Stanmore, UK

Alexander L. Dodds

Consultant Orthopaedic Surgeon, Imperial College Healthcare NHS Trust, London, UK

James Donaldson

Consultant Orthopaedic Surgeon, Royal National Orthopaedic Hospital, Stanmore, UK

Bassel El-Osta

Orthopaedic Specialist Trainee, St. George's Hospital, London, UK

Michael Fertleman

Consultant Physician, Imperial College Healthcare NHS Trust, London, UK

Chinmay M. Gupte

Consultant Orthopaedic Surgeon and Senior Clinical Lecturer, MSk Lab, Charing Cross Hospital, Imperial College London, London, UK
and
Imperial College Healthcare NHS Trust, London, UK

Cynthia Gupte

Consultant Radiologist, The Hillingdon Hospitals NHS Foundation Trust, Uxbridge, UK

Simond Jagernauth

Orthopaedic Specialist Trainee, The Royal London Hospital, Barts Health NHS Trust, London, UK

Sanam Kia

Rheumatology Specialist Trainee, Abertawe Bro Morgannwg University, Port Talbot, UK

Anita Khurwal

Orthopaedic Specialist Trainee, North West London Rotation, London, UK

Joshua KL Lee

Consultant Orthopaedic Surgeon, The Royal London Hospital, Barts Health NHS Trust, London, UK

Robert Lee

Consultant Orthopaedic Surgeon, Royal National Orthopaedic Hospital, Stanmore, UK

Shuli Levy

Geriatric Medicine Specialist Trainee, Imperial College Healthcare NHS Trust, London, UK

Georgina Meredith
Geriatric Medicine Specialist Trainee, Imperial College Healthcare NHS Trust, London, UK

David Metcalfe
Orthopaedic Specialist Trainee & NIHR Fellow, University of Warwick, and University of Oxford, UK

Jonathan Miles
Consultant Orthopaedic Surgeon, Royal National Orthopaedic Hospital, Stanmore, UK

Neel Mohan
Consultant Paediatric Orthopaedic Surgeon, St. George's Hospital, London, UK

Simon Mordecai
Orthopaedic Specialist Trainee, North West London Rotation, London, UK

Nadeem Mushtaq
Consultant Orthopaedic Surgeon, Imperial College Healthcare NHS Trust, London, UK

Dinesh Nathwani
Consultant Orthopaedic Surgeon, Imperial College Healthcare NHS Trust, London, UK

Mubeen Nazar
Orthopaedic Trainee, Epsom and St. Helier University Hospitals NHS trust, London, UK

Aamer Nisar
Consultant Orthopaedic Surgeon, Hull and East Yorkshire Hospitals NHS Trust, Hull, UK

Tom Quick
Consultant Orthopaedic Surgeon, Peripheral Nerve Injury unit, Royal National Orthopaedic Hospital, Stanmore, UK

Mike Rafferty
Orthopaedic Specialist Trainee, North West London Rotation, London, UK

Peter Reilly
Consultant Orthopaedic Surgeon, Chelsea and Westminster Hospital, London, UK

Philippa Rust
Consultant Orthopaedic Surgeon, NHS Lothian, Edinburgh, UK

Andrew Sankey
Consultant Orthopaedic Surgeon, Chelsea and Westminster Hospital, London, UK

Alex Shearman
Orthopaedic Specialist Trainee, North West London Rotation, London, UK

Ahsan Sheeraz
Locum Consultant Orthopaedic Surgeon, Barts Health NHS Trust, London, UK

Christian Smith
Orthopaedic Specialist Trainee, Guy's & St. Thomas' Hospitals, London, UK

Kapil Sugand
Surgical Research Fellow & Orthopaedic Specialist Trainee, MSk Lab, Charing Cross Hospital, Imperial College London, London, UK
and
North West London Rotation, London, UK

Hussein Taki
Orthopaedic Trainee, Addenbrooke's Hospital, Cambridge, UK

Bernard van Duren
Academic Orthopaedic Specialist Trainee, Yorkshire and Humber Deanery, UK

Jacqueline Waterman
Consultant Orthopaedic Surgeon, Hillingdon Hospital, London, UK

Sohail Yousaf
Orthopaedic Specialist Trainee, Ashford and St. Peter's Hospitals, Surrey, UK

Preface

Trauma and orthopaedics is a vast speciality covering the entire musculoskeletal and peripheral nervous systems. As it is a standard service in every hospital regardless of size or geography, it is considered a core topic within international medical education curricula. We have compiled a user-friendly reference guide to assist audiences in finding essential facts easily in an overview of everyday practice. This book will provide a framework for managing common conditions for use of junior doctors, general practitioners, medical students, physician's associates, physiotherapists, and other allied healthcare professionals. Since this book is the first of its kind for the ABC series, we would welcome feedback to consistently improve the content. Feel free to email your comments and feedback to ks704@ic.ac.uk.

Abbreviations

ACJ	Acromioclavicular Joint
ACL	Anterior Cruciate Ligament
ACPP	Anticitrullinated Peptide/Protein Antibodies
AFB	Acid Fast Bacilli
ALP	Alkaline Phosphatase
AIN	Anterior Interosseous Nerve
AIS	ASIA (American Spinal Injury Association) Impairment Scale
AS	Ankylosing Spondylitis
ASIA	American Spinal Injury Association
ATLS	Advanced Trauma Life Support
AVM	Arterio-Venous Malformation
AVN	Avascular Necrosis
BCIS	Bone Cement Implantation Syndrome
BMD	Bone Mineral Density
BMI	Body Mass Index
BOAST	British Orthopaedic Association Standards for Trauma
CAOS	Computer-Assisted Orthopaedic Surgery
CB	Conduction Block
CEO	Common Extensor Origin
CKD	Chronic Kidney Disease
CN	Cranial Nerve
COX	Cyclooxygenase
CRIF	Closed Reduction And Internal Fixation
CRP	C-Reactive Protein
CRPS	Complex Regional Pain Syndrome
CTPA	CT Pulmonary Angiogram
CTS	Carpal Tunnel Syndrome
CVA	Cerebrovascular Accident
CVS	Cardiovascular System
DAS	Disease Activity Score
DCO	Damage Control Orthopaedics
DDH	Developmental Dysplasia of Hip
DHS	Dynamic Hip Screw
DIP	Distal Interphalangeal (joints)
DMARD	Disease-Modifying Antirheumatic Drugs
DVT	Deep Vein Thrombosis
DXA/DEXA	Dual-Energy X-ray Absorptiometry

EA	Enteropathic Arthritis
eGFR	Estimated Glomerular Filtration Rate
EMG	Electromyography
ESR	Erythrocyte Sedimentation Rate
ETC	Early Total Care
EUA	Examination Under Anaesthesia
FBC	Full Blood Count
FCU	Flexor Carpi Ulnaris
FDP	Flexor Digitorum Profundus
FDS	Flexor Digitorum Superficialis
FRAX	Fracture Risk Assessment Tool
GI	Gastrointestinal
GUM	Genitourinary Medicine
HA	Hydroxyapatite
HBL	Horizontal Beam Lateral
HIV	Human Immunodeficiency Virus
HRT	Hormone Replacement Therapy Human
IBD	Inflammatory Bowel Disease
IgG	Immunoglobulin G
IM	Intramedullary
IMRT	Intensity-Modulated Radiation Therapy
IV	Intravenous
LCL	Lateral Collateral Ligament
LFCA	Lateral Femoral Circumflex Artery
LFT	Liver Function Test
LOAF	Lumbricals (1 and 2), Opponens Pollicis, Abductor Pollicis Brevis and Flexor Pollicis Brevis
MBD	Metabolic Bone Disease
MC	Metacarpal
MCL	Medial Collateral Ligament
MCP	Metacarpophalangeal (joints)
MFCA	Medial Femoral Circumflex Artery
MPFL	Medial Patellofemoral Ligament
MRI	Magnetic Resonance Imaging
MT	Metatarsal
MTC	Major Trauma Centre

MTP	Metatarsophalangeal (joint)		ReA	Reactive Arthritis
MUA	Manipulation Under Anaesthesia		RF	Rheumatoid Factors
			RICE	Rest, Ice Compression and Elevation
NCS	Nerve-Conduction Studies			
NICE	National Institute for Health and Care Excellence		SD	Standard Deviation
NOF	Neck Of Femur		SERM	Selective Oestrogen Receptor Modulator
NOGG	National Osteoporosis Guidelines Group		SLE	Systemic Lupus Erythematosus
			SPA	Spondyloarthropathy
OA	Osteoarthritis			
OPAT	Out Patient Antibiotic Therapy		TB	Tuberculosis
ORIF	Open Reduction and Internal Fixation		TFCC	Triangular Fibrocartilage Complex
			TFT	Thyroid Function Test
PCL	Posterior Cruciate Ligament		TKR	Total Knee Replacement
PET	Positive Emission Tomography		TNF	Tumour Necrosis Factor
PHILOS	Proximal Humerus Internal Locking System		TSA	Total Shoulder Arthroplasty
PICC	Peripherally Inserted Central Catheter			
PIPs	Proximal Interphalangeal (joints)		U&E	Urea and Electrolytes
PLC	Posterolateral Corner (knee)		UC	Ulcerative Colisis
PMMA	Polymethyl Methacrylate		UHMWP	Ultra-High-Molecular-Weight Polyethylene
PNI	Peripheral Nerve Injury		UKR	Unicompartmental Knee Replacement
POP	Plaster of Paris		USS	Ultrasound Scan
POSI	Position of Safe Immobilisation			
PsA	Psoriatic Arthritis		VAC	Vacuum-Assisted Closure
PTH	Parathyroid Hormone (rh prefix – recombinant human)		VMO	Vastus Medialis Oblique
			VTE	Venous Thromboembolism
RA	Rheumatoid Arthritis		WCC	White Cell Count
RANK	Receptor Activator of Nuclear Factor		WHO	World Health Organisation

CHAPTER 1

General Overview

Kapil Sugand[1,2], Anita Khurwal[2], and Chinmay M. Gupte[1,3]

[1]MSk Lab, Charing Cross Hospital, Imperial College London, London, UK
[2]North West London Rotation, London, UK
[3]Imperial College Healthcare NHS Trust, London, UK

OVERVIEW

- Orthopaedics is one of the oldest surgical practices since ancient civilisations.
- With an ever-growing and ageing population, there is a greater global clinical burden of trauma and elective orthopaedics.
- Fracture classifications can help with management plans, either nonoperative or operative treatment.
- Poor management of fractures and dislocations can lead to loss of function, long-term disability, and chronic pain, as well as deterioration in quality of life.

Introduction

Trauma and orthopaedics is an ancient practice of surgery. Records from Ancient Egypt, for example, document the splintage of fractures, wound care, and the reduction of shoulder dislocation. The art and skill of managing musculoskeletal injuries depends on adequate history, thorough examination, patient selection, and meticulous operative technique. Orthopaedic surgeons are trained not only to manage fractures but also to treat deep-seated infection, degenerative disease, tumours, and congenital deformities, as well as the repair of soft tissue like muscles, nerves, tendons, ligaments, and minimally invasive access surgery.

Epidemiology

There is an increasing demand for orthopaedic surgeons, owing to an ever-growing population. Immigration patterns and an ageing population have further contributed to the clinical burden worldwide. The World Health Organisation (WHO) predicts that by 2020, trauma will be the third most common cause for the global burden of disease, and that one in two people in the world will require at least one orthopaedic procedure in their lifetime. Trauma services have been centralised in more economically developed countries, where specialist centres manage complex trauma effectively. However, there is a discrepancy in the infrastructure of the trauma services in less economically developed countries, which leads to increased mortality and chronic disability rates, which are potentially avoidable. Furthermore, specific registries have collated information including demographics, indications and complications, in order to improve the orthopaedic service provided to patients.

Definitions

Trauma and orthopaedics, like any other speciality, has its own jargon and terminology. There are 300 bones in newborns and 206 in adults, divided into the midline axial skeleton (head, spine, ribs, and pelvis) and the appendicular skeleton (limbs), seen in Figure 1.1a. Movements of the body are seen in Figure 1.1b.

Some popular terms include the following:
- Trauma: any injury, bony or soft tissue
- Joint: articulation between two or more bones
- Arthro-: related to a joint
- Arthrocentesis: joint aspiration
- Arthroscopy: insertion of a minimally invasive camera into a joint
- Arthroplasty: joint reconstruction
- Arthrodesis: joint fusion
- Displacement: deviation of fracture fragment from original anatomical site
- Intra-/extra-articular: inside/outside joint
- Stable fractures: those able to withstand physiological loading, without further displacement (usually extra-articular and minimally displaced)
- Open fracture: bone breaching soft tissue and skin, to be in contact with outside environment (as opposed to closed)
- Revision surgery: successive surgical attempts at achieving the desired result

History

Taking a thorough history is the cornerstone of medical practice. It is important that as much information as possible about the patient's symptoms and medical background is ascertained, in order reach a

---

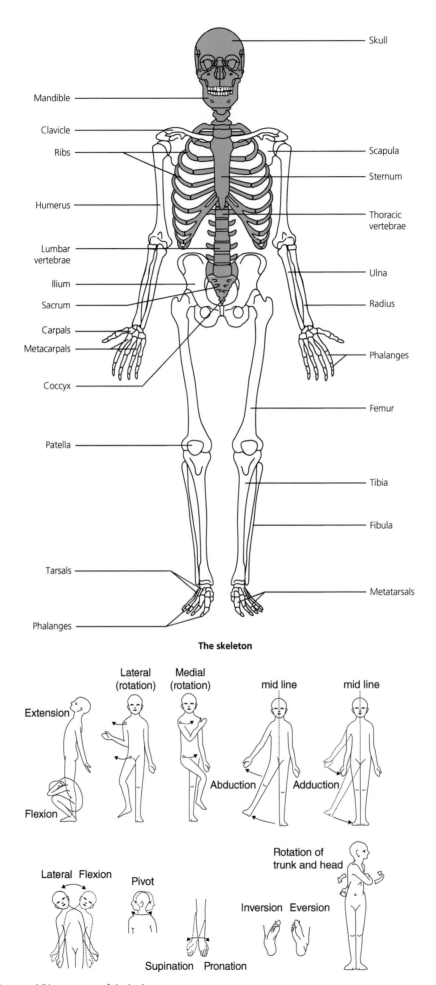

Figure 1.1 (a) Human skeleton and (b) movement of the body

Table 1.1 Orthopaedic history

- Age
- Occupation and dominant side
- Pain (mnemonic – SOCRATES)
  - Site
  - Onset – sudden vs. progressively worsening?
  - Character – sharp, dull, ache, stinging?
  - Radiation
  - Associations – any trauma, fever, swellings?
  - Timing – at rest, night pain, constant or intermittent?
  - Exacerbating/relieving factors – what position makes the pain better/worse?
  - Severity – grade out of 10?
- Associated symptoms
  - Stiffness, snapping, clicking, squeaking, deformity, numbness, weakness, locking, giving way, swelling
- Function
  - How far can patient walk on a flat surface?
  - Difficulty with stairs?
  - Need any walking aids?
  - Can patient participate in sports?
  - Is patient able to work?
- Past medical and surgical history
  - History of trauma
  - Other joints affected
  - Treatments already given (e.g. injection, physiotherapy etc.)
- Systems review
- Family history
- Social history

list of differential diagnoses and to offer optimal management options. It is said that 80% of the diagnosis is within the medical history. An orthopaedic approach to history taking is seen in Table 1.1.

Examination

A systematic examination is essential in orthopaedic practice. The impression gained from the history is tested and further information is ascertained. The management options, and whether surgical intervention is necessitated, depends on the extent of disease and its consequent functional limitation and quality of life. As the idiom goes, a good surgeon knows when to operate, but the best surgeon knows when not to operate. The general principles of examining in orthopaedics are to (1) look, (2) feel, and (3) move as well as any (4) special tests (Figure 1.2).

Reading radiographs

Regardless of speciality, all doctors and medical students are expected to interpret basic orthopaedic plain radiographs (do not refer to them as X-rays). Competency in reading radiographs is based on the following six points of information:

1 Anatomical site: which bone and which part of bone? Long bones are divided into proximal, middle, and distal thirds.
2 Number of fragments: simple (two-part) vs. multifragmentary (formerly referred to as comminuted).
3 Fracture pattern: transverse vs. oblique (>30°) vs. spiral.
4 Is the fracture displaced vs. undisplaced (Figure 1.3)?
5 Is the fracture translated/ angulated/ rotated?
6 Extent of displacement/angulation/rotation/tilt in X/Y/Z planes.

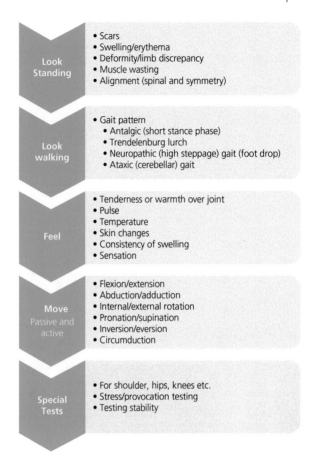

Figure 1.2 Orthopaedic examination

Look Standing
- Scars
- Swelling/erythema
- Deformity/limb discrepancy
- Muscle wasting
- Alignment (spinal and symmetry)

Look walking
- Gait pattern
  - Antalgic (short stance phase)
  - Trendelenburg lurch
  - Neuropathic (high steppage) gait (foot drop)
  - Ataxic (cerebellar) gait

Feel
- Tenderness or warmth over joint
- Pulse
- Temperature
- Skin changes
- Consistency of swelling
- Sensation

Move Passive and active
- Flexion/extension
- Abduction/adduction
- Internal/external rotation
- Pronation/supination
- Inversion/eversion
- Circumduction

Special Tests
- For shoulder, hips, knees etc.
- Stress/provocation testing
- Testing stability

Examples of presenting radiographs

Figure 1.4 is "*an AP and lateral radiograph of the right tibia and fibula of [patient name] taken on [date] at [time]. There is a two-part transverse fracture of the junction between middle and distal third of the tibia, with 15% anterolateral translation and 10° angulation in the x plane*."

Figure 1.5 is "*an AP and lateral radiograph of the right tibia and fibula of a skeletally immature (growth plates present and not fused) patient, named [patient name], taken on [date] at [time]. There is a displaced multifragmentary fracture of the fibula and a minimally displaced two-part oblique fracture of the tibia, both at the junction of middle and distal thirds of the diaphysis. Both have 20° valgus angulation and anterior tilt*."

Note that angulation and translation is always described of the distal fragment, relative to the proximal fragment. Look for fracture dislocations near joints. Valgus refers to deviation away from the midline in the coronal plane, whereas varus is *towards* the midline. Malrotation is more common in the shoulder, hip, and ankle.

An aide-memoire is va**L**gus is **L**ateral to midline.

Common fracture classifications

There are numerous fracture classifications (Table 1.2) to describe the severity of injury, energy of trauma, and to guide your management options. Each classification has an eponymous name, often of the surgeon who developed it. The ideal classification describes the

Displacement

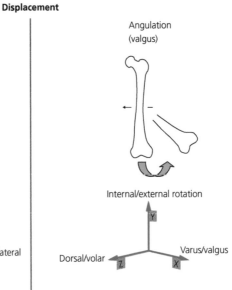

Figure 1.3 Displacement in three planes

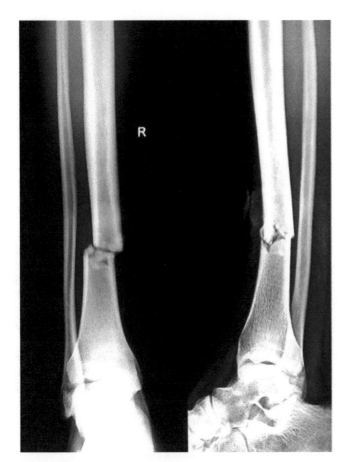

Figure 1.4 AP and lateral radiograph of the right tibia and fibula

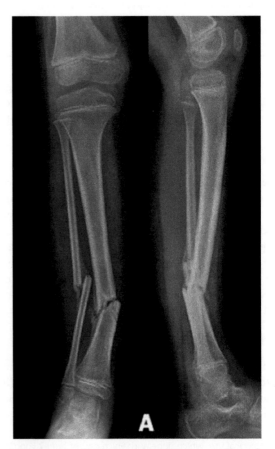

Figure 1.5 AP and lateral radiograph of the right tibia and fibula of a skeletally immature patient

severity of injury in terms of anatomy, displacement, stability, and prognosis. Since most fall short of this ideal, it is up to the orthopaedic surgeon to not simply follow guidelines but to deliver optimal healthcare with a patient-centred approach. It is the duty of every surgeon to offer the right treatment, to the right person, at the right time, and in the right place.

Principles of fracture fixation

An international community, known as AO (Arbeitsgemeinschaft für Osteosynthesefragen), has developed protocols, standards, and guidelines that have been adopted worldwide for the past half a century. There are four AO principles of fracture fixation:

Table 1.2 Common fracture classifications

Classification	Site
Salter Harris	Paediatric physeal plate
Neer	Proximal humerus
Tile	Pelvis
Garden	Intracapsular neck of femur
Weber	Distal fibula
Schatzker	Tibial plateau
Gustillo-Anderson	Open fractures
Denis	Spine
Tscherne	Soft tissue disruption

1 *Fracture reduction to restore anatomical relationships*

  Joints require their surfaces to be anatomically reduced to perfection.

  Bones require functional reduction by restoration of their length and alignment.

2 *Fracture fixation providing absolute or relative stability as the "personality" of fracture, patient, and injury requires*

  The goals are to maintain the reduction with or without metalwork and to achieve sufficient stability. Stability leads to less pain, early range of movement, and physiotherapy, to achieve full function. Two options for stability are absolute versus relative. Absolute stability is usually due to fixation with plates and screws and means that there is no movement at the fracture site, thereby bypassing the callus-formation stage of fracture healing, to allow direct bone healing. Relative stability is usually achieved by splinting, nailing, or bridging and means that there is some movement at the fracture site, which allows callus formation and indirect bone healing.

3 *Preservation of blood supply to soft tissues and bone*

  Fracture healing relies on biomechanics and biology, among other factors. The soft tissue envelope and blood supply to the fracture site need to be viable, to allow adequate fracture healing. If the soft tissue is heavily disrupted, then a staged procedure, with primary stabilisation (using external fixation), followed by secondary stabilisation (definitive fixation) ought to be considered. Elevation of the limb pre- and post-operatively is essential, to minimize swelling. Other postoperative instructions include offering (i) adequate analgesia, since the body does not heal if in pain, and (ii) venous thromboembolic prophylaxis (TED stockings and low molecular weight heparin).

4 *Early and safe mobilisation of the injured part and the patient as a whole*

  The management plan does not end as soon as the operation is over. The last step of any management plan is rehabilitation. The duty of the health care team is to restore patients to their premorbid level of functional ability, or to the closest scenario, using means such as physiotherapy.

Principles of fracture management

Fracture management consists of the 4Rs: Resuscitate → Reduce → Rest (hold) → Rehabilitate (Figure 1.6).

General principles

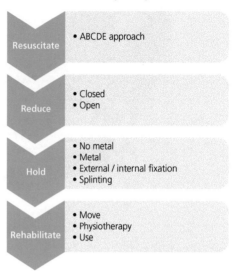

Figure 1.6 General principles of fracture management

Complications of fractures

Fractures can lead to multiple complications, both locally to the fracture site and systemically (refer to Chapter 16, Table 16.4). Systemically, venous thromboembolism and infection are the commonest complications. Other complications specific to the fracture site are myriad and can consequently lead to chronic pain, disability, and deformity. Complications can be divided into *general vs. specific* or *immediate vs. early vs. late*. Of particular note, there is a misconception that compartment syndrome tends only to occur in closed fractures, but it can also occur in open fractures.

Education and training

Trauma and orthopaedics is one of the most popular choices of surgical speciality, and the demand for these surgeons is increasing. However, there has been a dramatic change in the quality of education and demands of the career. Compared to previous generations, where their working week was usually over a 100 hours per week, current working restrictions set by the European Working Time Directive and Accreditation Council for Continuing Medical Education for North America have nearly halved the working week. This has also reduced the number of dedicated training hours in the operating theatre, to a predicted 80% reduction. Like general surgical specialities, there is a further inclination to adopt safer training practices to train future generations of surgeons, in a safe and controlled environment, while upholding patient safety. Some of this has been achieved by simulation, using virtual-reality simulators, multimedia online platforms, and holograms (Figures 1.7 and 1.8).

Future of trauma and orthopaedics

Orthopaedics has modernised after the implementation of technology. Computer-assisted orthopaedic surgery (CAOS) has aided implantation of prostheses in both hip and knee arthroplasty, with three-dimensional (3D) preoperative planning, for real-time, intraoperative use. Another method of improving

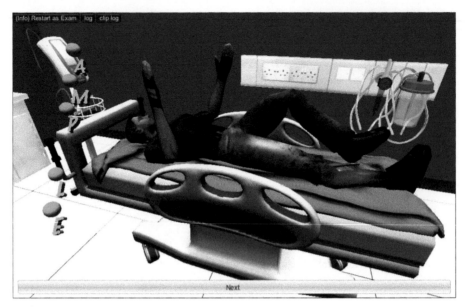

Figure 1.7 Multimedia online platform

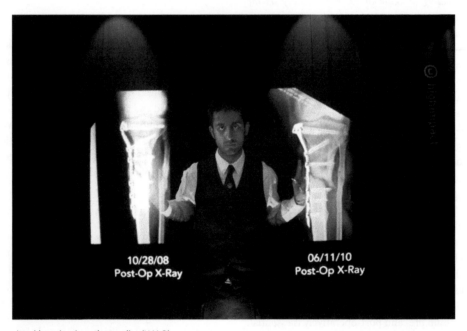

Figure 1.8 Holography-assisted learning in orthopaedics (HALO)

preoperative planning and patient satisfaction, is the use of 3D printing. Personalised models can be printed, using data from CT and MRI scans, to visually give the surgeon and patient a much more realistic understanding of the injury or disease process, prior to operating.

Currently, there are prostheses of differing sizes, but they often do not take into account anatomical variations. The next step in orthopaedic practice will be the use of patient-matched implants, to improve outcomes. 3D printing has created personalised implants in other surgical specialities. The better the implant fit, the longer the likely lifespan and the lower the likelihood of mechanical complications, including the need for revision surgery. Biological treatments are currently being developed and used in clinical trials, not only to heal diseased bone but to cure it. Stem cells harvested from bone marrow may have the potential to restore the integrity of the articular surface. The shape of joints can also be restored with the use of 3D biosynthetic scaffolding.

Further reading

Akhtar, K., Sugand, K., Sperrin, M., et al. (2015). Training safer orthopedic surgeons. *Acta Orthopaedica* 86: 616–621.

Bizzarro, J., and Regazzoni, P. (n.d.) *Principles of fracture fixation.* Davos, Switzerland: AO trauma.

Chikwe, J., De Souza, A.C., and Pepper, J.R. (2004). No time to train the surgeons. *British Medical Journal* 328: 418–419.

Cobb, J. et al. (2006). Hands-on robotic unicompartmental knee replacement: a prospective, randomised controlled study of the acrobot system. *Journal of Bone and Joint Surgery (Br.)* 88:188–197.

Sugand, K., Mawkin, M., and Gupte, C. (2015). Validating Touch Surgery™: A cognitive task simulation and rehearsal app for intramedullary femoral nailing. *Injury* 46: 2212–2216.

World Health Organisation. (2004). *Guidelines for Essential Trauma, Violence and Injury Prevention.* World Health Organisation. Geneva, Switzerland. Available at www.apps.who.int/iris/bitstream/10665/42565/1/9241546409_eng.pdf

CHAPTER 2

Epidemiology of Musculoskeletal Disease

David Metcalfe

University of Warwick, and University of Oxford, UK

OVERVIEW

- Musculoskeletal (MSk) disorders (involving bones, muscles, and joints) account for a substantial proportion of disability worldwide. One in two of us will need an orthopaedic intervention during our lives.

- In the United Kingdom, MSk disorders are the most common cause of illness; affecting over 8 million people, leading to 11 million lost working days, and costing over £3 billion per year.

- Both osteoporosis and osteoarthritis are increasing, a trend that is partly driven by population aging and lifestyle choices. It is estimated that an osteoporotic fracture occurs every 3 minutes in the United Kingdom.

- Novel and effective surgical interventions can improve the lives of patients but impose a significant resource burden.

Introduction

Trauma and orthopaedic surgeons treat a heterogenous group of musculoskeletal disorders that range from congenital deformity through tumours and fractures to joint diseases. The World Health Organisation (WHO) Global Burden of Disease study estimates that MSk disorders are the second biggest cause of *years lived with disability* globally. The most important musculoskeletal causes of disability worldwide are lower back and neck pain. However, the WHO does not categorise injuries within *musculoskeletal disorders*, and so this claim underestimates the burden of disorders that might require orthopaedic intervention. There is also good evidence that disability caused by musculoskeletal conditions is increasing: disability related to MSk disorders increased by 45% between 1990 and 2010. Although orthopaedic surgery is a broad specialty, these pages focus on the epidemiology of osteoarthritis and osteoporosis, which are particular challenges for the global orthopaedic community.

Osteoarthritis and joint replacement

The most common primary joint disorder is osteoarthritis (OA), which is characterised by degeneration of articular cartilage and subchondral bone. Its epidemiology can be difficult to describe because OA symptoms (pain, stiffness, loss of function) and radiographic features (joint space narrowing, subchondral sclerosis, subchondral cysts, osteophytes) do not always overlap. Incidence estimates therefore depend on how each study defines OA. The Framingham Osteoarthritis Study found that the prevalence of radiographic OA is around 44% among individuals aged over 70 years.

Theory of aetiology

The aetiology of OA is poorly understood, but potential contributors include (1) an inherited predisposition, (2) systemic factors, and (3) local insults to the joint. OA is often thought to result simply from excessive weight-bearing on articular surfaces. This view is supported by the observation that knee OA is associated with body mass index and by studies suggesting an association with specific physical activities such as elite football and long-distance running. Knee OA is also more prevalent amongst individuals whose jobs require kneeling and squatting.

However, the relationship with obesity may be more complicated than suggested by the popular term *wear-and-tear arthritis*. For example, obesity is associated with OA at the non–weight-bearing carpometacarpal joints of the hand but has – at best – only a weak association with hip OA. It has therefore been suggested that obesity might affect OA progression through an endocrine mechanism rather than simply increasing the load on weight-bearing joints. An endocrine mechanism is also implicated by the fact that females are more likely to develop OA, have more severe disease, and experience worsening OA around the time of the menopause. However, randomised trials have not

---

ABC of Orthopaedics and Trauma, First Edition. Edited by Kapil Sugand and Chinmay M. Gupte.
© 2018 John Wiley & Sons Ltd. Published 2018 by John Wiley & Sons Ltd.

found evidence that OA risk is attenuated by hormone replacement therapy.

Age is the strongest risk factor for OA at all joints. However, this tells us little about OA aetiology because age may simply be a proxy for cumulative exposure to other risk factors (e.g. weight-bearing, abnormal joint loading, and/or endocrine influences). Injury is also an important risk factor for subsequent development of OA. This may be because of direct injury to articular cartilage (e.g. an osseochrondral defect after an ankle pilon fracture), disruption of the articular surface (e.g. an intra-articular fracture that healed with callus), or a consequence of altered joint loading (e.g. malalignment to a mismanaged fracture fixation).

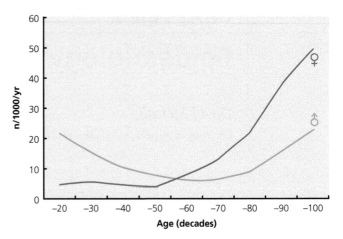

Figure 2.1 Epidemiology of fractures by age and sex (Court-Brown & Caesar, 2006)

TREATMENT OPTIONS

Unsurprisingly, given its association with age, activity, and obesity, OA incidence is increasing worldwide. Although a number of treatments are available, joint replacement (arthroplasty) is the most common intervention for end-stage OA. In addition to the increasing number of patients developing end-stage OA, the average age at which patients undergo arthroplasty is falling. Possible explanations for this trend include the following:

1 Ageing of the population
2 Increased physical demands as older patients are independent for longer
3 Prosthetic improvements, reducing the concern about implant longevity
4 Patient demand

Nevertheless, prosthetic joints may need to be revised in the future, particularly when implanted in younger patients who are more active and have many decades of life ahead of them. Hip and knee replacements have an annual failure rate of 0.5–1.0%, which means that there is a 15–20% chance that each implant will require revision within 20 years. Hip and knee replacements are some of the most cost-effective operations in any branch of surgery, but these factors suggest that primary joint disease and arthroplasty will account for an increasing proportion of orthopaedic practice in the future.

Most fractures have a bimodal incidence, as they predominantly affect young adults and the elderly. In reality, the peak fracture incidences occur at ages 15–24 for males (7% annual incidence) and >85 for females (8% annual incidence; Figure 2.1).

Gender differences

Young males are likely affected because of behavioural differences (e.g. contact sports), whereas the high incidence of fractures among elderly females can be explained by metabolic bone disease. The archetypal metabolic bone disease is osteoporosis, which results in reduced bone mass, disruption of bone architecture, and increased risk of fracture. An estimated 30% of post-menopausal women have evidence of osteoporosis (using WHO criteria), and this rises to 70% at age 80. One in three women (usually post-menopause) and one in five men will experience a fracture as a consequence of osteoporosis during their lifetime.

Osteoporosis, trauma, and fractures

Almost a billion people worldwide seek assistance for injuries every year, and five million are fatally injured. Unlike most other MSk disorders, there is evidence that the global burden of injuries is falling (but will still be the third largest contributor to global clinical burden and cause of disability by 2020 according to the WHO). This has been attributed to injury prevention (e.g. road safety laws), measures to reduce injury severity (e.g. crumple zones to protect passengers during road traffic collisions), and improvements in trauma interventions (e.g. trauma systems).

Incidence

The incidence of fragility fractures rises with age as bone mineral density decreases and the risk of falling increases. It is therefore unsurprising that the worldwide burden of fragility fractures is increasing as the global population ages. The worldwide incidence of hip fractures is projected to increase by approximately 280% by 2050. Hip fractures are increasing in the United Kingdom despite interventions (e.g. bisphosphonates) to improve bone health. It is estimated that 70,000 hip fractures occur in the United Kingdom annually, leading to £2 billion in total cost of care.

Further Reading

British Orthopaedic Association. Joint action – improving mobility. www.boa.ac.uk/wp-content/uploads/2016/11/Sponsorship-Pack-2016.pdf

British Orthopaedic Association. British Orthopaedic Association for Standards of Trauma one version 2. Patients sustaining a fragility hip fracture. www.boa.ac.uk/wp-content/uploads/2014/12/BOAST-1.pdf

Court-Brown, C.M., and Caesar, B. (2006). Epidemiology of adult fractures: a review. *Injury* 37 (8): 691–697.

Metcalfe, D., et al. (2012). Does endotoxaemia contribute to osteoarthritis in obese patients? *Clinical Science* (Lond.) 123 (11): 627–634.

Smith, E., et al. (2014). The global burden of other musculoskeletal disorders: estimates from the Global Burden of Disease 2010 study. *Annals of Rheumatic Diseases* 73 (8): 1462–1469.

Storheim, K., and Zwart, J.A. (2014). Musculoskeletal disorders and the Global Burden of Disease study. *Annals of Rheumatic Diseases* 73: 949–950.

Warming, L., Hassager, C., and Christiansen, C. (2002). Changes in bone mineral density with age in men and women: a longitudinal study. *Osteoporosis International* 13: 105–112.

Zhang, Y., and Jordan, J.M. (2010). Epidemiology of osteoarthritis. *Clinics of Geriatric Medicine* 26 (3): 355–369.

CHAPTER 3

Orthopaedic Investigations

Adil Ajuied[1], Christian Smith[1], and Cynthia Gupte[2]

[1] Guy's & St. Thomas' Hospitals, London, UK
[2] The Hillingdon Hospitals NHS Foundation Trust, Uxbridge, UK

OVERVIEW

- Orthopaedic surgeons utilise a large range of investigative techniques, including radiological, neurophysiological (nerve conduction test and electromyelography), and laboratory (blood, synovial fluid) tests, biopsy, and arthroscopy.
- Radiological techniques include:
  - Plain radiographs (X-ray)
  - Ultrasound
  - CT
  - MRI
  - Nuclear scan
  - Contrast arthrography
- The various forms of radiological imaging have different applications, and the most suitable modality must be chosen in conjunction with the clinical scenario.
- In the setting of suspected infection, adequate samples must be obtained before starting antibiotics. Early liaison with a microbiologist is strongly advised.
- Liaison with specialist centres should be undertaken in the setting of suspected musculoskeletal cancers. Biopsies should never be performed at nonspecialist centres.

Introduction

There are numerous forms of investigations utilised in orthopaedics. Their primary roles are to aid diagnosis, monitor disease progression, assist in the planning of operative interventions and assessing the outcomes of treatment.

Radiological imaging

Imaging is the most common form of investigation in orthopaedics, ranging from plain radiographs to complex MRI. Radiological assessments utilises three orthogonal planes (sagittal, coronal, and axial) for standardisation of views (Figure 3.1).

It is vital to obtain images in two orthogonal planes (i.e. at right angles to each other) to allow full assessment of bones and joints (Figure 3.2).

Imaging is important in assessing damage to bones or joints caused by trauma, aiding ambiguous clinical findings, monitoring disease processes (such as osteoarthritis), and planning treatments. Any nontraumatic bone or joint pain should be imaged if there is no obvious diagnosis to rule out sinister causes; this may require further, more complex imaging if simple techniques still do not offer any explanations. There tends to be a cross-over in imaging modalities depending on pathology. MSk Radiologists takes into account age of the patient, resources, radiation risk, differentials, pathology and clinical questions. Any ambiguous clinical scenarios may require a number of imaging modalities that will be reviewed in a MDT setting to determine the likely pathology.

More complicated investigations are often costly and can carry associated risks, such as increased radiation dose. These investigations need to be justified, and relevant clinical findings ought to raise significant concern to warrant them. Imaging should not need to be repeated unless there is progression of the disease process. Progression may include worsening pain, deformity, or loss of function.

Radiographs (plain X-rays)
Image generation
X-ray photon beams are emitted towards a patient positioned in front of a detector. Higher molecular weighted structures (e.g. bone) absorb and attenuate X-rays more effectively, preventing them from reaching the detector. A two-dimensional (2D) projected image is formed based on the contrast created by differing attenuated intensities of X-rays reaching the detector (Figure 3.3). Structures are differentiated with respect to density.

Morbidity potential
Ionising radiation can cause cellular damage, and repetitive high dose exposure may result in cell death, cancer, or infertility. Additionally, it may be teratogenic to unborn babies, so the

ABC of Orthopaedics and Trauma, First Edition. Edited by Kapil Sugand and Chinmay M. Gupte.
© 2018 John Wiley & Sons Ltd. Published 2018 by John Wiley & Sons Ltd.

pregnancy status of females needs to be confirmed beforehand. Otherwise, lead-based shields are used to reduce the risks of radiation to the gonads. Radiation doses for imaging modalities mentioned in this chapter are summarised in Table 3.1.

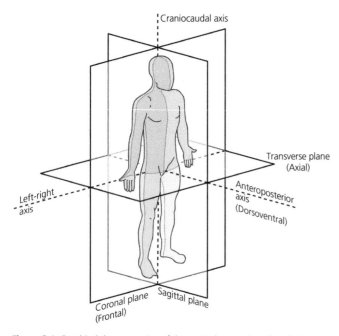

Figure 3.1 Graphical demonstration of the sagittal, coronal, and axial planes

Examples of orthopaedic applications

Assessment of bone and joint anatomy in a wide variety of elective and trauma situations, including fracture diagnosis, post-reduction and healing, osteoarthritis progression and assessment of metal work or prostheses. Antero-posterior (AP) and lateral view of joints, bones, and the joints above and below affected bones should be ordered at least. There are also special views (e.g. oblique) to highlight joints, bones and pathologies.

Dual energy X-ray absorptiometry (DXA)
Image generation

DXA (formerly DEXA) is used to estimate bone mineral density (BMD). Two X-ray beams of different energy levels are targeted at a specific region (normally the neck of the femur or lumbar vertebrae). Absorption of the X-rays by the bone can be used to determine the bone mineral content, once soft tissue absorption has been subtracted. The bone mineral content of the specific site is divided by the estimation of the bone volume calculated from its area, resulting in an approximation of the BMD.

Morbidity Potential

As for radiographs.

Examples of orthopaedic applications

Diagnosis and monitoring of osteopenia and osteoporosis. DXA is poor at predicting osteoporotic fractures risk, as it only measures the mineral content of bone and does not take the organic content into account.

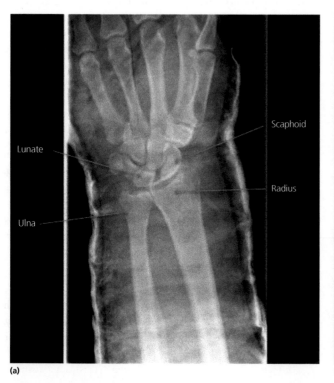

(a)

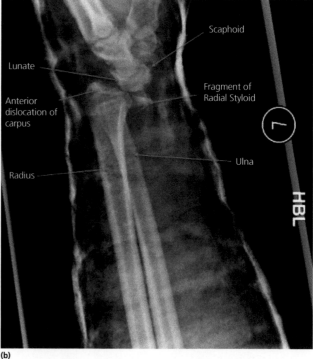

(b)

Figure 3.2a and b These AP and lateral radiographs of a wrist stress the importance of obtaining two views when assessing bones and joints. To the untrained eye the AP view (a) may not appear overtly abnormal, especially due to artefact from the plaster cast. The lateral view; (b) reveals that there is a fracture-dislocation of the wrist

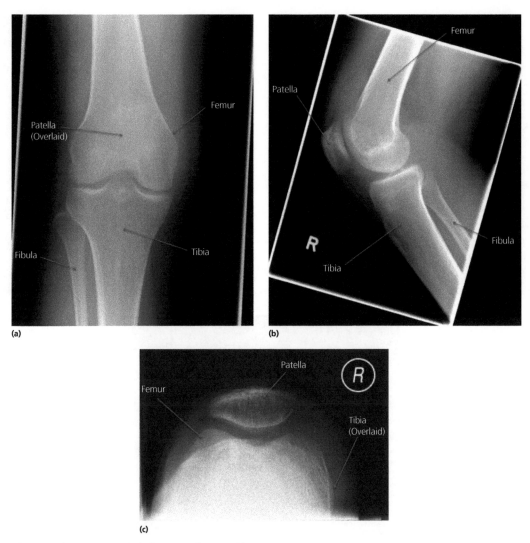

Figure 3.3a, b, and c An AP, lateral, and axial (skyline) view of a normal knee

Table 3.1 The effective radiation dose of various forms of imaging (values given in millisieverts (mSv))

Exposure	Effective radiation dose, mSv
135 g Brazil nuts	0.005
Chest (AP) radiograph	0.02
UK annual background	2.7
US annual background	6.2
20/day annual smoker	53
Radiographs:	
Hand/foot (AP and lateral)	0.001
Knee (AP and lateral)	0.02
Pelvis (AP)	0.7
Thoracic spine (AP and lateral)	0.7
Hip (AP)	0.83
Lumbar spine (AP and lateral)	1.0
Computed tomography:	
Pelvis	8.8
C-spine	3.6
Nuclear medicine:	
Bone scan	4.2
WBC scan	18.5
SPECT/CT scan	25–30

Computerised tomography (CT)

Image generation

Axial X-ray slice acquisitions are produced using an X-ray source that rotates around the patient. Detectors are positioned opposite the source and rotate in the same circle. 3D volumetric information is generated by software integration of the individual images. The volumetric data can be reconstructed in the three orthogonal planes, utilising X-ray attenuation as image contrast. The true plane of acquisition is the axial plane; thus, image resolution is greatest in this plane. Structures are differentiated with respect to density.

Morbidity potential

The morbidity associated with CT is a result of ionising radiation with doses significantly greater than those of plain radiographs (Table 3.1). Moreover, the same precautions mentioned for plain radiography certainly apply to a greater extent in CT scanning.

Examples of orthopaedic applications: CT is valuable in the assessments of bony anatomy and pathology, especially intra-articular fractures, the diagnosis of occult fractures and preoperative planning for spinal and tumour surgery (Figure 3.4).

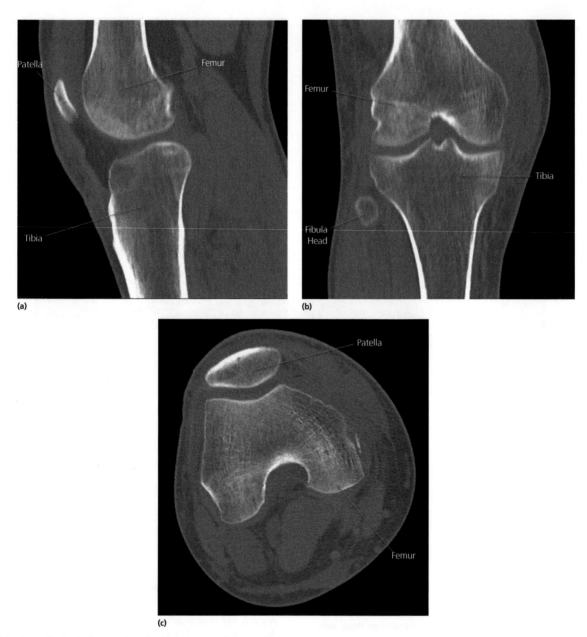

Figure 3.4a, b, and c Sagittal, coronal, and axial CT images of a normal knee

Magnetic resonance imaging (MRI)
Image generation
Hydrogen nuclei (usually contained in water in tissues) become aligned in large magnetic fields. A temporary electromagnetic pulse reverses the spin of the nuclei before they return to thermodynamic equilibrium. As they relax, a radiofrequency signal is generated, with the density of hydrogen nuclei determining the strength of the signal and thus image contrast. These signals are converted into 3D volumetric acquisition that can be reconstructed in the three orthogonal planes. Structures are differentiated with respect to signal intensity. Various MRI sequences can be used to emphasize certain types of tissues. Some of the most common are summarised in Box 3.1.

Morbidity potential
There is no clinically proven morbidity to MRI; however it may be contraindicated in patients with certain implants or foreign bodies (e.g. cardiac pacemakers, mechanical heart valves, shrapnel wounds, aneurysm clips). However, joint replacements and spinal implants are safe. A safety questionnaire is filled out by the patient and the clinician to ensure patient safety for the scan. Knowledge of the correct implant will also adjust for the type of MRI sequence e.g. MARS (metal artefact reduction sequence).

Examples of orthopaedic applications
MRI provides optimal assessment of soft and deep tissue, oedema, and inflammation (e.g. in osteomyelitis) compared to other forms of imaging (Figure 3.5). The sequence performed are tailor-made

depending on the clinical question, the radiologist and the differentials being considered.

Table 3.2 summarises specific joint pathologies that imaging can evaluate.

Arthrograms

Arthrograms involve taking a series of imaging (fluoroscopy, CT and MRI) before and after joint has been injected with a contrast medium (usually iodine-based). There is increasing use of MRI or

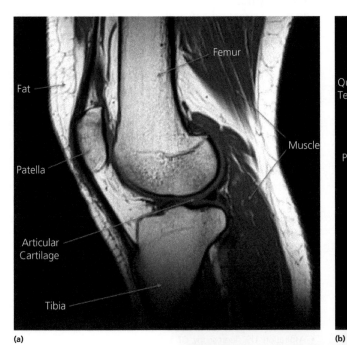

(a)

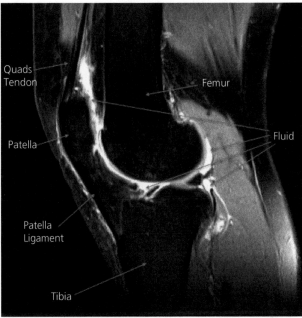

(b)

(c)

Figure 3.5a, b, and c Sagittal and coronal MRI images of a knee. Image (a) is T1-weighted, used to help differentiate fat from water. Image (b) is T2-weighted (fat suppressed), particularly efficient at demonstrating oedema and fluid. Image (c) is a also a T2 weighted fat suppressed coronal view. Please refer to Box 3.1

Table 3.2 The use of imaging to determine site-specific orthopaedic pathology

Anatomical Area	Pathology
Universal	Infections (especially osteomyelitis)
	Inflammation (e.g. tendinopathies, bursitis)
	Soft tissue and bone tumours
	Occult fractures
	Cartilage defects
Hip	Avascular necrosis
	Femoro-acetabular impingement
	Labral tears
	Transient osteoporosis of the hip
	Synovial osteochondromatosis
	Occult hip fractures (Gold standard)
Knee	Ligament rupture (ACL, PCL, MCL, LCL, postero-lateral corner)
	Meniscal tears
	Discoid meniscus
	Osteochondritis dissecans
	Patella tracking and dislocation
	Extensor mechanism disruption
Shoulder	Rotator cuff tears
	Labral tears
	Acromial morphology
	Hill Sachs lesion
Wrist/hand	Ganglion cysts
	Occult fractures (especially scaphoid)
	Giant cell tumours
	Triangular fibrocartilage complex (TFCC) tears
	Complex ligament instability/rupture
	Scapholunate advanced collapse (SLAC)
	Keinbock's disease
	Flexor tendon pulley injury
Spine	Cord compression (especially cauda equina)
	Discitis
	Disc disease and herniation
	Spinal deformity (e.g. scoliosis)
	Spinal canal or foraminal stenosis
	Neurofibromatosis

CT arthrograms but it depends on numerous factors including the clinical questions, radiation dose and risk, and available resources. Arthrograms are commonly used to evaluate the larger ball and socket or spheroidal joints like the hip, wrist (TFCC), and shoulder. They show defects of the joint capsule, ligaments, tendons, labral cartilage, and the position of joints in children. They also confirm correct placement of needles within a joint before injection of therapeutic substances such as anti-inflammatory corticosteroids for pain relief.

Ultrasound

Image generation

Linear arrays of acoustic transducers emit sound waves. As sound waves pass through one tissue to another a certain amount will be reflected in the form of an echo, depending on the material properties of the tissue on each side of the boundary. Reflected sound waves are detected by the transducer and turned into electrical signals visualised as slice acquisition image through the piezoelectric effect.

The amount of sound wave reflected depends on the difference in acoustic impedance of the two materials (i.e. the differences in the density and the conduction of sound). Transitions through boundaries between tissues of different acoustic impedance results in the contrast seen on the image. The greater the difference of acoustic impedance, the more waves will be reflected back; hence, gel is used on the transducer to reduce acoustic impedance by air and improve imaging quality. Structures are differentiated with respect to echogenicity.

Morbidity potential

Ultrasound scanning is safe, with no clinically proven adverse effects.

Examples of orthopaedic applications

Typical applications are the assessment of deep vein thrombosis, superficial tissue, and soft tissue masses, including abscesses. It is also excellent for dynamic soft tissue assessment e.g. muscle or tendon tears. Ultrasound is especially useful when investigating hip stability and feet deformities of babies under 12 months of age, as their bones have not ossified sufficiently to reveal much detail on radiographs. It is also helpful in paediatric cases since there is no radiation risk involved. However, ultrasound is not appropriate to assess internal derangement of joint or diffuse clinical symptoms. Ultrasound is the commonest modality used for a MSk Radiologist to perform joint injections.

Image guided interventions conducted by Radiologists:
- Joint injections: US, fluoroscopy, CT
- Aspiration: US, fluoroscopy, CT
- Dry needling of tendon: US
- Hydrodistension: US
- Biopsy: US, CT

Nuclear medicine

Body scans

Image generation

Radioactive labelled biological markers are administered intravenously. The radiation emission is captured by a gamma camera, producing a projectional image of the distribution and pooling of the marker (Figure 3.6). A variety of labelled markers can be used to highlight different pathologies (Table 3.3).

Morbidity potential

The amount of ionising radiation from nuclear medicine can vary significantly but is usually equivalent to years of background radiation (Table 3.1).

Examples of orthopaedic applications

Nuclear medicine studies are used for the diagnosis of stress fractures, Paget's disease, osteomyelitis, primary and secondary neoplasia, occult fractures, and infected prosthetic loosening.

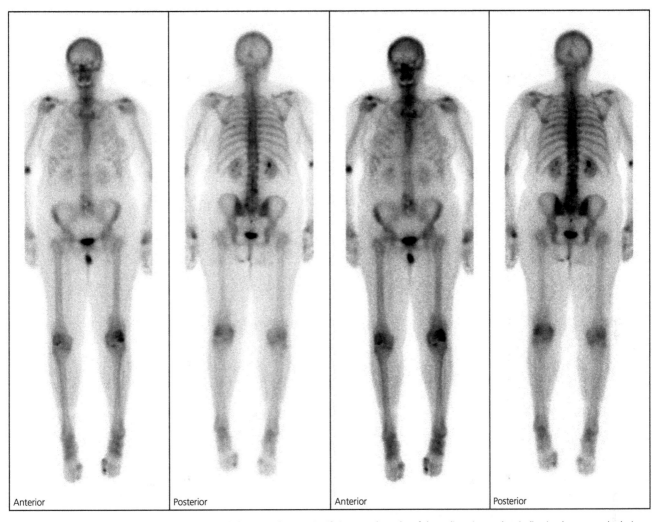

Figure 3.6 Nuclear medicine bone scan of the whole skeleton. Dark areas signify increased uptake of the radioactive marker, indicating hypervascular lesions or areas of increased osteoblastic activity. In this example, it is specifically seen in the left knee and right elbow, due to osteoarthritis

Table 3.3 Radioactive tracers and their biological markers used in nuclear medicine scans. Half-life is expressed in minutes (m), hours (h) or days (d)

Tracer	Biological marker	Half life	Pathology
Technetium-99 m (Bone scan)	Diphosphate	6.01 h	Hypervascular lesions Areas of increased osteoblastic activity (e.g. fractures, osteoarthritis, bone tumours, Paget's disease).
Indium-111 (WBC scan)	Patient's leucocytes	2.80 d	Acute infection (especially periprosthetic infections)
Gallium-67 (Gallium scan)	Citrate	3.26 d	Tumours Inflammation Chronic infection (especially osteomyelitis outside of spine)
Carbon-11 or nitrogen-13 or fluorine-18 (PET scans)	Fluorodeoxyglucose	20.3 m 9.97 m 109.8 m	Primary and secondary cancers

Single-photon emission computed tomography (SPECT)

SPECT scans are a special form of nuclear medicine imaging. Multiple 2D bone scan are acquired with a gamma camera and reconstructed to provide a 3D image on a similar principle to CT scans. SPECT scans can be further reconstructed with data from a CT scan to produce a SPECT/CT scan (Figure 3.7). Some indications include looking for infection, inflammation and loosening of implants.

Positron emission tomography (PET)
Image generation

A positron-emitting radionuclide tracer is injected into the body attached to a bioactive molecule, usually the glucose analogue fluorodeoygluose (FDG). FDG is taken up by metabolically active tissue. Positrons emitted as the tracer decays interact with electrons in the body, producing a pair of photons that move apart in opposite directions. The detection of photon pairs

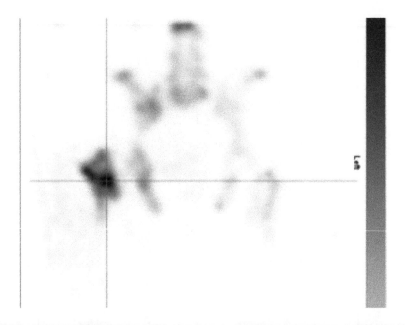

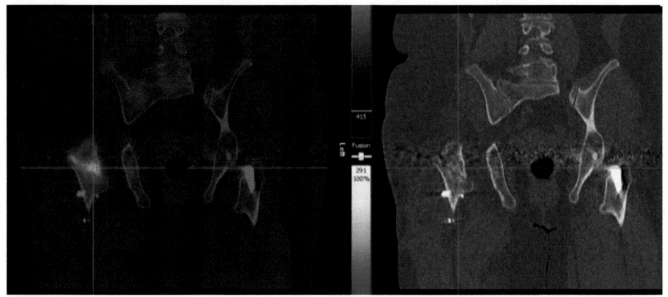

Figure 3.7 A bilateral hip SPECT/CT scan. The central image is reconstructed using data from the SPECT scan (top) and the CT scan (bottom)

moving approximately opposite to each other are filtered from photons not detected as divergent pairs. The origin of the photon pairs can thus be determined, and thus areas where FDG is concentrated.

Morbidity potential

See bone scans.

Examples of orthopaedic applications

PET scans are being used more frequently in assessing musculo-skeletal tumours. It is also able to evaluate the metabolism and function of deep tissues not applicable to neurophysiological testing. PET scans can also be reconstructed with CT scan data to produce a PET/CT scan, allowing precise anatomical localisation correlating to the functional imaging.

Neurophysiological tests

Nerve conduction studies

Nerve conduction studies examine the function of motor and sensory nerves. The speed of the action potential from the stimulus to the sensor (nerve conduction velocity in ms^{-1}), travel time (latency ms), and size of the response (amplitude mV or μV) are basic readings derived from studies.

Motor studies stimulate peripheral nerves and examine the response of the muscles it innervates. The innervating peripheral nerve can be stimulated at multiple sites to help determine the site of any pathology.

Sensory studies stimulate a peripheral nerve distally and record from a proximal sensory portion of the nerve. Amplitudes are generally smaller compared to motor nerve studies – thus are measured in μV.

F-wave studies determine the conduction velocity of a motor nerve between the limb and the spinal cord. The stimulating electrode causes an action potential to travel to the ventral horn of the spinal cord and back to the limb via the same nerve.

Hoffmann's (H)-reflex studies examine reflex arcs within a limb. Stimulation of an appropriate sensory nerve causes action potentials to travel to the spinal cord and return via motor nerves to the respective muscles.

Morbidity potential

Nerve conduction studies are noninvasive but can be uncomfortable due to the use of electrical currents. Metallic implants (pacemakers, permanent tissue stimulators, etc.) are not contraindications for the study; however, may require special precautions.

Examples of orthopaedic applications

Pathological conditions can cause changes in the conduction velocity, latency, or amplitude of the action potential. Generalised reduction of conduction velocity may represent demyelination (e.g. Charcot-Marie-Tooth disease). Specific reduction of sensory and motor latency at a specific site, such as across the wrist, may indicate a focal compression of the nerve (e.g. carpal tunnel syndrome). Slowing of all nerve conductions in multiple limbs may indicate a more systemic pathological process (e.g. diabetic neuropathy).

Electromyography (EMG)

Technically distinct from nerve conduction studies, EMG is often performed at the same time. EMG evaluates the electrical potential produced by skeletal muscles when they are activated. Electrodes are placed either topically or directly (via a cannulated needle and fine wire) into the target muscle.

Direct insertion usually causes electrical stimulation of the muscle, providing immediate feedback regarding the state of the muscle and its innervating nerve (M-wave). The muscle is studied when electrically inactive at rest, before assessment when electrically active during contractions. In normal muscle, electrical potentials should only be seen when the muscle is actively contracting (once the muscle has resumed a resting state after needle insertion).

The amplitude, shape, and frequency of electrical activity are examined. The electrode is retracted until information has been collected on at least 20 motor units. Topical electrodes are used when needle insertion is deemed inappropriate (e.g. non-neurologist outpatient clinic).

EMG studies aid in the diagnosis and monitoring of numerous neuromuscular pathologies. The characteristic of action potentials can differentiate between neuropathic and myopathic disease (Table 3.4).

Morbidity potential

This is the same as for nerve conduction studies, except direct electrode insertion can cause further pain and routes of infection.

Examples of orthopaedic applications

Used in conjunction with nerve conduction studies, EMG aids in the diagnosis of numerous neuromuscular pathologies (Box 3.2).

Table 3.4 Comparing the differences in EMG results for myogenic and neurogenic pathological processes

	Myogenic	Neurogenic
Amplitude of potential	Decreased	Increased
Duration of potential	Decreased	Increased
Number of motor units	Decreased (severe cases)	Decreased
Examples	Muscular dystrophy Lambert-Eaton Syndrome Myotubular Myopathy	Carpal tunnel syndrome Charcot-Marie-Tooth disease Motor neurone disease

Box 3.2 **Pathological processes EMG studies are useful in diagnosing and monitoring.**

- Brachial plexus injury
- Carpal tunnel syndrome
- Charcot-Marie-Tooth disease
- Mononeuropathy
- Myopathy
- Nerve dysfunction
- Neuritis
- Polymyositis
- Radiculopathy (e.g. sciatica)
- Spinal stenosis
- Spondylosis
- Ulnar nerve entrapment
- Muscular dystrophy (e.g. Duchenne's and Becker's)

Laboratory investigations

Microbiology

Microbiology concerns pathogen isolation, identification, and determination of antimicrobial sensitivities and resistances from fluid obtained intra-operatively or by arthrocentesis. The most frequently requested diagnostic microbiological investigation is microscopy, culture, and sensitivities (MC&S).

Orthopaedic infections involve soft tissue, bone (osteomyelitis), or joints (septic arthritis), with foreign material such as implants possibly acting as harbours or foci of infection. The majority of infections are spread through contiguous (direct inoculation through open wounds or local spread) or haematogenous (via the blood stream) mechanisms. Predisposing factors include indwelling urinary catheter, intravenous drug usage, sexually transmitted infection, and immunocompromised state. High extents of morbidity can result from orthopaedic infections; hence, prompt diagnosis and aggressive treatment is crucial.

Obtaining appropriate and adequate samples prior to commencing antibiotics is vital (e.g. aspirated joint fluid, deep periprosthetic tissue samples, blood cultures, etc). There is usually only one opportunity to obtain a sample uncorrupted by the administration of antibiotics, and failure jeopardises subsequent treatment. Sampling must be performed aseptically to minimise contamination and prevent secondary pathogens entering the tissue field.

Prompt transfer of samples to the laboratory for microbial analysis is important, especially if anaerobic bacteria are suspected. Fluid samples should be transported as a pure sample and, if possible, in culture media bottles.

Once samples are obtained, patients can be started on broad-spectrum antibiotics and more aggressive management may be considered (e.g. irrigation and debridement of infected tissue, wash-out or removal of in-situ metalwork). The choice of antibiotics will depend on the suspicion of the causative bacteria; *Staphylococcus aureus* is the most common cause of orthopaedic infections, and treatment may be tailored to this or more broad-spectrum antibiotics until sensitivities are deduced. Nevertheless, gram staining takes a few hours to aid antibiotic choice. Microbiologists are able to advise on sampling, interpretation of results, and appropriate antibiotic therapy, which could last for weeks through a peripherally inserted central catheter (PICC line).

Biopsy

Biopsy is a technique for tissue sampling of suspected soft tissue and bone cancers, deep infected tissue (e.g. periprosthetic), or inflammatory conditions. Ideal biopsy criteria are shown in Box 3.3.

The three types of biopsy techniques are summarised in Table 3.5.

With respect to cancer, biopsies should only be performed at specialist centres where they are frequently performed, expert pathologists are available for accurate diagnosis, and definitive treatment (surgery and adjuvant therapies) can all be performed. Management in nonspecialist centres is proven to have higher levels of misdiagnosis and associated morbidity and mortality. Table 3.6 shows details of history or physical examination that are suspicious of cancer.

Box 3.4 shows red and yellow flags seen in radiological investigations for cancer, warranting biopsy.

Histology

Histology is the microscopic analysis of tissue. It involves the fixing, embedding, sectioning, and staining of specimens, followed by light or electron microscopic analysis. There is a large variety of stains used, all specifically employed for different types of cells and different pathologies. The commonest use in orthopaedic practice is diagnosing suspected cancers.

Cytology

Cytology involves the examination of single cells or small cluster of cells. Fine-needle aspiration is used to sample fluid or harvest cells from tissue. Cytology has a role in confirming cancer diagnosis in conjunction with clinical and radiological findings, but open biopsy is utilised if there is any doubt. Cytology allows immediate interpretation, rapid oncological consultation and expedited chemotherapy or radiotherapy. Cytology is still readily used for fluid analysis, especially joint effusions. Table 3.7 shows the different results for synovial fluid analysis.

Blood tests

Although not exhaustive, Table 3.8 shows blood tests with a specific roll within orthopaedic practice. Generic preoperative tests (e.g. urea and creatinine as a marker of renal function) are not covered.

Box 3.3 The characteristics of an ideal biopsy

- The site and route of biopsy is carefully planned. For suspected cancer, the route should be in line with the proposed surgical incision to prevent seeding of tissue. These areas must also be excised should resection be necessary.
- An adequate volume is acquired, which is representative of the site biopsied.
- Minimal contamination of other tissues is caused, especially those in different fascial compartments to the biopsied lesion.
- Appropriate preparation facilities for the specimen in order to expedite accurate diagnosis.
- Expert pathologists, who are experienced in analysing musculo-skeletal tissue specimens, are available to examine the biopsies.

Table 3.5 Biopsy techniques employed in orthopaedic surgery

Biopsy technique	Comment
Excisional biopsy	Removal of an entire lump or tissue *en bloc.* E.g. suspected lipomas.
Incisional biopsy	A sample of the tissue is cut out of the lesion, preserving the histological architecture of the tissue. A wedge of tissue can be removed or a core can be taken using special biopsy needles such as Trucut biopsy needles.
Needle aspiration biopsy	Removal of tissue or fluid using a needle. Low pressure is created in the syringe and movement of the needle shears cells from tissues, which are sucked into the syringe.

Table 3.6 Specific details of history and examination that should arouse suspicion of cancer

History	Insidious onset
	Worsening of symptoms, especially pain or lump size
	Pain characteristics: night wakening, constant pain
	Systemic symptoms: weight loss, night sweats
	Past medical history: previous cancer, trauma, or radiotherapy in the area
	Family history of cancer
Examination	Anatomical site: Distal femur, proximal tibia, proximal humerus
	Size: >5 cm and increasing
	Deep to fascia
	Edge: Irregular
	Consistency: firm/hard
	Tender

Box 3.4 Features to note when describing space occupying lesions on plain radiographs

- Anatomical site: Distal femur/proximal tibia/proximal humerus
- Site within bone: Metaphyseal or intramedullary
- Size: <5 cm/>5 cm
- Zone of transition: Narrow/wide
- Pattern of bone destruction: Permeative/discrete/moth eaten
- Cortical response: Expanded/Scalloped/Destruction
- Periosteal reaction: Laminated/solid/vertical
- Matrix mineralisation: Ossous/chondral/fibrous

Table 3.7 Analysis results for normal synovial fluid, septic, inflammatory, haemorrhagic, and osteoarthritic effusions

	Normal	Septic	Inflammatory	Haemorrhagic	Osteoarthritic
Volume/mL	<3.5	>3.5	>3.5	>3.5	>3.5
Viscosity	High	Mixed	Low	Low	High
Clarity	Clear	Opaque	Cloudy	Mixed	Clear
Colour	Pale straw	Yellow/ Green	Yellow	Red	Straw/yellow
WBC/mm³	<200	>50000	5000-75000	As blood	<2000
Polymorphs	<25%	>70%	5070%	As blood	<25%
Gram stain	−ve	+ve	−ve	−ve	−ve

Table 3.8 Specific blood tests used in orthopaedic surgery

Test [Normal range]	Comment	Related Pathology
Haemoglobin (Hb) [Male: 13.8–18.0 g/dL] [Female: 12.1–15.1 g/dL]	The mean cell volume and haematocrit must be taken into account, as they may affect the reported level of Hb following fluid resuscitation. Ideally, repeat Hb should be taken 12–24 hours later.	Levels may be abnormally low following major surgery, trauma, or secondary to chronic infection (e.g. normocytic anaemia of chronic disease).
White cell count (WCC) [3.5–11 10⁹/L]		Increased levels: inflammation (usually due to trauma, infection or healing). Transient increases during pregnancy, myocardial infarction, and corticosteroid administration. Decreased levels: sepsis, old age, chronic use of steroids, and immunocompromisation.
Erythrocyte sedimentation rate (ESR) [Male: <Age/2 mm/hour] [Female: <(Age + 10)/2 mm/hour]	The height of stacked red blood cells (rouleaux formation) settling in a tube over a fixed time; correlated to extent of plasma protein concentration.	A raised ESR reflects an increase of large proteins within the plasma (such as fibrinogen), as a response to inflammation or infection. Physiologically, ESR increases naturally with age, more so in females, and also in patients with severe anaemia.
Complement-reactive protein (CRP) [<5 mg/L]	A protein synthesised within the liver during an acute phase response in response to inflammation. It usually begins to rise within 2 hours but may not reach its peak until 48 hours after the insult.	CRP is commonly elevated due to infectious or inflammatory causes and trauma (both accidental and surgical).
Urate/Uric acid: [Male: 3.6–8.3 mg/dL] [Female: 2.3–6.6 mg/dL]	Gout is a common differential diagnosis for patients with monoarthropathy, especially if recurrent. Urate levels are relative and must be considered within the whole clinical picture.	Elevated urate levels are not diagnostic of gout, and patients with gout may have normal urate levels.
Calcium: [1.03–1.30 mmol/L]		Increased levels: multiple myeloma, bone tumours or Paget's disease. Decreased levels: osteomalacia, osteoporosis secondary to hypoparathyroidism, chronic hypomagnesaemia or inadequate absorption.
Phosphate: [0.8–1.5 mmol/L]	Phosphate levels are intricately linked to calcium and are usually governed by the parathyroid glands.	Increased levels: osteomalacia, hypoparathyroidism or chronic renal failure. Decreased levels: hyperparathyroidism, hypophosphataemic rickets, malnourishment, alcoholism, or malabsorption syndromes.
Alkaline phosphatase (ALP): [Male 53–128 U/L] [Female 42-98 U/L]	Present in virtually all tissues, especially bones, ALP removes phosphate groups from many molecules by hydrolysis.	Increased specific to orthopaedics: Paget's disease, osteosarcomas, multiple myeloma, boney metastases (especially prostate cancer), fractures, renal osteodystrophy, osteomalacia, rickets, vitamin D deficiency.
Vitamin D: [50–125 nmol/L]	An important regulator of bone remodelling, calcium and phosphate levels. Low levels can be attributed to dietary insufficiency in conjunction with inadequate sunlight exposure.	Low levels can cause osteomalacia (rickets in children) and are commonly seen in patients with osteoporosis.
Rheumatoid factor (RF): [<20 U/mL]	An IgM autoantibody against IgG; RF is most relevant in orthopaedic practice in the diagnosis of rheumatoid arthritis.	Increased in rheumatoid arthritis. It may also be elevated in autoimmune diseases unrelated to rheumatoid arthritis and various infections (especially Epstein-Barr Virus (EBV)).
Anti-Cyclic Citrullinated Peptide Antibodies (Anti-CCP): [<20 EU]	As with RF, anti-CCP levels can correlate poorly with disease activity.	Autoantibodies frequently implicated in rheumatoid arthritis.
Anti-nuclear antibodies (ANA): [Depends on subtype]	Autoantibodies that attack the nucleus of native cells.	Increased levels: rheumatoid arthritis, Raynaud's phenomenon, fibromyalgia, juvenile idiopathic arthritis, and psoriatic arthritis.

Further reading

Glossary of Orthopaedic Diagnostic Tests. https://orthoinfo.aaos.org/en/treatment/glossary-of-orthopaedic-diagnostic-tests/

Wheeless Textbook of Orthopaedics. http://www.wheelessonline.com/ortho/lab_menu

Wheeless, C.R. (2012). *Wheeless' Textbook of Orthopaedics*. http://www.wheelessonline.com/ortho/extremity_tourniquets. Published 2012. Accessed September 22, 2017.

CHAPTER 4

Orthopaedic Trauma

Aamer Nisar[1], Chinmay M. Gupte[2,3], and Rajarshi Bhattacharya[3]

[1]Hull and East Yorkshire Hospitals NHS Trust, Hull, UK
[2]MSk Lab, Charing Cross Hospital, Imperial College London, London, UK
[3]Imperial College Healthcare NHS Trust, London, UK

OVERVIEW

- Trauma is a leading cause of death worldwide, according to WHO.
- ATLS has significantly improved management and outcomes of trauma victims by providing a system of prioritising and treating injuries in order of seriousness.
- Orthopaedic injuries form a significant proportion of the trauma victims' injuries.
- Fractures should be considered as soft tissue injuries with a broken bone.
- Radiological investigations help to identify musculoskeletal injuries in greater details.

Introduction

Trauma is a leading cause of disability and death across all age groups. It is important to have a clear understanding of basic principles of the assessment and management of this group of patients. This chapter gives a brief outline of the orthopaedic management principles of polytrauma and fractures.

Polytrauma

Trauma is a leading cause of death in individuals younger than 40 years of age. Three peak periods of death are known to occur in polytrauma patients:

1 *Immediate*: Occurs within seconds to minutes of injury. Death may happen on the scene and is generally related to severe brain or cardiac injury or damage to major blood vessels. The only effective way to reduce death in this period is prevention.

2 *Early*: Death usually occurs in the first few hours of injury. Causes include massive haemothorax or intra-abdominal visceral injury causing severe haemorrhage. This is the *"golden hour,"* and death in this period can be prevented by an effective ATLS approach.

3 *Late*: Usually from days to week after injury and related to sepsis or multiple organ failure.

A systematic approach to the polytrauma patients could prevent morbidity and avoid deaths through a multidisciplinary approach, which is based on ATLS principles.

Advance trauma life support

Advance trauma life support (ATLS) is a systematic approach to the management of high-energy trauma patients to prevent death and minimise morbidity. Now well known as the *ABCDE* approach, ATLS involves dealing with life-threatening injuries first, followed by less severe injuries to optimally stabilise the patient (Table 4.1).

Assessments are divided into primary (ABCDE) and secondary surveys. Patients are managed in a multidisciplinary fashion with several key personnel working in tandem and systematically (Figure 4.1). Secondary survey is carried out after the primary survey is complete and the patient has been resuscitated. Secondary survey could sometimes be delayed for many days. A complete head-to-toe examination is carried out, including complete neurological examination, which must be thoroughly documented.

Management of patients with multiple fractures in polytrauma

Basic principles of management of trauma patients include:
(1) pre-hospital recognition of major trauma and blue light (ambulance) transfer to major trauma centre,
(2) primary survey,
(3) management of life threatening injuries,
(4) secondary survey,
(5) transfer to definitive care (operating theatre and ward), and
(6) rehabilitation with MDT input.

A large number of polytrauma patients have multiple fractures (e.g. pelvic and long bone fractures) that may require definitive surgical treatment to avoid haemorrhaging, fat emboli and chronic disability.

Early total care versus damage control orthopaedics

There are two separate concepts that can be used in polytrauma management: (1) early total care (ETC), and (2) damage control orthopaedics (DCO). ETC used to be the mainstay of management until the 1980s and 1990s. It involved fixation of all the long bone fractures within the first 24 to 48 hours. The benefits include early stabilisation and mobilisation of the patients. However, not all patients are suitable for ETC

ABC of Orthopaedics and Trauma, First Edition. Edited by Kapil Sugand and Chinmay M. Gupte.
© 2018 John Wiley & Sons Ltd. Published 2018 by John Wiley & Sons Ltd.

due to multiple organ injuries and risk of pulmonary complications. Over the years, the understanding of the pathophysiology and immune response of the host to major trauma has also improved. Multiple traumatic injuries lead to systematic inflammatory response, the "first hit" for the patient. Surgery carried out within this time would be a "second hit," and could lead to multiple organ failure and early death. For this reason, definitive management of skeletal injuries is sometimes delayed for some days, generally 5–10 days. Therefore, in the early phase, minimal surgical intervention DCO is carried out for the most limb or life-threatening injury, and fractures can be immobilised temporarily with emergency surgery (i.e. external fixators), splints or plaster casts, until a suitable time for definitive fracture stabilisation.

Fracture pathology

Fracture is defined as a break in the continuity of a cortex. The bony injury is, however, only one component, and is often accompanied by significant soft tissue injuries, the management of which may sometimes be more difficult with more profound consequences than the actual fracture. Thus fractures should be considered as *soft tissue injury with a broken bone.*

Following a fracture, a series of events takes place at a microscopic level, as shown in Figure 4.2 and described as follows:

(a) Haematoma forms in the first few days.

(b) Acute inflammatory reaction occurs with migration of haemopoietic cells, which bring growth factors to the fracture site, leading to formation of soft callus over the first 2–4 weeks.

(c) The soft callus splints the fracture and is later replaced with bony callus, which is most prominent by 3 months.

(d) Through a combined action of osteoblasts (bone forming cells) and osteoclasts (bone removing cells), bone is remodeled over a period of many months to years, depending on age and extent of comorbidities.

Fracture healing is either primary or secondary. Primary healing occurs in fractures treated with absolute stability (rigid fixation e.g. plates) with direct bone healing. Primary healing will only occur when the two fractures' ends are in direct contact and there is no movement at the fracture site. Fractures treated with relative stability (nonrigid fixation such as plaster immobilisation or intramedullary nail) heal through responses in the periosteum with callus formation (secondary healing).

Fracture terminology

Description of fractures follows an internationally acceptable terminology for easy communication between health professionals. Fractures can be simple or complex, based on the fracture fragments. A fracture that has a single fracture line or two main fragments can be termed as a simple fracture, whereas a fracture that contains multiple fragments is termed as multifragmentary or comminuted fracture (Figure 4.3) from high-energy trauma.

Fractures can be described as undisplaced or displaced based on translation of bony fragments in antero-posterior or medio-lateral plane. Based on angulation of distal fragments, fractures can be angulated into varus (inward) or valgus (outward), or rotated on

Table 4.1 Primary survey in ATLS

A	Airway with cervical spine support	Assess and secure airway and apply cervical collar.
B	Breathing	Assess ventilation and oxygen saturation. Apply high-flow oxygen using a non-rebreather mask.
C	Circulation with massive hemorrhage control	Check capillary refill, central pulses, and BP. Insert two large-bore IV or intraosseous cannulation to send off bloods and venous blood gas. Apply pressure or tourniquet to achieve haemostasis and look for occult bleeding, splint pelvic, and long bone fractures.
D	Disability	Neurological examination (GCS), BM, pupils, limb deformity.
E	Exposure	Full exposure to assess the peripheries, assess abdomen, consider FAST scan, prevent hypothermia.

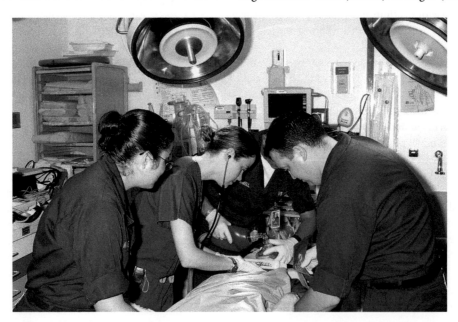

Figure 4.1 Trauma call being attended by multiple personnel

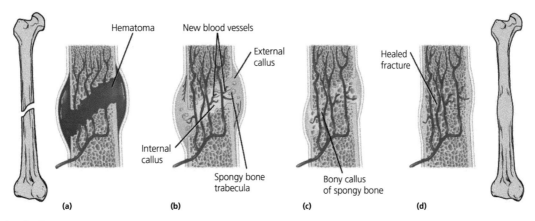

Figure 4.2 Fracture healing

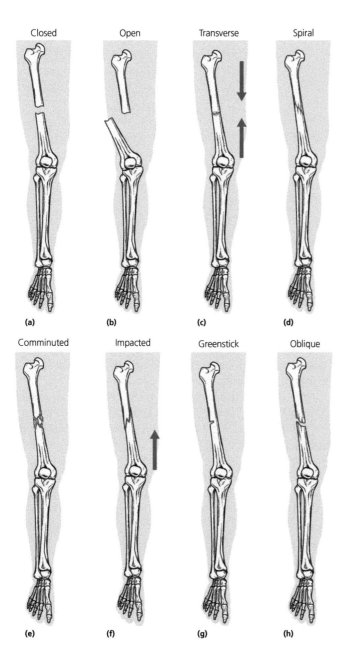

Figure 4.3 Fracture patterns

the long axis of the bone segment, internally rotated or externally rotated (Figure 4.3). It is also important to recognise the fractures occurring in the vicinity of the joints. Peri-articular fractures can be intra-articular or extra-articular. Intra-articular fractures could then be subdivided into simple articular (undisplaced) or complex articular (comminuted articular surface).

Joints can be described as dislocated if there is complete displacement of articulating surfaces, or subluxed if there is partial joint displacement. A dislocation is simple if there is no associated peri-articular fractures, which otherwise is termed as complex dislocation. A dislocated joint is an emergency and requires urgent reduction under appropriate analgesia, either in the resuscitation bay or in theatre.

A fracture can be open or closed. An open fracture has a bone exposed to the external environment, which would then increase the risk of infection, predisposing to fracture non-union, requiring repeat surgical procedures and increased patient morbidity. Open fractures are emergencies and require urgent management, including intravenous antibiotics, tetanus prophylaxis, and wound debridement besides fracture stabilisation. Guidelines on managing open fractures have been published under the British Orthopaedic Association Standards for Trauma (publication number 4).

Basic principles of fracture management

Management of any fracture becomes very simple if one takes a standardised approach. If ever in doubt, then always remember the four cardinal rules of Rs: resuscitate, reduce, rest (or hold – splinting followed by fixation using metal or no metalwork), and rehabilitation. There are some basic principles that apply to management of any fracture (Box 4.1).

Fracture assessment involves identifying whether it is open or closed, assessing damage to soft tissues like muscle contusions, tendon ruptures, and compartment syndromes. It is important to document the neurovascular status on initial assessment and then on regular intervals, especially after any intervention. A change in neurovascular status may necessitate emergent treatment of the fractures. Fractures can be a source of immense pain; therefore, adequate analgesia is important. Bear in mind that even anatomical

Box 4.1 **Basic Principles of Fracture Management**

1 **Assess**
   a Soft tissues (skin, muscles, tendons, compartments)
   b Bone and joints (appropriate radiographs)
   c Neurovascular status
2 **Pain relief** (IV, oral, nerve blocks)
3 **Immobilise temporarily**
   a Mode (backslab, plaster, splints)
4 **Definitive management** (nonoperative vs. operative)
   – Reduce
   – Immobilise
      a Duration (upper vs. lower limb, children vs. adults)
      b Method (various)
   – Rehabilitate (physiotherapy)

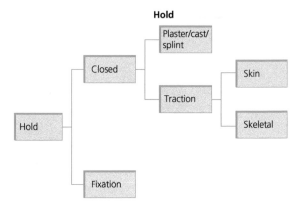

Figure 4.5 Principles of fracture holding

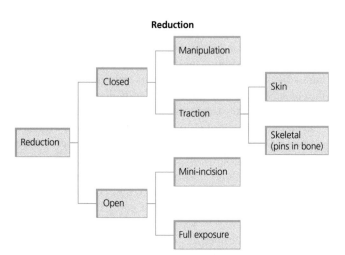

Figure 4.4 Principles of fracture reduction

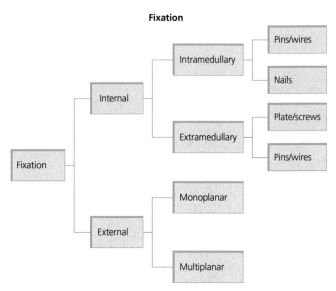

Figure 4.6 Principles of fracture fixation

reduction of fractures will provide pain relief. Subsequent management of fracture would depend on fracture type and associated injuries. Once the fracture has been treated definitively, the patient in general, and the fracture segment in particular, may require a course of rehabilitation. This is where a multidisciplinary approach is important right from the outset, with involvement of physiotherapists, occupational therapists, and specialist nurses.

Reduction (Figure 4.4) consists of closed techniques for functional reduction and relative stability, whereas the open technique achieves anatomical reduction for absolute stability.

Holding the fracture to avoid further displacement and to provide pain relief can be done as described in Figure 4.5.

Taking it one step further, once the fracture is held, the more definitive option is to fix the fracture using the options shown in Figure 4.6.

Stabilisation of fractures

Definitive management of fractures requires adequate stabilisation. A fracture can be treated with either absolute or relative stability. Absolute stability refers to anatomical reduction and rigid internal fixation. This can be achieved by inter-fragmentary compression with a screw or a compression plate. Absolute stability is generally

required in peri-articular fractures to prevent post-traumatic arthritis or occasionally in long bone fractures (e.g. in forearm fractures anatomic reduction is required to restore the bone length for optimal joint function). In fractures treated with absolute stability, there is minimal micromovement at the fracture and bone healing occurs with primary intention.

Extra-articular fractures can be treated with relative stability. This type of stabilisation is flexible and allows some micromovement at the fracture site. As a consequence the bone heals with secondary intention with formation of callus. Examples of fracture management with relative stability include plaster cast, intramedullary nails, or bridging plates. The choice of fixation device depends on the fracture personality (associated soft tissue injury, bone quality, and fracture orientation), patient, and surgeon factors.

Nonoperative versus operative management

One of the important questions that face an orthopaedic surgeon is whether a fracture requires an operation. A number of factors dictate the mode of treatment. Generally most undisplaced fractures can be treated in a plaster cast, duration of which is variable and depends on bone segment, fracture configuration, and patient's age.

Table 4.2 shows the average time taken by different bone segments to heal in children and adults.

A displaced, intra-articular, or peri-articular fracture may require surgery. A fracture is reduced and then stabilised. Reduction could be closed or open. Open reduction generally accompanies stabilisation with a plate or an intramedullary nail and here we go back to the concept of absolute or relative stability based on the fracture location and configuration. Occasionally, fractures are treated with an external fixator when soft tissues are damaged, and open reduction can lead to wound complications. Once again, it is important to remember that a fracture is a soft tissue injury with a broken bone and it is important to respect the state of soft tissues (Figure 4.7). Rehabilitation (Figure 4.8) is always the final treatment of fracture management. Regular exercises strengthen the adjacent musculature to take weight-bearing pressure of fractures while it continues to remodel. Weight bearing also propagates fracture remodelling (Wolff's law). Do not forget the age-old idiom in trauma and orthopaedics: "*If you don't use it, you lose it!*"

Special situations

Whereas basic principles of management of all trauma patients are same, certain special situations need to be considered. Fractures in children need special attention due to skeletal immaturity and potential for remodelling. Injury to growth plates and risk of deformity require close monitoring of physical injuries. Non-accidental injury should be considered in children less than 2 years of age who sustain fractures with referral to child safeguarding

services. Pregnant women with trauma should be considered special cases and use of radiographs should be limited in the first trimester. In polytrauma, obstetricians should be involved in the management of pregnant women with careful foetal monitoring instituted early. Elderly patients have multiple comorbidities, osteoporosis, preexisting arthritis, and are on multiple medications that may slow down rate of healing. Moreover, elderly patients have less cardiopulmonary reserves, thereby affecting their response to trauma.

Trauma radiology

Imaging is an integral part of orthopaedic and trauma investigations. Various modalities have different applications.

In polytrauma, trauma series radiographs of the following should be taken:
1 AP and lateral C-spine views, but this has been replaced with CT imaging to improve sensitivity and specificity
2 AP chest
3 AP pelvis
4 Any joints or long bones that are deformed or painful on secondary survey

Nowadays, with the care of polytrauma patients being centralised to major trauma centres (MTC), the trauma series radiograph is being superseded by CT scan of C-spine, chest, abdomen and pelvis, which

Table 4.2 Estimated median fracture healing time in children and adults

Bone segment	Fracture Union Time	
	Children	Adults
Radius/Ulna	4 weeks	6–8 weeks
Humerus	6 weeks	8–12 weeks
Clavicle	4 weeks	6–8 weeks
Femur	8 weeks	12–16 weeks
Tibia	8 weeks	12–16 weeks

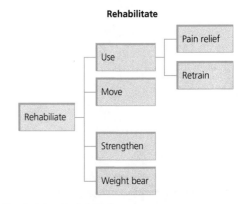

Figure 4.8 Principles of rehabilitation

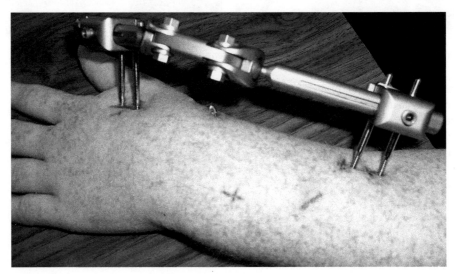

Figure 4.7 External fixator for wrist fracture

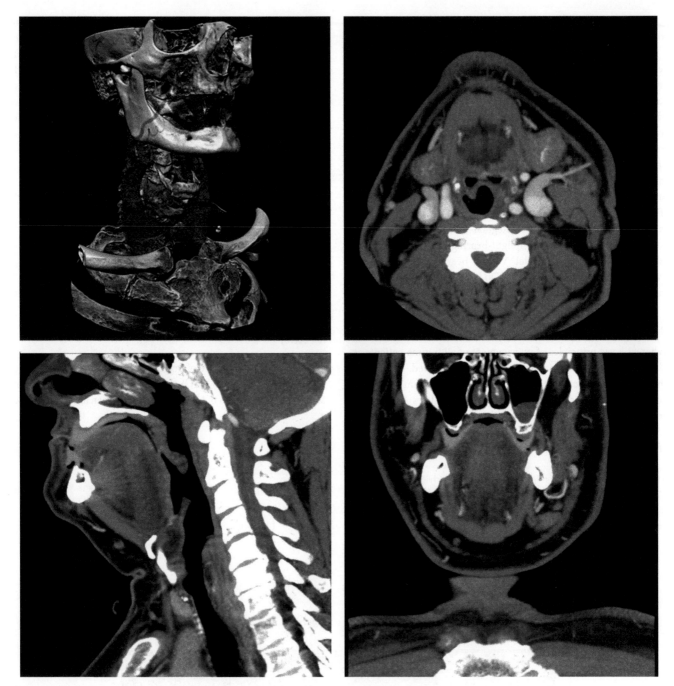

Figure 4.9 CT traumagrams showing base of skull and cervical spine with 3D reconstruction

is a fast and effective means of identifying any obvious fractures and organ injuries in the multiply-injured patient who is often either unconscious or intubated and hence difficult to examine. Focused assessment with sonography for trauma (FAST) scan is available in all major trauma centres, and is an important tool for detecting abdominal, pulmonary, and pericardial injuries at bedside. As a general principle, all radiographs for suspected fractures should have two views in orthogonal plane, AP and lateral, and include the joint above and below. Further imaging includes CT traumagrams, which is useful to study detailed bony anatomy in complex fractures. 3D CT reconstruction is now available for more detailed analysis (Figure 4.9). For soft tissue injuries or spinal trauma, MRI is generally a useful adjunct.

Further reading

Advanced Trauma Life Support. (2012). *ATLS Student Course Manual*, 9th ed. Chicago: American College of Surgeons.

Browner, B., Levine, A., Jupiter, J.B., et al. (2009). *Skeletal Trauma. Basic Science, Management and Reconstruction*, 4th ed. Philadelphia: Saunders.

Pape, H.C., Tornetta, P., III, Tarkin, I., et al. (2009). Timing of fracture fixation in multitrauma patients: the role of early total care and damage control surgery. *Journal of American Academic Orthopedic Surgery* 17 (9): 541–549.

Ruedi, T.P., Buckley, R.E., and Moran, C.G. (2007). *AO Principles of Fracture Management*. New York: Thieme.

Solomon, L., Warwick, D., and Nayagam, S. (2001). *Apley's System of Orthopaedics and Fractures*, 8th ed. New York: Arnold.

CHAPTER 5

Management of Adult Fractures

Aamer Nisar[1], Chinmay M. Gupte[2,3], and Rajarshi Bhattacharya[3]

[1] Hull and East Yorkshire Hospitals NHS Trust, Hull, UK
[2] MSk Lab, Charing Cross Hospital, Imperial College London, London, UK
[3] Imperial College Healthcare NHS Trust, London, UK

OVERVIEW

- A fracture is a discontinuity of bony cortex with an associated soft tissue injury.
- The general management of fractures comprises of the 4 **R**s: resuscitate (ABCDE), reduce (closed vs. open), rest (hold with traction vs. plaster vs. metal), and rehabilitate (physiotherapy).
- Treatment options include conservative (plaster/traction) or operative management (metal fixation).
- Operative management consists of internal (intra- vs. extra-medullary) vs. external fixation.
- Some fractures, such as of the pelvis and femur, can be life-threatening due to associated significant haemorrhage.
- Intra-articular fractures are at risk of early degenerative change and more commonly require anatomical reduction and fixation.
- Open fractures are considered as an orthopaedic emergency that requires urgent treatment due to risk of infection, pain, and loss of function.

Causes

Fractures can be caused by traumatic, stress, and pathological aetiologies. Most fractures occur due to energy from trauma or injury causing a breech in the continuity of bone. However, in some cases (e.g. tumours or osteoporosis), there is an inherent weakness in the substance of the bone that predisposes to a fracture. These are known as pathological fractures. In contrast, stress fractures occur when abnormal repetitive stresses are applied to normal bone that result in a fracture (e.g. during marathon running or marching).

Upper-limb fractures

Clavicle

These fractures can be subclassified according to the part of clavicle that is involved, splitting it into thirds, from medial to lateral. Middle third fractures are the most common (Figure 5.1) and the majority can be treated non-operatively in a broad arm sling. This provides support for the elbow and prevents downward displacement of the lateral part of the fracture with the shoulder. Operative intervention may be necessary in clavicle fractures that show significant shortening (greater than 2 cm compared with the other side) or those that involve the lateral third, as they have a higher risk of nonunion.

Proximal humerus

These are usually associated with osteoporotic bone often resulting from falls in geriatric patients (see Chapter 6). In the younger patient, however, these are often due to high-energy trauma. Fractures of the proximal humerus can be classified using the Neer classification system (Figure 6.10). These fractures can often be managed conservatively, with the angle of the humeral head and its position over the shaft determining whether further reduction is necessary. Operative options include open reduction and internal fixation or replacement. Better outcomes are achieved if the decision to leave, fix or replace are made early (i.e. within the first 2 weeks).

Shoulder dislocation (Chapters 6 and 14.3) can occur in the young as well as older age groups. Although, recurrence is greater in younger patients. Fractures of the proximal humerus may occur during the reduction of a dislocated shoulder itself (iatrogenic), or a fracture dislocation can occur at the time of injury, and these require judicious expertise in management. In all cases of shoulder injury, it is important to document the status of skin sensation provided by the axillary nerve over the upper lateral arm, otherwise known as the sergeants badge area or regimental patch.

Mid-humerus

Mid-humeral fractures are most likely traumatic but may also be pathological (osteoporosis and bone tumour). Coaptation splint followed by functional humeral brace is indicated in the majority of cases. Acceptable alignment consists of angulation (<30°) and length (<3 cm shortening). Operative fixation through ORIF is reserved for open fracture, injury to neurovascular structures, ipsilateral forearm fracture (i.e. floating elbow) and compartment syndrome. Intramedullary nailing is reserved for polytrauma, segmental, and pathological (including prophylactically for bone tumours) fractures.

ABC of Orthopaedics and Trauma, First Edition. Edited by Kapil Sugand and Chinmay M. Gupte.
© 2018 John Wiley & Sons Ltd. Published 2018 by John Wiley & Sons Ltd.

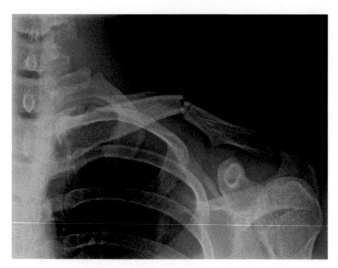

Figure 5.1 Clavicle fracture with shortening

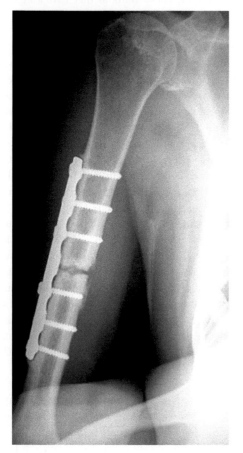

Figure 5.2 ORIF of mid humerus with plates and screws

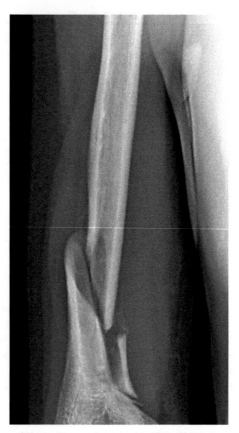

Figure 5.3 Holstein-Lewis fracture of the distal humerus

Distal humerus

These can involve the shaft of the distal humerus or the elbow joint. The neurovascular structures around the distal humerus lie in very close relation to the bone, and therefore thorough neurological assessment is essential in such fractures, particularly as further injury may occur during the treatment process. Fractures that extend into the joint are more likely to require fixation with plates and screws (Figure 5.2). Stiffness is a common post-injury complication.

The radial nerve runs in the spiral groove 7–14 cm proximal to the elbow directly on the posterior aspect of the humerus. This can be damaged at the time of a distal humeral fracture or can get trapped as the fracture reduces or is manipulated. This fracture pattern is known as a Holstein-Lewis fracture (Figure 5.3).

Intra-articular fractures of the elbow can impinge upon any of the surrounding neurovascular structures, including the ulna nerve, as it runs in very close proximity to the posterior aspect of the medial epicondyle.

Wrist

Fractures of the distal radius and carpus are the most common upper limb injury and present across all age groups (see Chapter 7). From distal buckle or greenstick fractures in children to high-energy intra-articular fractures and scaphoid fractures in adults to the osteoporotic dinner fork (Colles') type fractures (Figure 5.4a and b) of the elderly falling on an outstretched hand. It is important to be able to differentiate between Colles' and Smith's wrist fractures (Table 5.1).

The bony anatomy of the wrist consists of the distal ends of both the radius and ulna. These articulate with each other and with the hand at the proximal row of carpal bones. Appreciating the shape of the normal distal radius is essential to understand the management of the most common fractures that are encountered. Three main measurements follow the rule of 11 (Figure 5.5) to guide need for surgery.

Management of distal radial fractures in the elderly is still controversial. Frykman classification has been used historically

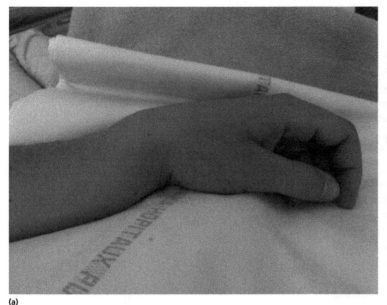

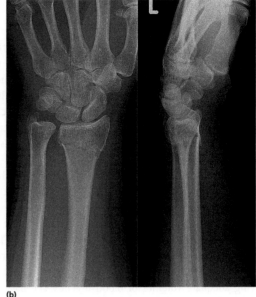

(a)   **(b)**

Figure 5.4 Colles' fracture: a) clinically and b) radiologically (or more accurately a dorsally tilted distal radius fracture)

Table 5.1 Colles' vs. Smith's fractures

Colles	Smith
Commoner	Less common
Fall on outstretched hand	Fall on flexed wrists or direct blow
Extra-articular	Extra-articular
Stable (can be reduced)	Unstable (closed reduction unlikely)
If reduced, unlikely to need surgery	More likely to need surgery (ORIF)
Dorsal tilt, dorsal angulation, dorsal displacement leading to dinner fork deformity	Volar angulation – referred to as reverse Colles
Put into a Colles' (dorsal) positioned backslab	Put into neutral positioned backslab

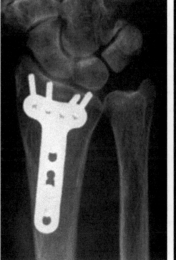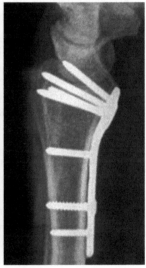

Figure 5.6 Wrist ORIF

fractures result in loss of carpal sagittal balance and therefore require surgery.

The management of dorsally displaced fractures is more controversial, with much evidence to suggest that restoring normal anatomy with manipulations and surgery may have little effect in improving functional outcome. The mainstay of treatment for dinner-fork deformities of the wrist following a distal radial fracture is manipulation into a better position and then cast immobilisation. This can be done with a haematoma block (injecting local anaesthetic directly into the fracture haematoma at the wrist).

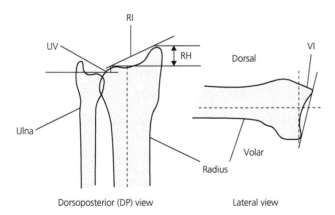

Dorsoposterior (DP) view   Lateral view

Figure 5.5 Rules of 11 for wrist joint: Anatomical relationships to observe around the distal radius. UV (ulnar variance = neutral), RH (radial height = 11 mm), RI (radial inclination = 22°), VI (volar inclination = 11°)

to describe distal radial and ulnar fractures, but this has become outdated. When reviewing the patient and their radiographs, it is important to identify whether the fracture is displaced in a dorsal or volar direction. The majority of volar displaced

Fixation can be achieved by using percutaneous wires or formal open reduction with plates and screws (Figure 5.6). Children often require manipulation under anaesthesia for forearm and wrist fractures before being placed in plaster. In severely comminuted fractures, external fixators may provide a useful alternative.

Lower-limb fractures

Pelvis

Fracture of the pelvic girdle can be subdivided into those of the pelvic ring and those that just involve the acetabulum (see Chapter 8). Two major classifications exist: (1) Tile and (2) Young-Burgess. After initial resuscitation and stabilisation they should be managed and treated by pelvic trauma specialists in regional centres. Both are associated with high-energy trauma and the multiply-injured patient. They may have associated organ injury such as bladder or urethral disruption.

Fractures of the pelvic ring are associated with a high risk of bleeding most commonly from damage to the extensive venous plexus that lies on the inner table of the pelvis. These damaged veins continue to bleed slowly and persistently after the injury, unlike arterial bleeding that might cease from spasm. The potential volume of the haemorrhage to expand into the retroperitoneal space is vast. Recognising this early in the acute trauma setting and giving adequate volumes of blood urgently can have a dramatic effect on outcomes. Pelvic binders are also used in the resus setting before a CT traumagram can identify the site and pattern of the fracture.

Acetabular fractures are complex and difficult to fix; however, they are less commonly life-threatening. They involve the hip joint and a significant proportion will develop post-traumatic arthritis late in life and require hip replacement. Occasionally, they can be managed conservatively with a plan to perform early joint replacement once the fracture has healed and the soft tissues have settled. Acetabular fractures can be classified using the Judet and Letournel classification system (Figure 8.15).

Hip

Fractures around the hip are the most common injury of the lower limb in the elderly (see Chapter 9). Neck of femur fractures can be divided into extracapsular or intracapsular, in which intracapsular fractures has historically been classified using Garden's classification system (Figure 9.8). Previously Garden's classification was used for intracapsular neck of femur fractures but more recently this has been simplified to either being displaced or undisplaced. They are often associated with fragility (osteoporotic) fractures. These elderly patients with neck of femur fractures usually have significant comorbidities and should be treated urgently with a view to early mobilisation to prevent systemic complications associated with immobility. As treatment of osteoporosis becomes more advanced and widespread, we are beginning to see the emergence of other fracture patterns associated with the relatively newer antiosteoporotic drugs like bisphosphonates. Alendronate induced fractures occur in the sub-trochanteric region and are pathological in nature due to the altered biology and architecture of the bone. They present further challenge in treatment, as they tend to occasionally progress to nonunion due to the abnormal bone biology already present.

Femur

Fractures of the femoral shaft are most commonly associated with high-energy trauma. It is possible to lose over two units of blood into the thigh after a femoral shaft fracture. Immediate management

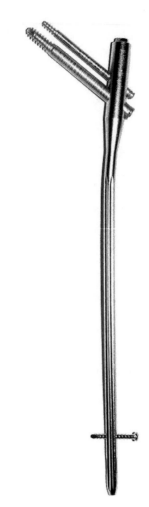

Figure 5.7 Intramedullary nail

would involve splinting of the limb to control bleeding and replacement of the lost volume. Over 50% of the circulating blood volume can pool in the compartments of the thigh with bilateral femoral fractures. 10% of shaft fractures have an associated femoral neck fracture. Treatment of femoral shaft fractures is most commonly with an intramedullary nail, along with a neck screw through the nail if there is a concomitant fracture (Figure 5.7).

Knee

Distal femoral fractures occur in high-energy injuries, in osteoporotic bone or around joint replacements (see Chapter 10). They often involve the articular surface of the knee and therefore require anatomical reduction to prevent post-traumatic arthritis as seen on an AP and lateral (horizontal beam lateral, HBL) knee radiographs.

Patella dislocation is most commonly seen in teenagers and young adults. The pathology behind these dislocations is multifactorial. Simple first-time dislocations can be treated with a period of immobilisation in a brace (2–6 weeks) and then physiotherapy. Recurrent dislocations are more complicated in their management and require referral and investigation by a knee sub-specialist.

Tibiofemoral knee dislocations (discussed in Chapter 10) are not common and are associated with high-energy injuries. They are always associated with ligament damage to the knee. Up to 25% of knee dislocations have an associated vascular injury. These may not present initially with distal pulses present in the limb, but there may be an intimal tear within the artery that clots off the vessel at a later point. Therefore, vascular imaging (e.g. CT angiogram) is essential when a dislocation is recognised. Further treatment depends on the nature and combination of ligaments injured. Compartment syndrome, another orthopaedic emergency, is also a recognised complication, so neurovascular observations are necessary.

Tibia

Fractures of the tibia can be intra-articular (fracture line enters knee or ankle joints) or extra-articular (tibial shaft fracture). Fractures of the proximal tibia (plateau) involve the knee joint and often require reduction and fixation (Figure 5.8). They can involve the lateral or medial plateau (associated with knee dislocations) or both. Schatzker classification is used for tibial plateau fractures (Figure 5.9). As these fractures involve the articular surface, there is a risk of early osteoarthritis, especially if the fracture remains unreduced (>2 mm step in articular surface). The main aim of treatment is to reduce the articular surface and align it appropriately with the tibia, using a plate and screws. Undisplaced fractures may be managed conservatively with either above-knee plaster or a special below-knee patellar tendon bearing plaster known as a Sarmiento cast while remaining non–weight-bearing with the use of crutches. Most displaced fractures require operative treatment. Most commonly, this involves closed reduction with insertion of intramedullary nail near the superior aspect of the tibia; on occasion, plates and screws can also be used, especially in intra-articular fractures.

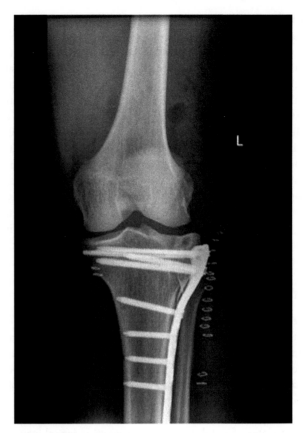

Figure 5.8 Tibial plateau ORIF

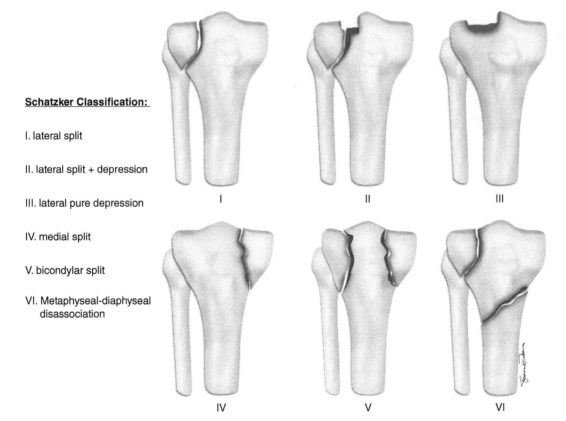

Schatzker Classification:

I. lateral split

II. lateral split + depression

III. lateral pure depression

IV. medial split

V. bicondylar split

VI. Metaphyseal-diaphyseal disassociation

Figure 5.9 Schatzker classification for tibial plateau

Ankle

The distal tibia (medial malleolus) and distal fibula (lateral malleolus) create the ankle joint and they articulate with the talus (see Chapter 11). Ankle injuries can be soft tissue alone or associated with a fracture of either or both malleoli (Figure 5.10). Lateral malleolar fractures can be classified using Weber's classification system (Figure 11.10). Assessment in the emergency situation can utilise the Ottawa ankle rules to indicate requirement for plain radiographs (Table 5.2). The degree to which the ankle is injured determines how it is treated, ranging from simple weight-bearing cast immobilisation to open reduction and fixation. Minimally displaced ankle fractures are managed with below-knee plaster, non–weight-bearing, for 4–8 weeks. Displaced fractures that involve shift of the talus in the ankle mortise require open reduction and fixation with plate and screws. Fractures that disrupt the inferior tibiofibular syndesmosis also require fixation.

Others

Spine

Fractures of the spinal column can be traumatic or osteoporotic (fragility) fractures and the management varies greatly between the two (see Chapter 12). These fractures are classified using the Denis 3-column classification system (Figure 12.12). Traumatic spinal fractures may be associated with neurological changes and will require urgent investigation and management by the spinal surgeons. The presence of sacral sparing following a neurological injury is a good prognostic indicator.

Osteoporotic vertebral body fractures cause a wedge deformity of the anterior column of the spinal column and are often associated with little or no trauma. Traditionally, they are managed with rest and analgaesia as required, but techniques of kyphoplasty and vertebroplasty to restore the height and inject bone cement to reduce the pain are increasingly being used.

Open fractures

British Orthopaedic Association Standards for Trauma (BOAST) guidance (number 4) for open fractures is changing the way open fractures are managed. Lower-limb shaft fractures are associated with high-energy trauma and have a high incidence of being open injuries due to the poor overlying soft tissue cover (Figure 5.11). Gustilo and Anderson provided the basis for a classification system (Table 5.3) that is used commonly to determine the management of open fractures. True classification occurs intra-operatively after exploration. All open fractures, which are recognised as an orthopaedic emergency, require management with broad-spectrum antibiotics, inspection and/or debridement of tissues (within 24 hours), and stabilisation of the fracture. The grade often changes after the initial debridement once an accurate assessment of the soft tissues can be made. All grade 3 and some grade 2 injuries are now ideally transferred to the major trauma centre, for definitive care, after initial resuscitation of the patient and temporary fracture stabilisation.

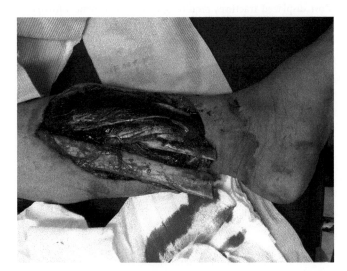

Figure 5.11 Open fracture of leg

Table 5.3 Gustilo Anderson classification of open fractures

Grade 1	Wound less than 1 cm; minimum contamination, soft tissue injury and bone comminution
Grade 2	Wound greater than 1 cm; moderate contamination, soft tissue injury and bone comminution
Grade 3	Associated with degree of soft tissue loss (wound larger than 10 cm), high energy mechanism of injury, periosteal and vascular injury
3A	Adequate bone periosteal coverage with extensive soft-tissue injury
3B	Extensive soft-tissue loss, periosteal stripping and bone damage ± massive contamination requiring soft tissue reconstructive procedure for closure (call Plastics team)
3C	Associated with major vascular injury requiring repair for limb salvage (call Vascular team)

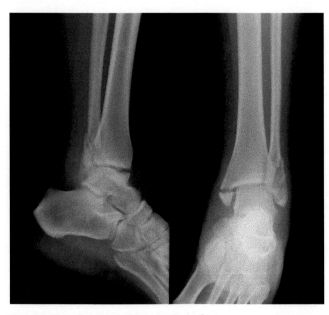

Figure 5.10 Radiograph showing trimalleolar fracture

Table 5.2 Ottawa ankle rules

- Bony tenderness in the distal 6 cm of the tibia or posterior fibula
- Bony tenderness at the tip of either malleolus
- Inability to bear weight immediately after the injury or four steps in the emergency department
- Bone tenderness at the base of the fifth metatarsal (avulsion fractures)
- Bone tenderness at the navicular bone (risk of AVN – Kohler's disease)

The management of these open fractures requires the involvement of a multidisciplinary approach involving orthopaedic, plastic, and vascular surgeons. Fractures where there is significant soft tissue disruption, either from open fractures or periosteal stripping, are at risk of nonunion and postoperative infection. In this situation, external fixation may be used either as a short-term emergency measure or as definitive fixation using a circular frame (Ilizarov frame, Figure 5.12).

Compartment syndrome (*see Chapter 14.6*) is commonly associated with long bone fractures but can occur in any closed tissue compartment of the body. The muscles of the leg are contained within four discrete compartments around the tibia, with a tough fibrous fascial layer enclosing them. If the pressure in one of these compartments rises (e.g. due to muscle swelling after injury), this creates a viscous cycle of poor venous return, poor oxygenation, and muscle necrosis followed by further swelling. To break the cycle, the compartment must be decompressed with fasciotomies (Figure 5.13).

Peri-prosthetic fractures

The number of ageing patients in our communities with joint replacements in situ is increasing and with it the potential trauma around these prostheses. They can happen around any implant but are most common around the hip and knee, as these are the most commonly replaced joints. The Vancouver classification is used to locate the fracture (Figure 5.14). The management of such fractures

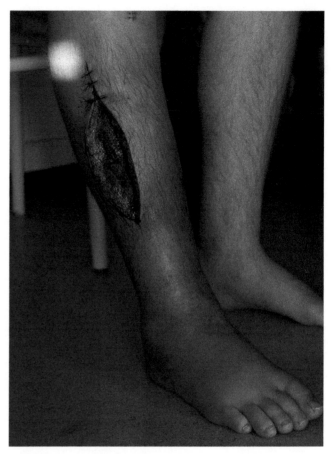

Figure 5.13 Leg fasciotomy wound

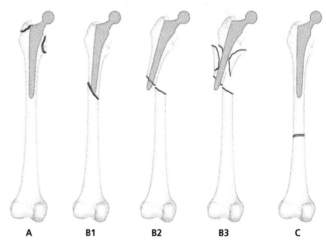

A   B1   B2   B3   C

Figure 5.14 Vancouver classification of femoral periprosthetic fracture

is complex and requires the input of specialists with the ability to either fix the fracture or revise the replacement as necessary.

Stress fractures

Repetitive or unusual actions can cause enough trauma to a bone to create stress (or incomplete) fractures. These are most commonly seen in the metatarsals of the feet (march fractures in soldiers), in anorexia nervosa, and in the tibia and the femoral neck in high-level athletes.

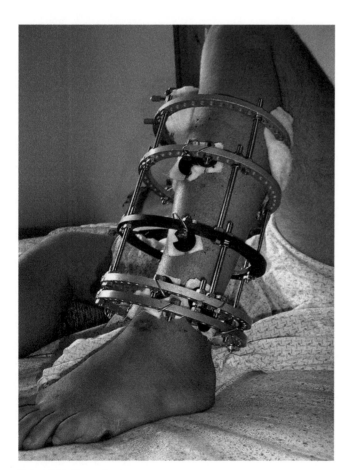

Figure 5.12 Ilizarov frame

Further reading

Brinker, M.R. (2013). *Review of Orthopaedic Trauma*, 2nd revised ed. Springhouse Publishing Co.

British Orthopaedic Association Standards for Trauma (BOAST) 4: guidelines for open fractures. https://www.boa.ac.uk/wp-content/uploads/2017/12/BOAST-Open-Fractures.pdf

British Orthopaedic Association Standards for Trauma (BOAST) (2012). Guidelines for hip fractures. www.boa.ac.uk/wp-content/uploads/2014/12/BOAST-1.pdf.

NICE guidelines for hip fracture management. www.nice.org.uk/guidance/cg124.

Solomon, L., Warwick, D., and Nayagam, S. (2001). Apley's System of Orthopaedics and Fractures. 8th Edition. New York: Arnold.

CHAPTER 6

Shoulder and Elbow

Andrew Sankey and Peter Reilly

Chelsea and Westminster Hospital, London, UK

OVERVIEW

- Shoulder pathology can be divided into:
  - Trauma, degenerative, sports injury
  - Bony and soft tissue pathology
- Loss of passive external rotation in the absence of trauma is usually frozen shoulder or osteoarthritis.
- Inadequate shoulder radiographs lead to missed posterior dislocation.
- Reduction of dislocations with an associated fracture may lead to displacement of fracture fragments.

Anatomy of proximal humerus

The proximal humerus be divided into four parts: the articular surface or head, the greater and lesser tuberosities, and the shaft of the humerus (Figure 6.1). There are anatomical and surgical necks. The subscapularis inserts into the lesser tuberosity whereas the other three rotator cuff tendons insert into the greater tuberosity. The blood supply consists of anterior and posterior humeral circumflex arteries and is innervated by the axillary nerve as well as other branches from the brachial plexus.

History

It is important to establish the patient's age, hand dominance, occupation, and recreational interests. Degenerate rotator cuff tears and osteoarthritis are conditions of older patients, impingement and frozen shoulder present in middle age, and instability tends to present in the younger sporting patient. These are not hard and fast rules, as young patients can develop post-traumatic arthritis or acute traumatic cuff tears, for example. However, this is less common.

Symptoms

Pain can emanate from several sources: the cervical spine, scapulo-thoracic and parascapular muscle region, acromio-clavicular joint (ACJ), subacromial space, and gleno-humeral joint (GHJ).

It is useful to distinguish the character and site of the pain. Shooting and burning pain is often neurological (C5) and may radiate below the elbow (C6-T1). Superior pain often emanates from the ACJ. Posterior pain may be myofascial. Diaphragmatic pain can refer up to the shoulder tip. However, the vast majority of times, shoulder pain is poorly localised to the lateral deltoid region as a consequence of referred pain from an inflamed subacromial bursa (Figure 6.2).

Weakness is characteristic of a rotator cuff tear, yet pain may inhibit movement and be perceived as lack of strength.

Stiffness is due to a physical restriction of movement of the GHJ (active and passive) due to adhesive capsulitis or osteoarthritis. Pain inhibition in other conditions may give the appearance of stiffness.

Examination

Like all joint examinations, it is important to "look, feel, and move." On *inspection,* there may be muscle wasting secondary to either a longstanding rotator cuff tear (Figure 6.3) or deltoid paralysis from an axillary nerve lesion.

The lateral end of the clavicle will be very prominent after an ACJ dislocation. Infection will present with redness, swelling, and occasionally a draining sinus. Scars tell a story of previous surgery. A biceps bulge in the distal aspect of the upper arm (Popeye sign) indicates a long head of biceps (LHB) rupture (Figure 6.4).

This should not be confused with acute pain and bruising of the anterior aspect of the elbow, associated with proximal retraction of the entire biceps, consistent with a distal biceps tendon rupture, which may cause more problems in the longer term (Figure 6.5).

Palpation has limited value in examination of the shoulder joint. The exceptions are the ACJ and LHB. The ACJ is easily identifiable and superficial, and tenderness may indicate underlying arthritic change. The bicipital groove is anteriorly placed at the proximal aspect of the humerus. Tenderness is indicative of LHB tendinitis.

Movement must be examined actively and passively and against resistance. Full active movement requires an intact rotator cuff (supraspinatus, infraspinatus, teres minor, and subscapularis) and

---

ABC of Orthopaedics and Trauma, First Edition. Edited by Kapil Sugand and Chinmay M. Gupte.
© 2018 John Wiley & Sons Ltd. Published 2018 by John Wiley & Sons Ltd.

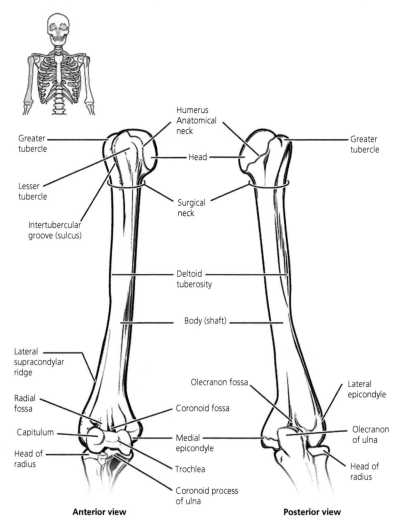

Figure 6.1 Bony anatomy of proximal humerus

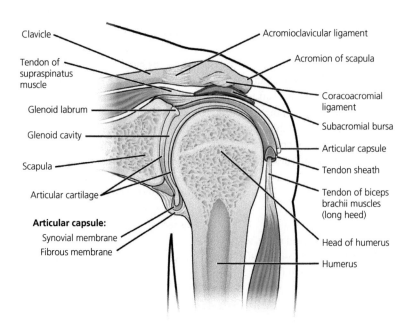

Figure 6.2 Musculoskeletal anatomy of the shoulder

compliance of the capsule of the GHJ. Passive movement will be normal in all conditions except OA and adhesive capsulitis including rotator cuff tears (Figure 6.6). Weakness of external rotation suggests a tear of infraspinatus and possibly teres minor, internal rotation subscapularis, and abduction due to supraspinatus pathology.

Special tests are specific to individual conditions and will be mentioned later in the chapter.

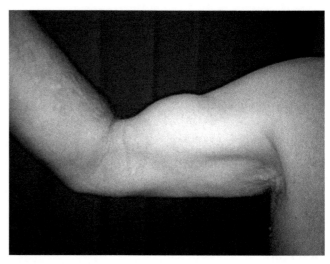

Figure 6.4 Popeye sign

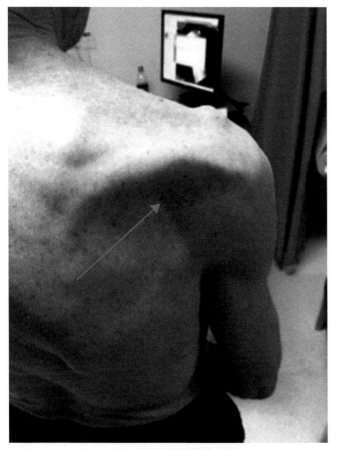

Figure 6.3 Muscle wasting secondary to chronic rotator cuff tear

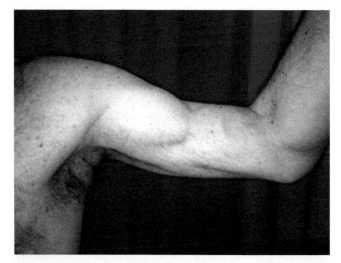

Figure 6.5 Distal biceps tendon rupture

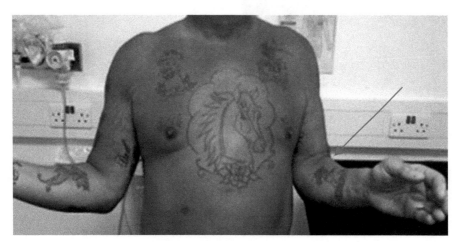

Figure 6.6 Reduced external rotation

Investigations

Unless the patient is to have an MRI scan, plain radiographs should always be performed (AP shoulder, GHJ view, axial). The combination of views will demonstrate pathology of the ACJ, OA of the GHJ, calcific deposition within the rotator cuff, and any acute trauma resulting in fractures or dislocations. Even patients with pain and their arm immobilised in a sling can have an axial radiograph, performed as a Velpeau or Stripp view.

Ultrasound scan (USS)

USS is a quick and relatively inexpensive tool for diagnosing subacromial bursitis, impingement, ACJ synovitis, and rotator cuff tears. It has the added advantage of accurate placement of diagnostic and therapeutic injections into the subacromial space or GHJ.

MRI scan

MRIs should be reserved primarily for the diagnosis of instability and labral tears (performed with the adjunct of an arthrogram) and to aid in the decision-making process for repair of rotator cuff tears (Figure 6.7). They should not be used as a routine tool in primary care because they are time-consuming and expensive and usually give no further information than can be gleaned from plain radiographs and USS.

Subacromial impingement

Subacromial impingement presents with pain based laterally in the shoulder, associated with above-shoulder-height movement, reaching behind one's back, and the pain often wakes the patient at night. The superior rotator cuff (supraspinatus) is pinched during arm abduction between the undersurface of the acromion and the humeral head. The subacromial bursa becomes inflamed (bursitis), as may the supraspinatus (tendinitis). It affects 20% of people at

some time of their life. Range of motion is not restricted, and there is a painful arc on abduction between 60° and 120°. Pain is reproduced with forward flexion and internal rotation (Figure 6.8). Radiographs should be normal – a USS will confirm the diagnosis. Primary treatment involves injection of steroid into the subacromial bursa and physiotherapy.

Calcific tendinitis

Calcific tendinitis presents in a similar way to subacromial impingement, except with a sudden and severe onset. Resorption of the calcium, which is most commonly situated within the supraspinatus tendon, leads to pressure build-up within the tendon and an associated bursitis. Radiographs confirm the diagnosis (Figure 6.9).

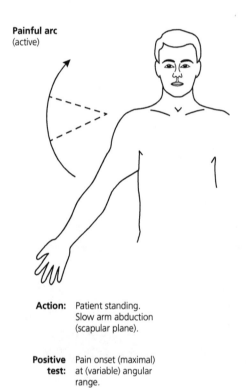

Painful arc
(active)

Action: Patient standing. Slow arm abduction (scapular plane).

Positive test: Pain onset (maximal) at (variable) angular range.

Figure 6.8 Painful arc in shoulder abduction

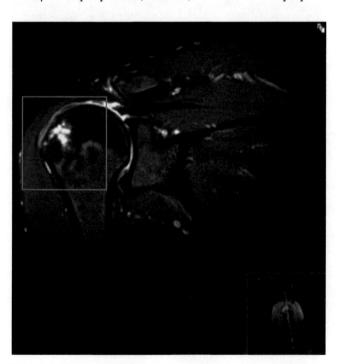

Figure 6.7 MRI scan of supraspinatus tendon tear

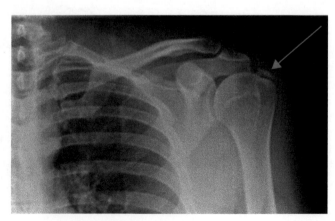

Figure 6.9 Calcific tendinitis

Needling and aspiration of the calcific deposit under USS (barbotage), and injection of steroid into the subacromial bursa often leads to rapid resolution of symptoms.

Rotator cuff tears

A common pathology is the development of degenerate rotator cuff tears – in particular, the supraspinatus tendon – in patients over 60 years of age. Examination may reveal wasting of the infraspinatus and supraspinatus muscles. The LHB is prone to rupture due to the proximity of the torn rotator cuff as the tendon exits the shoulder joint (Figure 6.3). It rarely requires acute intervention, as symptoms of pain and weakness are minimal.

Symptomatic tears can be treated conservatively with steroid injection into the subacromial space and physiotherapy to strengthen the remaining cuff muscles and parascapular muscles. Surgery is indicated if these measures fail. Many tears are amenable to repair (either arthroscopic or open); however, larger and more chronic tears with tendon retraction and muscle atrophy are often irreparable. This is a difficult situation for which there are several treatment options that have varying degrees of success. Young patients may be best treated with a tendon transfer (latissimus dorsi and teres major for supraspinatus and infraspinatus tears). Newer experimental treatments not supported yet by medium or long-term outcome data include balloon interposition arthroplasty and superior capsular plication. Yet, in the presence of cuff arthropathy (proximal migration of the humeral head towards the acromion followed by glenohumeral chondrolysis and humeral head collapse), the only viable option is reverse geometry total shoulder arthroplasty.

Supraspinatus tear

A supraspinatus tear clinically presents as resisted abduction in the plane of the scapula, with the arm internally rotated (Jobe's test), which will uncover weakness and reproduce pain. Passive range of movement should be full, but actively the range may be reduced, although the deltoid may compensate for chronic tears. Resisted external rotation tests are for tears of infraspinatus and teres minor, and the belly press test and lift-off test in internal rotation test are for the subscapularis. USS and MRI are helpful for confirmation of the diagnosis and planning treatment.

Adhesive capsulitis (frozen shoulder)

Adhesive capsulitis occurs in the fifth and sixth decades, more commonly in women, and is associated with diabetes and other endocrine disorders. It presents with pain consistent with bursitis (lateral deltoid) that is worse with movement, and at night, and the GHJ becomes progressively stiff over weeks and months. The capsule of the GHJ thickens, thereby restricting range of motion. Active and passive external rotation is most severely affected. Radiographs rule out OA as a differential diagnosis, and further imaging is unnecessary.

The diagnosis is clinical and is seen in three stages:
1 *Freezing phase*: Progressive loss of ROM from increasing pain lasting anywhere between 2 and 9 months.
2 *Frozen phase*: Worsening ROM (up to 50%) even if pain improves, lasting for 4 to 12 months.
3 *Thawing phase*: A gradual return to normal ROM and functionality over the next 12 to 42 months.

It is a self-limiting condition that will resolve with no treatment within 2 years in the vast majority of patients. Treatment consists of pain relief in the form of analgesics and steroid injection. Hydrodilatation (injection of 20–30 mL of saline, steroid, and local anaesthetic into the GHJ under image guidance) is often successful in treating symptoms. Surgical interventions such as manipulation under anaesthetic or capsular release are appropriate for resistant cases that are affecting function.

Instability

Introduction

Instability is a condition of young adults. There are two broad categories: traumatic and atraumatic. The direction of dislocation is anterior in 97% of cases, posterior in 2% (falling forward in seizures or in electrocution) and inferior (luxatio erecta) in 1% (from hyperabduction of GHJ).

Examination

Examination helps to diagnose the direction of instability. The position of apprehension in anterior instability is in abduction and external rotation. The relocation test relieves apprehension by applying a posterior force on the proximal humerus. Combined flexion, adduction, and internal rotation reproduces posterior apprehension.

Traumatic

Trauma to the arm in an abducted and externally rotated position leads to translation of the humeral head in an anterior direction, leading to detachment of the antero-inferior labrum (Bankart lesion) and anterior dislocation. The shoulder usually requires relocation with analgesia with sedation. Recurrent dislocations require surgical stabilisation.

Nerve palsy

There is an association between anterior dislocations and axillary nerve palsy, presenting with loss of sensation in the regimental badge area of the lateral deltoid and weakness of the deltoid muscle. The palsy commonly resolves spontaneously over a period of weeks.

Atraumatic

Atraumatic instability may be multidirectional and has an association with increased joint laxity. Both shoulders may be affected, and the patients are often capable of relocating the joint themselves. Surgery is rarely indicated and physiotherapy is the main treatment option.

Other

A third, much less common, group of patients with muscle patterning may present to Emergency Department with an acute dislocation. Patients can lose normal neuro-muscular control and dislocate involuntarily. The shoulder is structurally normal. MR arthrogram is indicated if the diagnosis is unclear, and to determine whether surgery is indicated, and should be ordered by the treating shoulder specialist.

Proximal humeral fractures

Fractures of the proximal humerus is common, especially among the geriatric population who sustain falls. They are usually associated with osteoporotic bone. These fractures are classified using the Neer classification system (Figure 6.10), which looks at displacement and angulation on plain radiographs. Most proximal humeral fractures are managed nonoperatively in a Lancaster polysling, hanging cast, or a U-slab. Follow-up in clinic, analgesia, and physiotherapy can return the patient to almost full function within months. Noncompliant patients

may be suitable for a shoulder spica. There must be a balance between the benefits and risks of surgery, especially on geriatric patients with comorbidities and pre-morbid low-functional state. Alternatively, surgical options are reserved for severely displaced or angulated fractures, comminuted fractures, fracture dislocation, open fractures, and polytrauma, and consist of ORIF with plate and screws (Proximal Humerus Internal Locking System [PHILOS] plate, Figure 6.11) or total versus hemiarthroplasty (Figure 6.12).

Glenohumeral osteoarthritis

Osteoarthritis may affect the shoulder joint, which can cause expected symptoms of pain, stiffness, and reduced functionality affecting activities of daily living. Chronology of management options consist of analgesia, physiotherapy, (image-guided), joint

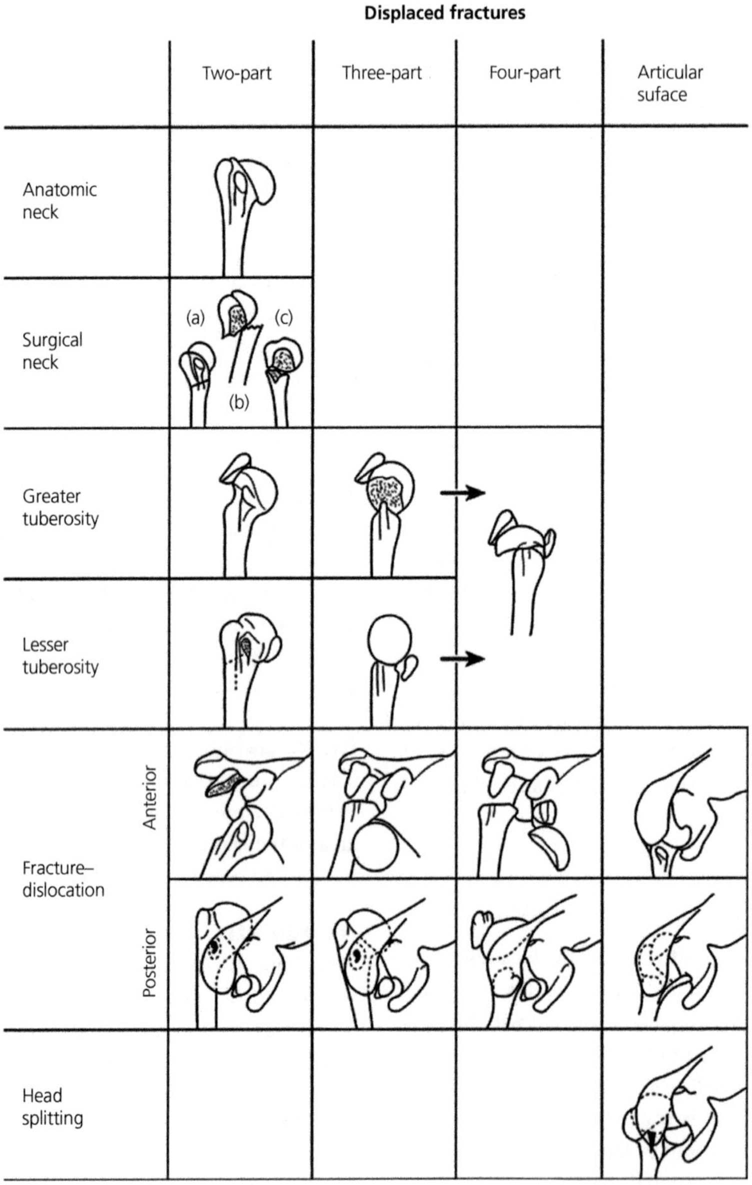

Figure 6.10 Neer classification for proximal humeral fractures

injections, and finally, joint replacement. Arthroplasty options are (1) resurfacing or stemless prosthesis (ideally younger patients), (2) hemiarthroplasty, (3) total shoulder arthroplasty (TSA; need an intact rotator cuff), or (4) reverse polarity total shoulder replacement (usually > 70 years with low functional demand, rotator cuff arthropathy, late-stage disease (including acetabularisation), but deltoid muscle must be functional). The bigger the procedure, the more restricted is post-operative range of movement (e.g. 90° abduction/flexion for reverse TSA, which is enough to reach your mouth, face, and head), and (5) arthrodesis.

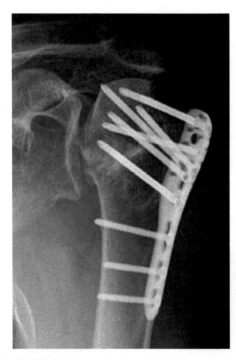

Figure 6.11 PHILOS plate

Elbow conditions

Tendinopathies around the elbow account for the majority of presentations of elbow pain.

Tennis elbow (lateral epicondylitis)

The common extensor tendon origin (CEO) is vulnerable to repeated stress from activities such as racquet sports and gardening. The tendon becomes degenerate and accumulates micro-tears, culminating in pain situated 1 cm distal to the lateral epicondyle of the distal humerus (Figure 6.13). Resisted wrist and finger extension recreates the pain. Radiographs are typically normal and the diagnosis may be confirmed on USS. Treatment consists of rest, physiotherapy, counterforce bracing, and dry needling of the CEO (under USS). Surgery to release the CEO is reserved for patients who fail to improve after conservative measures.

Golfer's elbow (medial epicondylitis)

This condition is similar to tennis elbow, except that it affects the common flexor tendon origin on the medial aspect of the elbow. Resisted wrist and finger flexion provokes pain, and treatment options mirror those of tennis elbow.

Distal biceps tendon rupture

Distal biceps tendon rupture occurs suddenly on lifting. There is immediate bruising of the ante-cubital fossa, and the biceps retracts proximally on resisted elbow flexion (Figure 6.5). The tendon cannot be palpated distally. Significant weakness of supination and flexion are a direct consequence, and therefore, unlike LHB tendon rupture at the shoulder, urgent surgical referral for discussion of acute repair is indicated.

Olecranon bursitis

Olecranon bursitis presents as a fluid-filled collection at the posterior aspect of the elbow, superficial to the proximal ulna.

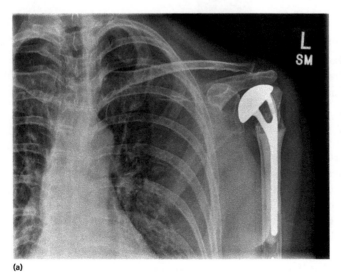

(a)

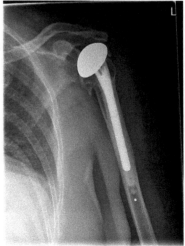

(b)

Figure 6.12a & b Shoulder replacement (arthroplasty)

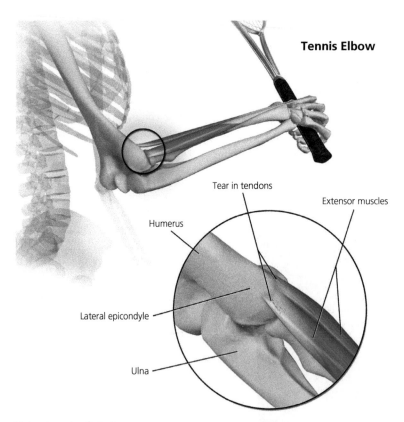

Tennis Elbow

Tear in tendons

Extensor muscles

Humerus

Lateral epicondyle

Ulna

Figure 6.13 Area of tenderness with tennis and golfer's elbow

Recurrent trauma from leaning on the elbow is usually the cause – hence the name *student's elbow*. It is important when examining to look closely for stigmata of gout. The range of motion of the elbow is preserved.

The inflammation of an acute bursitis will cause warmth and redness that will respond to nonsteroidal anti-inflammatory drugs (NSAIDs) and avoidance of pressure on the elbow. It may be difficult to distinguish from an infected olecranon bursitis, which presents with spreading cellulitis and raised inflammatory blood markers. Aspiration has a high incidence of recurrence and sinus formation, and should only be performed for chronic cases, using strict antiseptic technique.

A patient with septic arthritis of the elbow joint will be unwell, have a raised temperature, swelling, and redness not isolated to the posterior aspect of the elbow, and will have a marked restriction in range of motion due to severe pain. An infected joint needs urgent surgical washout.

Arthritides

Osteoarthritis and inflammatory arthritis (e.g. rheumatoid or psoriatic arthritis) of the elbow present with pain, restriction in range of motion, and possibly deformity. Loose bodies, with osteoarthritis in particular, lead to symptoms of locking and can be successfully removed arthroscopically (Figure 6.14). End-stage disease may need surgical treatment to debride and release the joint capsule in the presence of stiffness or require total joint replacement when symptoms of pain and stiffness are uncontrolled.

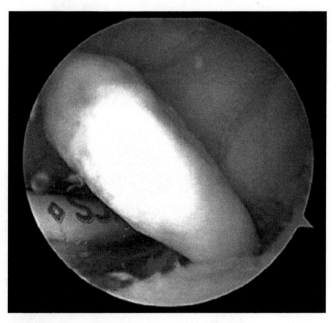

Figure 6.14 Arthroscopic view of loose body elbow joint

Cubital tunnel syndrome

Cubital tunnel syndrome presents with symptoms secondary to irritation and compression of the ulna nerve (ulna neuritis) at the level of the elbow as it passes behind the medial epicondyle. Mild cases cause intermittent paraesthesia in the medial (ulnar) 1½ fingers.

Table 6.1 Diagnostic algorithm of common shoulder conditions

History and Examination	Primary investigations	Abnormal?	Secondary investigations	Diagnosis
Acute trauma, pain and weakness	X-ray	Y		Fracture/dislocation
		N	USS	Acute Rotator cuff tear
Pain and tenderness ACJ	X-ray	Y		ACJ arthritis
Gradual onset pain, painful arc +/– weakness	X-ray	N	USS	Impingement
				Rotator cuff tear
Sudden onset pain, no trauma, painful arc	X-ray	Y	USS	Calcific tendinitis
		N		Impingement
Pain and Stiffness	X-ray	Y		Osteoarthritis
		N		Adhesive capsulitis
Recurrent dislocation or apprehension	MRA	Y		Traumatic instability
		N		Atraumatic instability

Severe compression leads to weakness of the small muscles of the hand, leading to weakness and difficulty with fine motor function. Wasting of the first dorsal interosseous muscle and abductor digiti minimi are most obvious clinically, and Tinel's testing over the cubital tunnel recreates the patient's symptoms of paraesthesia. Nerve conduction studies confirm the diagnosis and level of nerve compression. Surgical release is required in severe cases.

Further reading

Rees, J.L. (2008). The pathogenesis and surgical treatment of tears of the rotator cuff. *Journal of Bone and Joint Surgery (Br.)* 90 (7): 827–832.

Robinson, C.M., and Dobson, R.J. (2004). Anterior instability of the shoulder after trauma. *Journal of Bone and Joint Surgery (Br.)* 86 (4): 469–479.

Solomon, L., Warwick, D., and Nayagam, S. (2010). *Apley's System of Orthopaedics and Fractures*, 9th ed. Boca Raton, FL: CRC Press.

CHAPTER 7

Hand and Wrist

Issaq Ahmed[1] and Philippa Rust[2]

[1] Royal Infirmary of Edinburgh, Edinburgh, UK
[2] NHS Lothian, Edinburgh, UK

OVERVIEW

- Hands are vital for daily life, both for activities and communication, and as such, patients often fear loss of function.
- Good function depends on sensation, mobility, and strength without pain.
- Hands are commonly injured, at home, during sports, and at work.
- Hand therapy is essential to maximise postoperative results.
- The thumb accounts for half of total hand function.

General clinical assessment

The treatment goal is to restore function not only to the affected area but also the whole upper extremity. The history begins by carefully determining the patient's main complaint (Table 7.1). Enquiring about the occupational and recreational activities are also paramount to a successful outcome in the management of both chronic conditions and acute trauma.

Elective conditions

In nontraumatic conditions, focus very closely on the exact site of the problem after taking a thorough history of onset, progression, functional limitations, and interventions. An understanding of what helps to relieve and aggravate their symptoms is essential in determining treatment (Table 7.2). Information about patients' underlying medical conditions such as gout, rheumatoid arthritis, or generalised osteoarthritis, as well as the presence of diabetes, thyroid dysregulation, heart disease, or other illnesses help in making the diagnosis and formulating a treatment strategy.

Traumatic conditions

The history ought to elicit the mechanism of injury, time of injury, and the environment in which this occurred. Patients can often present late, especially following closed wrist injuries, and it is important to note the evolution of the patient's problems, what

treatments have occurred, and what the current functional losses are. Many of these patients can later become involved in compensation, and therefore, it is essential to have clear documentation (Table 7.2).

Physical examination

The assessment of the hand and wrist typically follows the standard musculoskeletal assessment of look, feel, and movement, followed by special tests, assessment of the neurovascular status, and detailed functional evaluation. The physical examination begins with range of movement of the neck, shoulder, and elbows, as the hand is useful only if it can be positioned in space. Observation of the resting hand should include the posture of the hand and digits, and comparisons should be made to the opposite side (Table 7.3). These movements of the digits can be seen in Figure 7.1.

When feeling for tenderness, localise the patient's pain as anatomically accurate as possible to help define the diagnosis. An understanding of the surface anatomy is critical to this. As stiffness has a significant effect on hand function, range of movement should be recorded carefully for later comparison testing. Specific range of movement and ligament testing should be tailored depending on patients' complaints.

Vascular status

Vascular function can be determined by evaluating capillary refill or a Doppler ultrasound evaluation of pulses distal to the laceration. The patency of the palmar arch can be verified by the Allen's test, which involves occluding the radial and ulnar arteries (70% supply to hand) with manual pressure while the patient makes a fist several times. Pressure is released from one artery, and capillary refill should be noted in the fingertips within 5 seconds.

Neurological status

Where nerve laceration or compression is suspected, a detailed neurological function should be tested. The sensory supply of the hand is tested by light touch (Figure 7.2). Light touch is easy to test in clinic, but two-point discrimination or Semmes-Weinstein

---

Table 7.1 Common causes of hand or wrist pain

	Younger patients	Older patients
Finger pain	• Carpal tunnel syndrome • Cubital tunnel syndrome	• Carpal tunnel syndrome • OA DIP joint
Hand pain	• Inflammatory arthritis • Carpal tunnel syndrome	• Trigger finger
Radial-sided wrist pain	• de Quervain's tenosynovitis • Acute scaphoid fracture or nonunion • Distal radius/styloid (Chauffeur's) fracture	• OA base of thumb joints • OA post scaphoid (fracture) nonunion advance collapse (SNAC) or chronic scapholunate [ligament injury] advance collapse (SLAC) • STT (scapho-trapezial-trapezoidal) joint pain
Mid-dorsal wrist pain	• Kienbock's (lunate avascular necrosis) • Wrist ganglion • Scapholunate ligament instability • Mid carpal instability	• SLAC/SNAC grade 3 or 4
Ulnar sided wrist pain	• Triangular fibro-cartilage complex (TFCC) tear • Lunotriquetral instability • Distal radial ulna joint instability • Extensor carpi ulnaris tendonitis • Hamate fracture nonunion	• Distal radial ulna joint OA • Ulna impaction syndrome • Pisiform triquetral joint OA

Table 7.2 Essential history for hand surgery patient

All	Elective	Trauma
Age	Pain history	Mechanism of injury: cut, crush, or traction
Hand dominance	Impact on activities of daily living	Time since injury
Occupation and hobbies	Family history	Time since last meal
Past medical history	Investigations and interventions	Tetanus status
Drugs and allergies, including analgesia	Does patient have someone to take him/her home after surgery?	
Social history, including smoking		

Table 7.3 Examination of the hand

Look at general appearance of the hands	Nails	Clubbing, splinter haemorrhages, pitting, leuconychia
	Skin	Colour, i.e. palmar erythema
		Skin conditions, i.e. dermatitis, psoriasis, scars
		Lesions, i.e. skin cancers (basal cell carcinomas)
	Joints	Any abnormality in shape or size, i.e. finger deformity, joint deformity, or swelling
	Muscles	Wasting of thenar or hypothenar eminences
Feel	Nerves	Test sensation and motor function of median, ulnar, and radial nerves
	Circulation	Vasculitis, Allen's test
	Temperature, Palmar fascia, muscle, and bone	Lumps, i.e. ganglion or Dupuytrens, joint tenderness, muscle wasting
Move	Function and grip	Gross movements, i.e. "make a fist," "open hand"
	Active and passive range of movement	Wrist – flex and extend, supinate and pronate thumb – oppose to each finger and extend flexion and extension at each finger joint

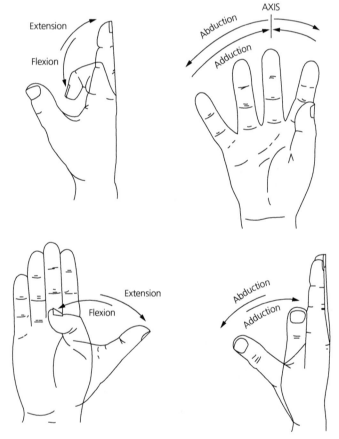

Figure 7.1 Movements of the fingers and thumb

monofilament threshold testing can also be used. Motor testing for the main peripheral nerves is shown in Table 7.4.

In trauma cases, examination of hand function distal to wounds can usually determine what structures are injured. The function of flexor digitorum superficialis (FDS) and profundus (FDP) tendons should be assessed, as shown in Figure 7.3. The integrity of the radial and ulnar digital nerve to each finger can be assessed by

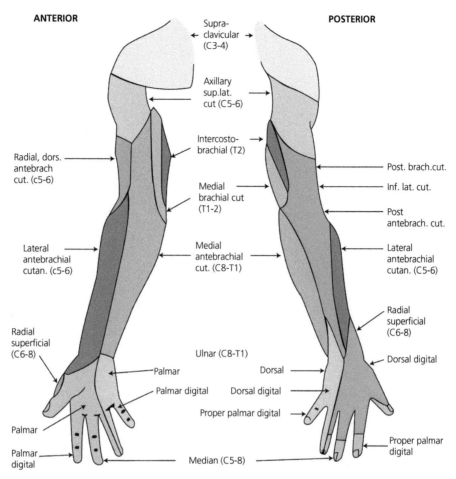

ANTERIOR

POSTERIOR

Supra-
clavicular
(C3-4)

Axillary
sup.lat.
cut (C5-6)

Intercosto-
brachial (T2)

Radial, dors.
antebrach
cut. (c5-6)

Medial
brachial cut
(T1-2)

Post. brach.cut.

Inf. lat. cut.

Post
antebrach. cut.

Lateral
antebrachial
cutan. (c5-6)

Medial
antebrachial
cut. (C8-T1)

Lateral
antebrachial
cutan. (C5-6)

Radial
superficial
(C6-8)

Radial
superficial
(C6-8)

Dorsal digital

Ulnar (C8-T1)

Palmar

Palmar digital

Dorsal

Dorsal digital

Proper palmar digital

Palmar

Palmar
digital

Median (C5-8)

Proper palmar
digital

Figure 7.2 Innervation of hand and wrist

Table 7.4 Neurological testing motor function of the hand

Median – LOAF muscles	Lateral two lumbricals, opponens pollicis, abductor pollicis brevis, and flexor pollicis brevis
	Look at thenar muscles
	Test thumb abduction (abductor pollicis brevis)
Ulnar – other small muscles of hand	Look at hypothenar and web spaces
	Abduct fingers (dorsal interossei)
	Adduct fingers (palmar interossei)
Radial nerve – extensors	Extend fingers
	Extend thumb (extensor pollicis longus)
Generalised – all small muscles of the hand	Look for guttering (wasting)

testing sensation on each side of each finger pulp. Careful observation for swelling and palpation of each bone will guide towards specific radiographic views to obtain fracture diagnosis.

Nerve compression syndromes

Carpal tunnel syndrome
Anatomy
Carpal tunnel syndrome (CTS) is the most common cause of nocturnal hand paraesthesia and should be suspected in any patient with this symptom, whatever the age. It results from compression of the median nerve at the wrist within the carpal tunnel, an anatomical compartment bounded by the bones of the carpus and the transverse carpal ligament (Figure 7.4). The flexor retinaculum contains four FDSs, four FDPs, FPL, FCR, and the median nerve.

Aetiology
Causes are primary (idiopathic), RA, acromegaly, post-trauma (e.g. Colles' fracture), diabetes, and pregnancy.

Presentation
The hallmark symptoms are tingling, numbness, and pain in the median nerve distribution, which can wake the patient from sleep or occur during the day with hand elevation and gripping (e.g. driving). Symptoms are sometimes relieved with hanging the affected hand over the side of the bed or shaking it off.

Examination findings
In more advanced stages, patients may develop weakness of the hand and drop objects, with atrophy of the thenar musculature seen on examination (Figure 7.5). Examination is shown in Table 7.5.

Investigation
Nerve conduction studies are useful to document the degree of slowing median nerve conduction at the wrist.

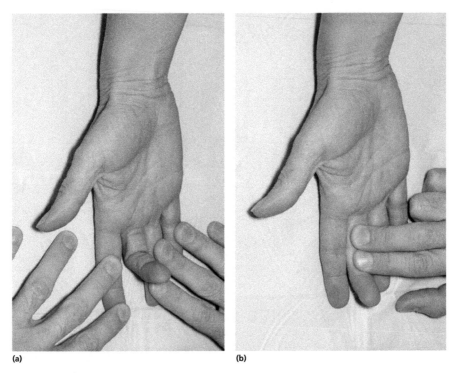

(a)   **(b)**

Figure 7.3 (a) Testing for FDS; (b) Testing for FDP

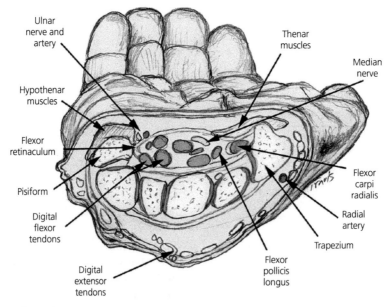

Ulnar nerve and artery
Thenar muscles
Median nerve
Hypothenar muscles
Flexor retinaculum
Pisiform
Digital flexor tendons
Flexor carpi radialis
Radial artery
Trapezium
Digital extensor tendons
Flexor pollicis longus

Figure 7.4 Cross section of the carpal tunnel

Management

- *Nonoperative*: Initial treatment is a neutral angle splinting at night. This may help with diagnosis and can alleviate mild symptoms. The first-line treatment where there is a temporary cause, such as in pregnancy, is a steroid injection into the tunnel (not the nerve). This can also be helpful where the diagnosis is unclear; however, relief of symptoms is usually temporary.
- *Operative*: Open carpal tunnel decompression, performed as an outpatient case under local anaesthesia, is considered as the definitive treatment. Be careful not to damage the palmar cutaneous and the recurrent branch of the median nerve (i.e. the "million-dollar

nerve"). Although it provides a permanent cure in most cases, it is not without complication. These include infection, sensitive scarring, stiffness and complex regional pain syndrome, pillar pain, and recurrence (around 10%). True recurrence, after successful initial surgery, is rare and is mostly attributable to misdiagnosis, failure to fully divide the transverse carpal ligament completely, and delay of treatment to a point when median nerve function is beyond recovery. Endoscopic methods of carpal tunnel decompression have been popular in recent years, with reduced time to return to work, although long-term outcomes do not differ significantly between these methods.

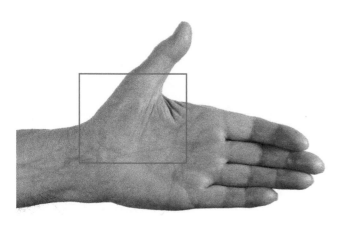

Figure 7.5 Atrophic thenar eminence

Table 7.5 Examination and tests for carpal tunnel syndrome

Physical examination	Test description	Findings
Phalen's sign	Symptoms are reproduced by holding the wrist in maximal flexion for a minute or less	61% sensitive and 83% specific
Combined compression test (i.e. Durkan's test)	Pressure is placed over the carpal tunnel and the wrist is held in flexion	82% sensitive and 99% specific
Tinel's sign	Tapping over the median nerve at the wrist crease elicits paraesthesia in a median nerve distribution	74% sensitive
Thumb abduction	Strength of APB should be tested	Reduced in severe CTS
Sensory evaluation should be documented	Median, ulnar, and radial nerve areas	Reduced in median nerve area in longstanding CTS

Cubital tunnel syndrome

Cubital tunnel syndrome, or compression of the ulnar nerve at the elbow, is the second-most common compressive neuropathy.

Presentation

Patients present with numbness and tingling in the small finger and the ulnar half of the ring finger and frequently complain of elbow pain. Symptoms are often worse at night or after long periods in which the elbow has been flexed.

Examination findings

Physical examination findings include a positive elbow flexion test where full flexion of the elbow for more than 30 seconds reproduces symptoms, a positive Tinel's sign over the ulnar nerve and behind the medial epicondyle, and in some cases, subluxation of the ulnar nerve out of the condylar groove when flexing the elbow. Distally, there is usually reduced sensation in an ulnar nerve distribution. In advanced cases, weakness to finger abduction or even intrinsic atrophy can be present. In the Froment's test, the patient is required to pinch a card between the thumb and index finger using

adductor pollicis, which is innervated by the terminal branch of the motor branch of the ulnar nerve. The test is positive when the patient cannot strongly pinch the card and flexes the IPJ of the thumb recruiting FPL to hold the card.

Differentials

The main differential diagnoses include cervical radiculopathy, thoracic outlet syndrome, and distal ulnar nerve compression (at the wrist).

Investigations

Nerve conduction studies and an EMG can be helpful to differentiate between these sites, but it may be negative even in moderately advanced stages of cubital tunnel syndrome.

Management

- *Nonoperative*: Treatment usually starts with extension splinting, activity modification, and anti-inflammatories.
- *Operative*: If symptoms do not resolve in 3–6 months or if patients develop significant atrophy, an ulnar nerve decompression with or without an anterior transposition of the ulnar nerve (to reduce risk of recurrence) can be helpful in relieving symptoms and stopping progression.

Ulnar clawing and ulnar nerve paradox

A high ulnar nerve lesion at the elbow causes weakness of FDP to little and ring fingers in addition to weakness of the intrinsic hand muscles, including little and ring finger lumbricals. This results in complete weakness of the ulna side of the hand. Following repair of such a proximal injury, the nerve end regenerates, reinnervating the proximal muscles first. This results in return of function of FDP muscles and flexion of the ring and little fingers, but loss of balance in the hand as the intrinsic muscles remain weak. Thus, ulnar clawing develops as the lesion moves from proximal to distal, and this is the *ulnar paradox*.

Tendon compression syndrome

Stenosing tenosynovitis
Pathology

In stenosing tenosynovitis, the tendon segments become thickened within the tendon tunnel or sheath, with myxoid degeneration of the tendon.

Presentation

Patients initially present with pain and eventually develop problems with gliding motion and sometimes even develop frank catching or triggering of the tendon as it passes through its retinacular tunnel. These problems are more common with diabetes and renal failure. They are sometimes felt to be due to overuse; however, most of the time the underlying cause is unknown.

Trigger finger
Population

Trigger finger usually occurs in middle-aged females affecting the ring, middle finger, and thumb.

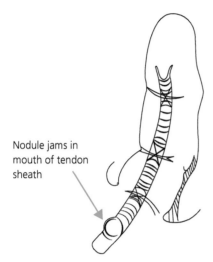

Figure 7.6 Trigger finger pathology

Nodule jams in mouth of tendon sheath

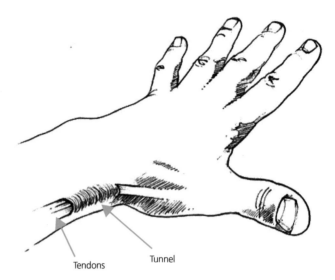

Figure 7.7 de Quervain's pathology

Tendons   Tunnel

Pathology

The most common of these tendon disorders is trigger finger, in which the flexor tendons are entrapped underneath due to nodular thickening and stenosis of the A-1 pulley of the flexor tendon sheath at the MCP joint level (Figure 7.6).

Risks

Primary (idiopathic), RA, diabetes mellitus, and amyloid deposition from renal dialysis.

Presentation

Patients will often end up with locking and clicking of the finger in flexion requiring a prying open of the digit with a palpable and sometimes visible pop as the finger fully extends.

Management

Some cases resolve with time without any intervention. Initial treatment may consist of splinting in extension or corticosteroid injection (80% success rate). If symptoms recur or persist, a surgical release of the A-1 pulley under a local anaesthetic is indicated.

de Quervain's tenosynovitis
Pathology

Abductor pollicis longus (APL) and extensor pollicis brevis (EPB) tendons become constricted in the first (out of six) dorsal compartment of the wrist (Figure 7.7). This is especially common in mothers with small children (i.e. diaper thumb) where overuse aggrevates the pain.

Examination

Hallmark physical findings are significant tenderness over the first dorsal compartment at the radial styloid and a positive Finkelstein's test, in which the thumb is gripped in the palm and wrist are placed into ulnar deviation eliciting severe pain. Pain may also be reproduced on resisted thumb extension.

Management

Treatment options include anti-inflammatory medications, corticosteroid injections, splinting/bracing (which must include the thumb and wrist), and if these fail, surgical release of the first dorsal compartment (but avoid damage to superficial branch of radial nerve).

Other tendon compression syndromes

Other less common tendon compressions around the wrist include tendinitis of the flexor carpi radialis (FCR) tendon, which can be associated with scapho-trapezoid-trapezium (STT) joint OA, extensor carpi ulnaris (ECU) tendon (see Table 7.1), and extensor carpi radialis brevis (ECRB) and extensor carpi radialis longus (ECRL) tendons (i.e. intersection syndrome). Treatment of these conditions follows similar methods to that of de Quervain's tenosynovitis.

Dupuytrens disease
Population

The disease is particularly common in older men of Celtic and Scandinavian origin, suggesting a hereditary component to the process.

Risk factors

Male, age, smoking, alcohol, and diabetes.

Pathology

This disease involves changes in the palmar fascia with normal fibroblast cells transforming into myofibroblasts, which thicken and contract. The normal fascial bands, "anchoring" the fat and skin of the palm, thicken and contract, pulling the digits (especially ring and little fingers) into flexion contractures and cause web space narrowing (Figure 7.8).

Presentation and examination

Over time, this causes a functional problem. Patients complain of sticking their finger in their eye when they wash or having difficulty putting on a glove. The contractures can become so severe that patients cannot place their hands flat on a table (Hueston's tabletop test).

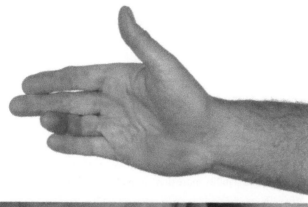

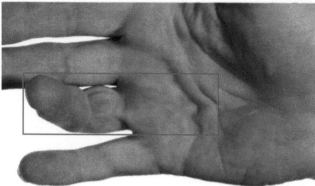

Figure 7.8 Dupuytren's contracture

Table 7.6 Arthritis in the hand

Type of arthritis	Common site affected	Investigation of choice
Osteoarthritis	Base of thumb, DIPJ	Radiography
Rheumatoid arthritis	Wrist, MCPJ, PIPJ	CCP antibody, radiography
Psoriatic arthritis	PIPJ	Radiography, skin biopsy
Gout	Wrist, thumb	Urate blood test, joint aspirate for crystals
Reactive arthritis	Previous fracture/ trauma to joint	Radiography, inflammatory markers

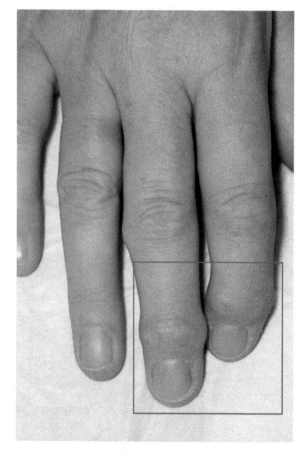

Figure 7.9 Digital osteoarthritis

The usual presentation starts as a nodule in the palm. Over time, it will often progress into a painless cord along the digit, following the fascial bands, pulling the MCP and/or PIP joint into a flexion contracture.

Management

Hand therapy and splinting have shown no effect on the progression of the disease. The mainstay of treatment at this time is surgical excision. Traditional treatment in the United Kingdom is a fasciectomy, which carries a 50% risk of recurrence of the disease in a digit that has had cords removed at 5 years.

The use of *C. histolyticum* collagenase injection in the treatment of palmar form of Dupuytren's disease is a recent advance in the treatment of Dupuytren's. Although, emerging studies show good results in the short and medium term, its use is still contentious. It is a simple and minimally invasive treatment, which is performed as a two-stage procedure under local anaesthetic. Patients should be well informed about local reactions, including swelling, bruising, and skin tears following injection.

Degenerative conditions

Arthritis of the hand and wrist is a common problem (Table 7.6), and as it becomes progressively severe, patients can experience marked limitation in hand use due to pain or loss of function.

Osteoarthritis

Nodal osteoarthritis (OA) is the most common form of arthritis that develops in the hand.

Presentation and examination

The joint swells and becomes inflamed and painful, but the pain may subside over a few years, leaving behind bony osteophytes (Herbenden's nodes at DIPJ, which is most frequently affected, Figure 7.9). The PIP joints can also become involved (Bouchard's node) and can develop significant angular deformity.

Management

- *Nonoperative*: Treatment starts with local anti-inflammatory gels, oral analgesia, splintage and intra-articular steroid injections, which are best carried out under fluoroscopic guidance.
- *Operative*: Surgical management in severe PIP and DIP joint OA causing persistent pain or deformity involves fusion or replacement of the joint.

First carpometacarpal (CMC) joint
Population
The prevalence of this condition increases with age and is greatest in postmenopausal women.

Presentation and examination
Patients with OA of the base of the thumb (trapezio-metacarpal joint) commonly present because of pain and loss of pinch grip function. The diagnosis can often be made by the patient's description of symptoms alone with most complaining of pain on resisted pinch grip activities such as turning a key. Physical examination often shows a "shouldering at the base of thumb" causing z-shaping (Figure 7.10) with tenderness at the trapezio-metacarpal

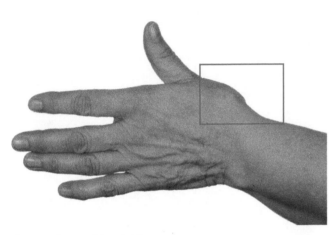

Figure 7.10 Base of thumb OA

joint and a positive grind test here. Plain radiographs confirm the diagnosis in nearly all cases but may underestimate disease (Figure 7.11).

Management
- *Nonoperative*: Similar nonoperative treatments should be tried first and corticosteroid injections can ameliorate symptoms and delay surgery.
- *Operative*: Trapeziectomy gives positive results 85% of the time. Arthrodesis may be a better option where the arthritis is limited to the trapezio-metacarpal joint, for patients who require strength and stability more than mobility, such as younger manual workers.

Posttraumatic OA
Posttraumatic OA can occur following joint injury, which results in increased cartilage wear and secondary arthritis formation. In the hand, PIP joints are most commonly affected. In the wrist, it follows the altered biomechanics after SNAC or untreated scapholunate ligament injury (i.e. SLAC), which results in abnormal wear patterns. Treatment options depend on symptoms and the stage, nonoperative then operative, as for other sites of OA.

Rheumatoid arthritis
Pathology
Rheumatoid arthritis often manifests itself in the hand (Figure 18.2). This disease is a systemic problem. In the hand, soft tissues become chronically inflamed with pannus that can destroy ligaments, causing joint deformity and bone erosions.

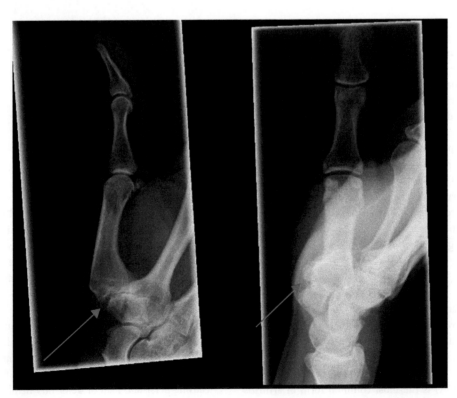

Figure 7.11 Radiograph showing base of thumb OA

Presentation and examination

Tendons may be infiltrated by disease, causing rupture and resulting in loss of function. In the wrist, the ligament damage can cause volar and ulnar subluxation of the carpus on the radius and a radial deviation deformity of the wrist. The MCP joints of the fingers usually drift into an ulnar deviation, further compromising hand function. The PIP joints may develop severe synovitis that can lead to either a Boutonnière or swan-neck deformity. The DIP joints are usually spared.

MANAGEMENT

A multiple disciplinary approach is essential for optimum patient care.
- *Nonoperative*: Initial treatment is focused on medical management, and disease modifying agents may control inflammation and prevent deformity. Accompanying hand therapy and splinting can be useful adjuncts for maintaining strength.
- *Operative*: For patients for whom medical treatment fails to control disease progression, individual problems can be addressed and many surgical treatments are available, ranging from tenosynovectomy and resection of bony protrusions to replacement arthroplasty and fusion.

Ganglion

A ganglion is a mobile cystic swelling in tortuous continuity with a joint or tendon sheath through a connecting duct. They are usually painless until they impose mass effect. A ganglion is filled with clear, viscous fluid rich in hyaluronan and is thus transilluminable. Imaging is usually not required. As the natural history is often for

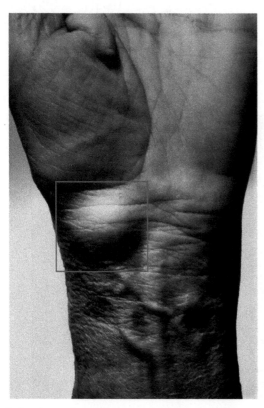

Figure 7.12 Palmar wrist ganglion presenting between the flexor carpi radialis tendon and the radial artery

these to resolve spontaneously, the risks of surgical resection, with variable recurrence rates of 5–10%, may exceed the benefit (Table 7.7). Needle puncture and aspiration may avoid the need for surgery, but beware of high risk of recurrence.

Inflammation and infection

Flexor sheath tenosynovitis is a surgical emergency (Table 7.8). The operation entails incision, exploration of the wound and sheath, sampling of turbid fluid, washout, and review for washout in 48–72 hours with IV antibiotics and elevation. Delayed treatment leads to the risk of further tracking, fibrosis, and contracture to reduce range of movement and function. Late surgical reconstruction is staged with long-term disability.

There is a high risk of infection related to human and animal bites (Table 7.9). Some hospitals tend to wash out the wound sooner rather than later, and some tend to waitfully watch and operate if the infection does not respond to IV antibiotics and elevation or if a collection has developed. If a cellulitis, ascending lymphangitis or

Table 7.7 Ganglia occur in four locations and account for half of all hand swellings

Location	Underlying association	Treatment
Dorsum of the wrist	Scapholunate joint	Aspiration (20% recurrence)
Volar wrist adjacent to the radial artery	Scaphotrapezial joint	Care with aspiration as close to radial artery
Volar base of the finger	Flexor tendon sheath	May resolve spontaneously
Dorsum of the finger, proximal to nail fold	DIP joint	With excision of mucous cyst, nail groove resolves

Table 7.8 Flexor sheath infection

History	Examination	Consequences	Treatment
Penetrating injury (e.g. rose-thorn bush)	Kanavel's signs: **1** Fusiform swelling **2** Tenderness over flexor sheath **3** Semiflexed posture **4** Pain to passive extension	• Spread to palmar or thenar space • Widespread infection • Stiff finger	• Urgent open surgical drainage and washout • Intravenous antibiotics • Elevation • Hand therapy

Table 7.9 Human/animal bites include fight bites

Type of bite	History	Bacteria	Treatment
Human	Fight-bite: metacarpal strikes a tooth	*Eikenella corrodens*	Surgical debridement – healing by secondary intention
		S. aureus α-haemolytic *Streptococcus*	Antibiotic (co-amoxiclav)
Dog and cat bites	Patient may delay seeking treatment until infected	*Pasteurella multocida* *S. aureus* α-haemolytic *Streptococcus*	Appropriate surgical debridement Antibiotic (co-amoxiclav)

abscess develops the patient is at risk of sepsis. Ensure the erythema is outlined daily to observe for regression with treatment.

Hand trauma

Careful history and examination are vital as seen in Tables 7.2 to 7.4.

1 *Fingertip injuries (Figure 7.13)*: aim of treatment to result in a painless fingertip with durable, sensate skin. If pulp loss only, with no bone exposed consider treatment with dressings and healing by secondary intention. Subungual haematoma may cause a throbbing pain in which nailplate trephination or removal of nailplate for decompression is possible. Any nail bed injured should be repaired and if there is soft tissue loss with exposed bone this should covered with a local flap or the finger terminalised. Distal phalanx crush fractures (i.e. tuft fracture) should be managed as open fractures regardless, with splinting and augmentin. The nailplate can be discarded and the patient needs to be counselled that the nailplate will regrow in layers that can take up to 6 months. The new nailplates may not be of the same quality, colour, and thickness as the other uninjured nailplates. Hand therapy is very important, as with all trauma cases, to prevent stiffness.

2 Tendon and ligament injuries require careful assessment. Open injuries should be referred to the local surgical team early.

  a *Closed mallet* fingers with loss of active extension of the DIP joint (from rupture of the extensor tendon insertion) should have a radiograph. If there is a fracture, this should be reduced and held either in a splint for 6 weeks or operated on, depending on fragment size and position. Tendinous mallet should be treated in a hyperextension (mallet) splint immediately from injury for 8 weeks.

  b *Boutonniere deformity* results from rupture of the central slip at PIP joint, and this can be traumatic. After a radiograph excludes a significant fracture, these are treated in a PIPJ extension splint.

  c *Rugger jersey* finger is the avulsion of the FDP tendon from the distal phalanx. This needs urgent surgical assessment and repair due to the avascularity of the flexor tendon.

3 Ligament injuries

  a *Skier's/Gamekeeper's thumb* is when the ulna collateral ligament tears. Assess for weak pinch grip and tenderness on the ulnar side of MCP joint opening on stressing UCL compared with other side. Radiograph looks for an avulsion fracture from forced

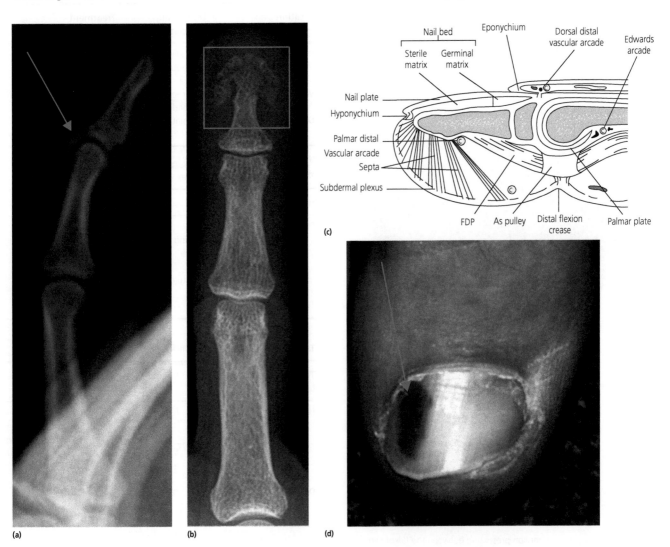

Figure 7.13 Finger tips: (a) radiograph of bony mallet injury: (b) tuft fracture; (c) nail anatomy; and (d) subungual haematoma

abduction. Treat partial ligament injuries in a cast or thumb spica, but complete ligament injuries need surgical repair.

b PIP joint dislocations results in volar plate +/− collateral ligament injury. They require reduction and check radiograph to ensure joint reduction and that no fracture involves greater than 25% of the articular surface. Where these criteria are met, the finger can be treated in a dorsal blocking splint and hand therapy to prevent stiffness.

Hand fractures

After careful assessment of the hand and the position and alignment of the fracture, the majority of hand fractures are minimally displaced, stable, extra-articular fractures that can be treated with buddy strapping (in the absence of rotational deformity). These include most fifth metacarpal neck (boxer's) fractures. Unstable fractures require referral, which include phalangeal, intra-articular, and comminuted fractures. The most common splint is position of safe immobilisation (POSI; also known as the Edinburgh splint), where the wrist is in 0–30° of extension, MCP joints in 70–90° of flexion, and IP joints in full extension.

Common sites for intra-articular fractures (Figure 7.14) include base of first metacarpal (Bennett's fracture dislocation), Rolando (comminuted with at least three fragments) and fifth metacarpal base (reverse Bennett's), and PIP joint. Treatment of these follow orthopaedic principles of joint reduction and maintenance of this until healing is sufficient to start mobilisation. However, as function of the hand is reliant on movement, controlled motion is started earlier, with removable thermoplastic splints.

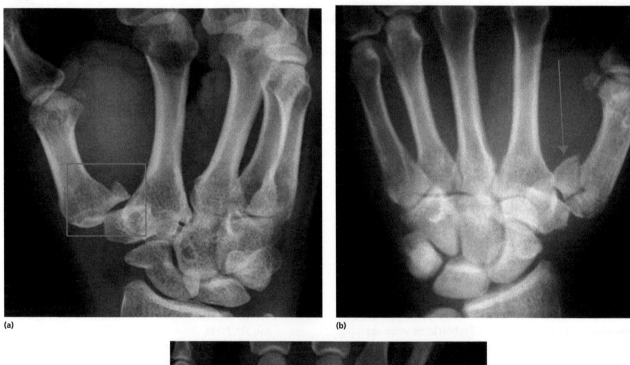

(a)

(b)

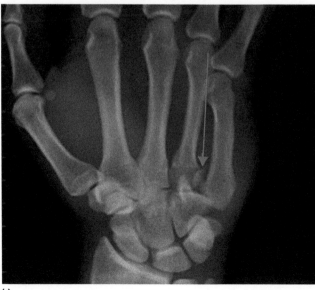

(c)

Figure 7.14 Radiographs showing (a) Bennett's fracture; (b) Rolando fracture; and (c) reverse Bennett's fracture

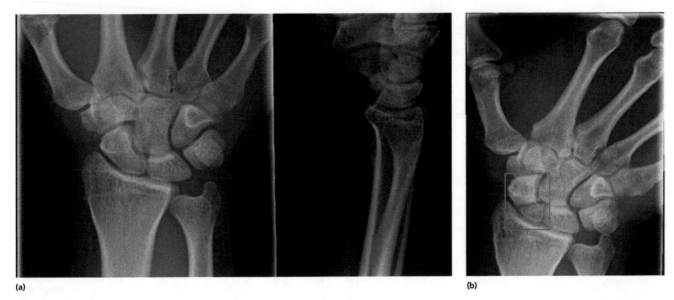

(a)   (b)

Figure 7.15 Radiographs of scaphoid fracture (a) at initial injury; and (b) 6 months later showing nonunion

Wrist injuries

Scaphoid fractures
Background
Scaphoid fractures are the most common type of carpal bone fracture and occur frequently in young men. The typical mechanism is a fall on the outstretched hand. Early diagnosis and treatment for these fractures is critical to avoid scaphoid nonunion (SNAC) and irreversible avascular necrosis.

Examination
There are no reliable clinical tests to confirm the diagnosis of a scaphoid fracture. An observable swelling of the anatomic snuffbox (bounded by APL, EPL, and EPB) increases the chance of a scaphoid facture, but this is a subtle sign. Pain when applying pressure on the anatomic snuffbox or the scaphoid tubercle, or when applying axial pressure on the first metacarpal bone, are positive findings for a scaphoid fracture.

Investigations
Initial radiographs can be negative, and further assessment and imaging (CT or MRI scan) may be necessary to make the diagnosis. Radiographs with specific scaphoid views can also be repeated in 10–14 days to better demonstrate the fracture line.

Management
The aim of the treatment is to achieve fracture healing and functional recovery whilst avoiding complications such as avascular necrosis (AVN), non- or mal-union (Figure 7.15). Due to the retrograde blood supply (from distal to proximal) from the radial artery, a scaphoid fracture can lead to AVN. The more proximal the fracture, the higher likelihood of AVN. Therapeutic options consist of immobilisation in a scaphoid cast or operative treatment if greater displacement.

Further reading

Adebajo, A., ed. (2010). Chapter 1: Pain in the hand and wrist. *ABC of Rheumatology*. Hoboken, NJ: Wiley-Blackwell Publishers.

Anakwe, R.E., and Middleton, S.D. (2011). Osteoarthritis at the base of the thumb. *BMJ* 343: d7122.

Bland, J.D.P. (2007). Carpal tunnel syndrome. *BMJ* 335: 343.

British Society for Surgery of the Hand website: www.bssh.ac.uk

Leversedge, F., Goldfarb, C., and Boyer, M. (2010). *A Pocket Manual of Hand and Upper Extremity Anatomy Primus Manus*. Philadelphia: Lippincott, Williams, and Wilkins: 24–29.

Solomon, L., Warwick, D., and Nayagam, S. (2001). *Apley's System of Orthopaedics and Fractures*. Hodder Publishing.

Wolfe, S., Pederson, W., Hotchkiss, R., et al. (2016). *Green's Operative Hand Surgery*. Volume 1 & 2. Churchill Lovingstone. Elsevier.

CHAPTER 8

Pelvis and Acetabulum

Hani B Abdul-Jabar and Jasvinder Daurka

Imperial College Healthcare NHS Trust, London, UK

OVERVIEW

- Pelvic fractures can be divided into:
  - Low versus high energy
  - Stable versus unstable
  - Life-threatening or non-life-threatening
- Low-energy pelvic fractures are more common amongst the elderly and can be the result of a trivial fall.
- High-energy pelvic fractures are less common and are usually the result of high-speed road traffic accidents.
- Mortality rate is 15–25% for closed fractures and as much as 50% for open fractures where haemorrhage remains as the leading cause of death.
- Associated injuries are present in over two-thirds of these patients, especially those involved in high-energy injury, and include: long bone fractures, sexual dysfunction, head injury, abdominal injury, and spinal fractures resulting in a high prevalence of poor functional outcome and chronic pain.
- Stabilisation of the pelvis can be achieved through binder, ExFix, and definitive operations.
- Acetabular fractures are secondary to high-energy trauma and are usually caused by indirect trauma transmitted through the femur.
- In the elderly, these are typically low-energy injuries from simple falls.
- Associated hip dislocation must be reduced urgently and an assessment of its stability needs to be recorded.
- The neurovascular status before and after reduction must be documented and skeletal traction should be applied.
- A delayed or poorly managed acetabular fracture can lead to accelerated osteoarthritis or hip dysfunction.

The pelvis

Fractures of the pelvic ring can be classified as either low-energy or high-energy. Low-energy pelvic fractures are more common and are usually the result of a simple fall. The incidence increases with age, peaking in patients above 90 years. A high BMI and being male are usually protective factors of pelvic fractures. Mortality following a pelvic fracture is high and increases in an incremental fashion;

it is 10% at 1 year, 20% at 2 years, and up to 50% at 5 years. Prognosis is worse in females, in the presence of dementia and advanced age. High-energy pelvic fractures are less common and are usually due to high-speed road traffic accidents. Two-thirds of these patients also have other musculoskeletal injuries and more than half have multiple system injuries.

Anatomy

The pelvis is a made up of three bones (Figure 8.1): the sacrum and two innominate bones, each comprising the ilium, ischium, and pubis. The innominate bones join the sacrum posteriorly at the two sacroiliac (SI) joints. Anteriorly, these bones join to form the pubic symphysis. During weight bearing, the symphysis acts as a strut to maintain the structure of the pelvic ring.

Physical stability of the pelvis is largely dependent on the combined properties of both the ligaments and the bones that together form the osseo-ligamentous ring (Figure 8.2). Major blood vessels are embedded within the pelvic cavity. These arteries and their associated veins can all be injured during pelvic disruption. The superior gluteal is most frequently injured in unstable posterior injuries, and both pudendal and obturator vessels are most commonly injured from anterior ring injuries. Understanding of pelvic anatomy will help the orthopaedic surgeon recognise which fracture patterns are more likely to cause damage to these major vessels and could result in significant retroperitoneal bleeding leading, potentially, to death.

Imaging
Radiographs

1. *AP pelvis* (Figure 8.3): Look for asymmetry, rotation, or displacement of each hemipelvis as well as specific lines to exclude fractures.
2. *Inlet view:* Ideal for visualising A/P translation or internal/external rotation of the hemipelvis and widening of the SI joint (Figure 8.4).
3. *Outlet view:* Ideal for visualising vertical translation, flexion/extension of the hemipelvis, and disruption of sacral foramina (Figure 8.4).

ABC of Orthopaedics and Trauma, First Edition. Edited by Kapil Sugand and Chinmay M. Gupte.
© 2018 John Wiley & Sons Ltd. Published 2018 by John Wiley & Sons Ltd.

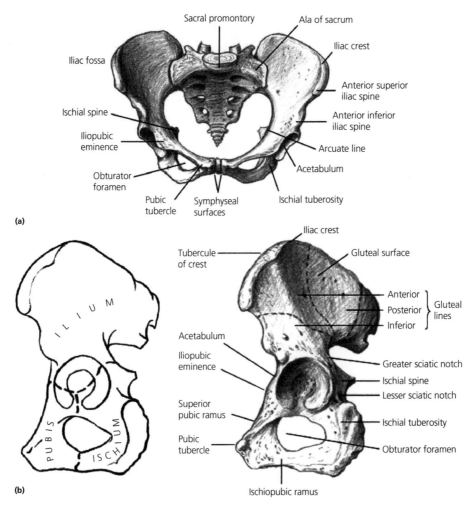

Figure 8.1 Anatomy of the bony pelvis: (a) anterior and (b) lateral

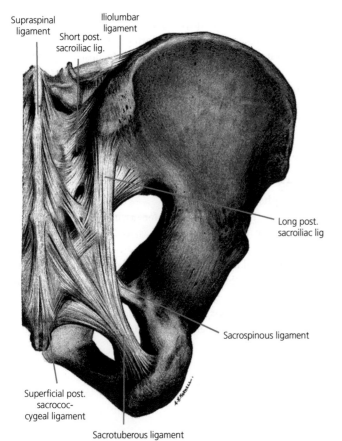

Figure 8.2 Ligaments in the pelvis

Figure 8.3 AP radiograph of the pelvis: Normal AP radiograph of the pelvis: Several important lines and structures are annotated on the left. Unannotated counterparts can be seen on the right. Purple lines = sacral arcuate lines; blue line = iliopectineal line; red line = ilioischial line; orange line = "Shenton's line"; green line = anterior acetabular wall; yellow line = posterior acetabular wall; solid black lines = compressive trabeculae of the femoral neck; dotted black lines = tensile trabeculae of the femoral neck; diagonal arrows = obturator fat stripe; dotted arrow = gluteus (minimus) fat stripe; solid horizontal arrow = iliopsoas fat stripe; OF = obturator foramen

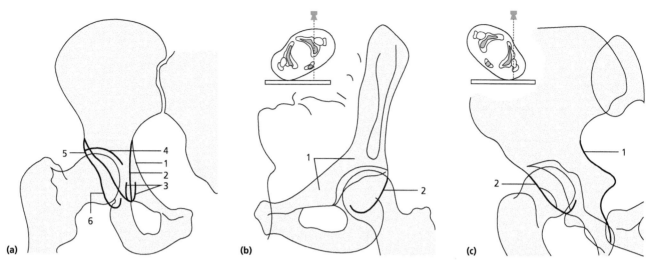

(a)   **(b)**   **(c)**

Figure 8.4 (a) Radiographic landmarks of the acetabulum on the anteroposterior view of the pelvis. 1, iliopectineal line; 2, ilioischial line; 3, teardrop; 4, roof; 5, anterior rim of the acetabulum; 6, posterior rim of the acetabulum. The iliopectineal line, the anterior rim, and teardrop are landmarks of the anterior column; the ilioischial line and posterior rim are landmarks of the posterior columns. (b) Obturator oblique view of the hemipelvis, obtained by turning the injured side 45° toward the X-ray beam. The obturator ring is seen en face, and the iliopectineal line is also present. 1, Area of the anterior column; 2, posterior rim of the acetabulum. Posterior wall fractures are best seen on this view. (c) Iliac oblique view, obtained by rotating the injured side away from the X-ray beam. The iliac wing is seen en face, and fracture lines extending into the iliac wing are often best seen on this view: 1, the greater sciatic notch is seen on this view, and represents the posterior column; 2, the anterior rim of the acetabulum is best seen on this view

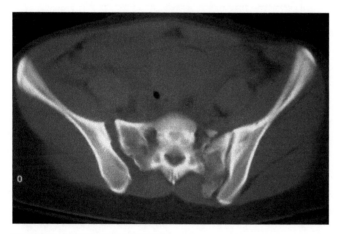

Figure 8.5 Axial CT view of the pelvis

Radiographic signs of instability

1 Greater than 5 mm displacement of posterior SI complex
2 Presence of posterior sacral fracture gap
3 Avulsion fractures: ischial spine, sacrum, and transverse process of fifth lumbar vertebrae

CT

CT allows better characterisation of posterior ring injuries and helps define degree of comminution, fragment size, and rotation (Figure 8.5).

Classification of pelvic injuries

The Tile, and Burgess and Young classifications are the most widely used descriptive systems for pelvic injury patterns.

The Tile classification system is based on the integrity of the posterior SI complex.

1 *Type A injuries*: In these patients the SI complex is intact. They are stable fractures and can be managed nonoperatively.
2 *Type B injuries*: These are caused by either external or internal rotational forces. They involve a partial disruption of the posterior SI complex. They are often unstable and often require operative treatment.
3 *Type C injuries*: These are characterised by complete disruption of the posterior SI complex. They are both rotationally and vertically unstable. Operative treatment is required.

The Burgess and Young classification system (Figure 8.6) is based on mechanism of injury. The forces involved are lateral compression (LC), anteroposterior compression (APC), vertical shear, or a combination.

Avulsion injuries

Fractures that occur at the sites of muscle attachments due to forceful muscle contractions in the pelvis and hip can be seen in Figure 8.7. Complications include nonunion, chronic pain, and osteonecrosis. Management options consist mainly of conservative management or surgical fixation as a last resort (in case of failed conservative treatment, non-unions and displaced fracture).

Emergency department tests

1 Serial Hb and Hct measurements to monitor ongoing blood loss
2 Urinalysis may reveal gross or microscopic haematuria
3 Pregnancy test indicated in females of childbearing age
4 Cross match and massive transfusion protocol as required
5 Clotting screen, glucose, U&E, and LFTs
6 Urethrogram/cystogram

Treatment of pelvic injuries

An overview of the treatment options is outlined in Figure 8.8. The early management of patients with mechanically unstable pelvic injuries is in accordance with ATLS principles. The initial

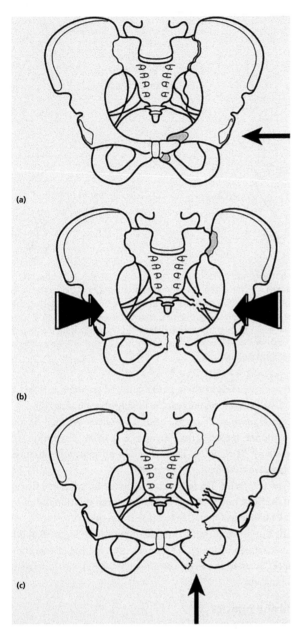

Figure 8.6 The Burgess and Young classification system: (a) Lateral compression fracture. (b) Open book fracture – anterior-posterior compression. (c) Vertical sheer fracture

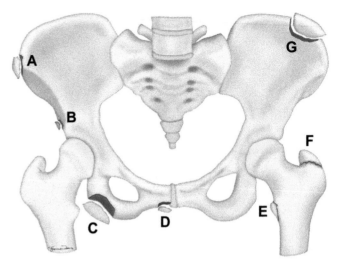

Figure 8.7 Avulsion fractures: (A)=ASIS (sartorius origin); (B)=AIIS (rectus femoris origin); (C)=ischial tuberosity (hamstrings origin); (D)=parasymphyseal pubis (hip adductors origin); (E)=femoral lesser trochanter (iliopsoas insertion); (F)=femoral greater trochanter (gluteus minimus and medius insertions); (G)=iliac crest (abdominal obliques attachments)

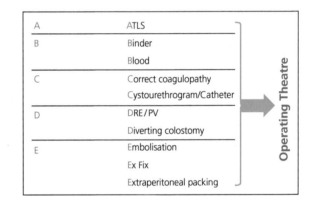

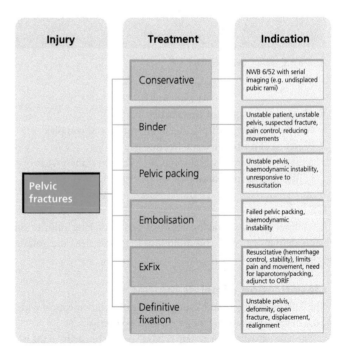

Figure 8.8 ABC Pelvic Assessment Protocol and treatment options

assessment of the injuries in conjunction with a review of the accident provides valuable information of the degree of energy dissipated and expected pattern of associated injuries. Injuries that result in an increase in intrapelvic volume can cause massive haemorrhage. Reducing the intrapelvic volume is required to assist in the formation of clot and its tamponade effect.

Pelvic binders

The use of external fixators in the emergency department has diminished in favour of pelvic binders. Whether improvised or commercially available, these are easy to apply and seem very effective. A degree of caution must be used in their use as they can recreate injury forces such as in lateral compression injuries and have also occasionally been associated with skin necrosis. The pelvic binder should be applied over the greater trochanters with the legs held in extension and internal rotation (Figure 8.9).

Angiography/embolisation

The use of angiography/embolisation in haemorrhage control (related to pelvic fracture) is controversial and based on multiple variables including: protocol of institution, stability of patient, proximity of angiography suite, and availability and experience of interventional radiology staff.

Associated urological trauma

Haematuria in a trauma patient may suggest a pelvic fracture. A haematoma over the ipsilateral flank, inguinal ligament, proximal thigh, or in the perineum also raise the suspicion of pelvic injury. Signs of urethral injury in males include a high-riding or boggy prostate on rectal examination, scrotal haematoma or blood at the urethral meatus. Retrograde urethrography is indicated in these patients and also in female patients in whom a Foley catheter cannot easily pass on gentle attempts.

Bladder ruptures and bladder neck injuries usually require laparotomy and direct repair. The early involvement of a urological surgeon is advised.

Open injury

The presence of an open injury to either the skin or mucosal membranes usually precludes the use of internal fixation and often requires a defunctioning colostomy. It is important to monitor the stoma to ensure no faecal contamination of the orthopaedic wound. The emergency care of pelvic fractures is very much priority driven using both ATLS and pelvis specific protocols (Figure 8.8).

External fixation (ExFix)

External fixation (ExFix) is reserved for pelvic ring injuries with a rotational component that causes instability (Figure 8.10). This is a temporary fixation technique prior to definitive reconstruction with the aim of decreasing the pelvic volume and aiding in the formation of clots in a bleeding venous plexus. Multiple pins are inserted into the supracetabular bone and superior iliac crests prior to performing a laparotomy for defunctioning colostomy.

Definitive reconstruction

The definitive management of pelvic fractures relies on the surgeon having an understanding of the osseo-ligamentous anatomy (Figure 8.2) of the pelvic ring and the structures that have been compromised by a particular fracture pattern. Low-energy pelvic

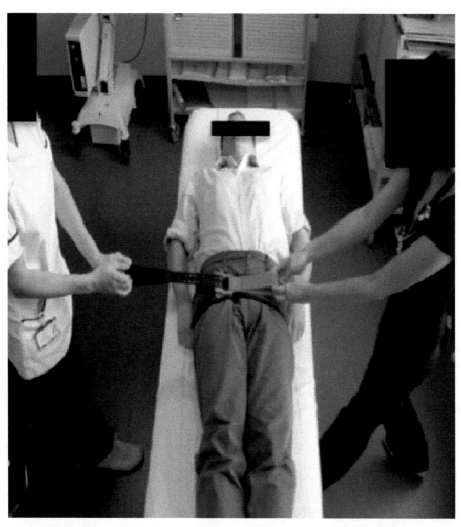

Figure 8.9 Correct placement of pelvic binder

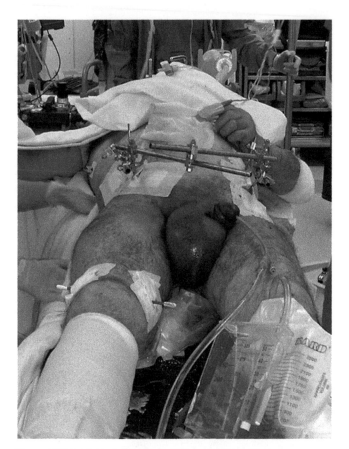

Figure 8.10 Pelvic binder replaced with anterior external fixator

fractures in the elderly rarely require operative stabilisation as the posterior SI and pelvic floor ligamentous structures are intact and provide inherent stability to resist physiological loading. Definitive treatment strategies for unstable pelvic fractures are aimed at providing stability and restoring function. Other factors to consider include preventing disability from leg length discrepancy, sitting imbalance, and postural instability. The pelvis is highly vascular and likely to heal in whatever position the fracture fragments come to rest. Ligamentous instability, however, is less likely to heal. The association between residual displacement and outcome as far as pelvic fractures is concerned is difficult to quantify, since the worse injury patterns are associated with higher rates of neurological, bladder, urethral, and vascular injury. Conservative management usually consists of non-weight bearing for 6 weeks with serial radiographs.

Indications for operative treatment include:
1 A symphysis diastasis > 2.5 cm (Figure 8.11)
2 SIJ displacement > 1 cm
3 Sacral fracture with displacement > 1 cm
4 Displacement or internal rotation of a hemi-pelvis > 160°
5 Open fracture

Prognosis

Pelvic fracture is a life-changing injury. Patient follow-up should occur in specialist pelvic units to ensure full advice is available for the pain, physical, urological, and sexual disabilities, which are common outcomes. There is a high prevalence of thrombotic events, and long-term prophylaxis may be required.

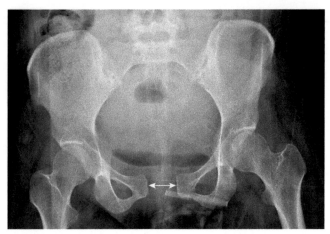

Figure 8.11 A radiograph demonstrating a symphysis diastasis of greater than 2.5 cm

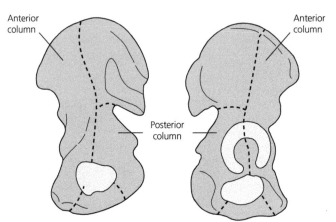

Figure 8.12 The inverted Y two-column acetabulum

Acetabulum

The incidence of acetabular fracture is estimated at three displaced fractures per 100,000 per year. The majority occur in males (70%) with a mean age of 40 years, but there is a growing incidence of fractures in the elderly. The management of acetabular fracture is aimed at preventing post-traumatic osteoarthritis and long-term disability, by restoring and maintaining the congruity and stability of the hip joint. It is important to understand the fracture pattern and classification so that the appropriate approach and fixation technique is selected.

Anatomy

The acetabulum is formed from all three bones of the innominate pelvis: the ilium, ischium, and pubis. The two-column theory advocates that the acetabulum is supported by two columns of bone to form an "inverted Y" construct connected to the sacrum through the sciatic buttress (Figure 8.12).

The Corona Mortis, an anastomosis of external iliac (epigastric) and internal iliac (obturator) vessels, is usually at risk with lateral dissection over superior pubic ramus during acetabular operative fixation (Figure 8.13).

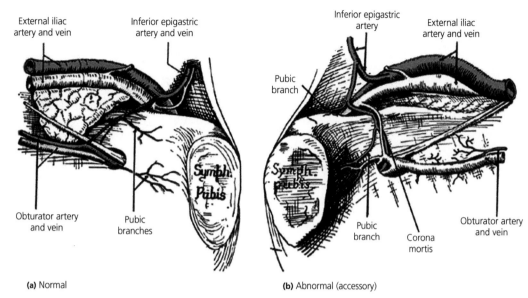

(a) Normal   **(b)** Abnormal (accessory)

Figure 8.13 Corona Mortis: Illustration of the commonly occurring small calibre anastomoses between the obturator and external iliac systems (a). Illustration of the true *corona mortis,* aberrant origin of the obturator artery from the external iliac system (b). (Reproduced from Grant, J.C.B. (1972). Grant's atlas of anatomy (6th edition). Williams & Wilkins, Baltimore, MD.)

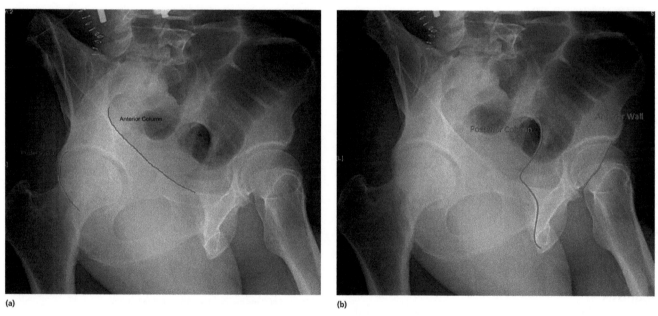

(a)   (b)

Figure 8.14 Plain radiographs demonstrating (a) obturator oblique and (b) iliac oblique

Imaging
Radiographs
An AP view of the pelvis should be obtained as part of the trauma series.

Six radiographic lines are assessed for loss of continuity (Figure 8.4):
1 Iliopectineal line
2 Ilioischial line
3 Radiographic tear drop
4 Roof
5 Anterior rim
6 Posterior rim

Judet views (Figure 8.14): these are oblique radiographic views of the acetabulum with the pelvis tilted at 45 degrees to the beam. The two views are named obturator oblique and iliac oblique. Specific bony anatomical areas are highlighted by each view (Table 8.1).

Table 8.1 Anatomical inclusions within Judet views

Obturator oblique	Iliac oblique
Anterior column	Posterior column
Posterior wall	Anterior wall

CT
CT scanning of the pelvis and acetabulae assists greatly in comprehending fracture pattern and surgical planning. CT can identify acetabular fractures not visible on plain radiographs, and enables the orientation of the fracture line to be understood.

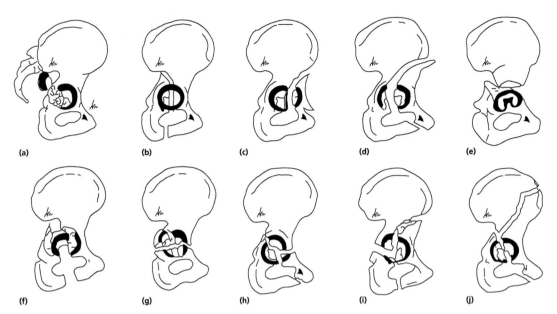

Figure 8.15 Judet-Letournel classification of acetabular fractures: There are 10 fracture types, divided into five elementary patterns and five associated patterns. The elementary patterns are: (a) posterior wall; (b) posterior column; (c) anterior wall; (d) anterior column; (e) transverse. The associated patterns are as follows: (f) posterior column and posterior wall; (g) transverse and posterior wall; (h) T-shaped; (i) anterior column (or wall) with associated posterior hemitransverse; (j) both-column

Classification

The Judet-Letournel classification describes five elementary or *simple* patterns and five complex, or *associated* patterns. Associated fractures include at least two of the elementary forms (Figure 8.15).

Treatment

- *Nonoperative*: protected weight bearing for 6–8 weeks is indicated in minimally displaced fracture (<2 mm) and in fractures involving < 20% of the posterior wall.
- *Operative*: ORIF is indicated if the displacement of the roof (>2 mm), posterior wall fracture involving more than 40–50%, intra-articular loose bodies or irreducible fracture-dislocation. Open reduction and internal fixation with acute total hip arthroplasty is indicated if significant osteopenia and/or significant comminution is present.

Prognosis

Post-traumatic degenerative changes within the hip joint is the most common complication. This can be minimised by urgent anatomical reduction to establish articular congruency. Heterotopic ossification has the highest incidence with extensile surgical approaches and should be treated with either indomethacin or low-dose external radiation.

Further reading

British Orthopaedic Association Standards for Trauma (BOAST 3). (December 2008). Pelvic and Acetabular Fracture Management, at www.boa.ac.uk/wp-content/uploads/2014/12/BOAST-3.pdf.

Butterwick, D., Papp, S., Gofton, W., et al. (2015). Acetabular Fractures in the Elderly: Evaluation and Management. *Journal of Bone and Joint Surgery (Am.)* 97: 758–768.

Daurka, J., Rankin, I., Jaggard, M.K., et al. (2015). A priority-driven ABC approach to the emergency management of high-energy pelvic trauma improves decision making in simulated patient scenarios. *Injury* 46: 340–343.

Guthrie, H.C., Owens, R.W., and Bircher, M.D. (2010). Fractures of the pelvis. *Journal of Bone and Joint Surgery* 11: 1481–1488.

Hill, R.M., Robinson, C.M., and Keating, J.F. (2001). Fractures of the pelvic rami. Epidemiology and five-year survival. *Journal of Bone and Joint Surgery* 83: 1141–1144.

CHAPTER 9

The Hip

Simond Jagernauth and Joshua KL Lee

The Royal London Hospital, Barts Health NHS Trust, London, UK

OVERVIEW

- Hip pain may also be referred from other sites such as lumbar spine or sacroiliac joints, and it is important to exclude these causes when examining patients.
- Hip fractures and osteoarthritis contribute to a substantial clinical burden to the NHS and mortality rates in the elderly.
- The main blood supply to the femoral head in the adult is from the retinacular vessels that run within the hip capsule.
- Disruption of the blood supply in hip fractures guides surgical management.
- Surgical management for hip fractures include (1) hip repair with cannulated screws or a dynamic hip screw and (2) hip replacement with hip hemiarthroplasty or total hip replacement.
- Hip osteoarthritis is usually treated by total hip replacement if conservative management has been exhausted. Occasionally resurfacing may be performed.

Anatomy

MSk anatomy

The hip joint is the largest synovial joint in the body consisting of a ball and socket articulation between the femoral head (ball) and acetabulum (socket). The acetabulum is formed by the fusion of the ilium, ischium, and pubis and normally takes place by the end of teenage years. The hip capsule is a fibrous structure lined by synovium that attaches proximally to the acetabulum and inserts into the intertrochanteric line anteriorly and approximately 1 cm proximally to the intertrochanteric crest posteriorly (Figure 9.1). It is composed of three strong ligaments: iliofemoral (the strongest), ischifemoral, and pubofemoral.

Vascular supply

In adults, the blood supply to the femoral head is from three sources: the retinacular vessels, nutrient artery (through the medullary cavity), and the artery of the ligamentum teres (Figure 9.2). The main arterial supply arises from the retinacular vessels, which pierce the capsule and run along the femoral neck to the head.

Retinacular vessels originate from the medial femoral circumflex artery (supplies approximately 70% of vascular supply to femoral head vs. lateral femoral circumflex artery) stemming from the profunda femoris artery that travels within the capsule along the femoral neck from distal to proximal. This is of relevance to hip fractures, as certain types can compromise the blood supply to the femoral head resulting in avascular necrosis.

History

A well-taken history should explore the patient's symptoms, the functional demands of the patient and how their symptoms impact on their lifestyle (Table 9.1). This will help to direct the examination, subsequent investigations, and treatment. It is important to remember that hip pain can occasionally present as isolated knee pain. A history should include the following:

Clinical examination

The clinical examination can be very reliable in detecting a hip joint problem. The spine should also be examined to exclude lumbar or radicular pain that may mimic hip pain. A hip examination should adopt a systematic approach, encompassing the "look, feel, move, special tests" principle (Figure 9.3, Table 9.2). With displaced fractures, the patient may have a shortened and externally rotated leg. Both sciatic nerve function and peripheral pulses should be checked and clearly documented.

General conditions

Be on the lookout for the following differential diagnoses according to age groups as seen in Table 9.3.

Hip fractures

Clinical burden

There are approximately 70,000–75,000 hip fractures in the United Kingdom each year with a cost to the NHS of £2 billion (NICE and BOAST 1 guidelines). With an ageing population, these figures are

---

ABC of Orthopaedics and Trauma, First Edition. Edited by Kapil Sugand and Chinmay M. Gupte.
© 2018 John Wiley & Sons Ltd. Published 2018 by John Wiley & Sons Ltd.

Frontal section through the right hip joint

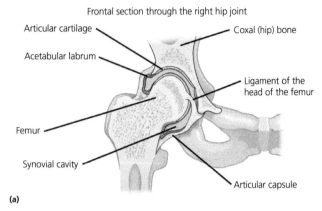

(a)

Anterior view of right hip joint, capsule in place

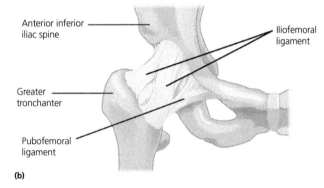

(b)

Posterior view of right hip joint, capsule in place

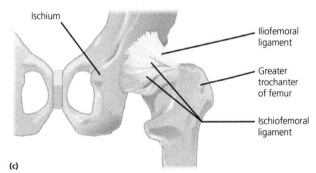

(c)

Figure 9.1 Hip anatomy

projected to increase in the future. Mortality rates are 10% within the first month of injury and 33% at one year. Elderly hip fracture patients often have significant comorbidities and a multidisciplinary approach to their care is essential to provide the best opportunity to achieve a full recovery.

Mechanism of injury

The mechanism of injuries is low-energy in the elderly (e.g. fall from standing), but require a significantly high-energy mechanism in young adults (e.g. road traffic accident or fall from a height).

Diagnostic imaging

AP pelvis and lateral radiographs of the hip should be performed to diagnose the injury. Look for the loss of Shenton's line (Figure 9.4). In cases where there is a high index of suspicion of hip fracture that is not visible on radiographs, an MRI should ideally be performed to confirm the diagnosis, but CT scans may also be an option. Any fractures that involve the shaft distal to the trochanters or when there is a suspicion of a pathological fracture (e.g. metastatic bone disease) require radiographs of the whole femur.

Hip fractures can be broadly classified into extracapsular and intracapsular injuries (Figures 9.5 and 9.6).

Extracapsular hip fractures

These consist of per-trochanteric (or intertrochanteric) fractures between greater and lesser trochanter, and subtrochanteric fractures distal to lesser trochanter. Unlike intracapsular fractures, the blood supply to the femoral head is preserved, and therefore, they

Table 9.1 History of hip symptoms

- Pain: rest, night time, activity-related
- Walking distance
- Functional restrictions: cutting toenails, climbing and descending stairs, limping
- Stiffness
- Clicking
- Instability
- Referred pain from spine or to knee

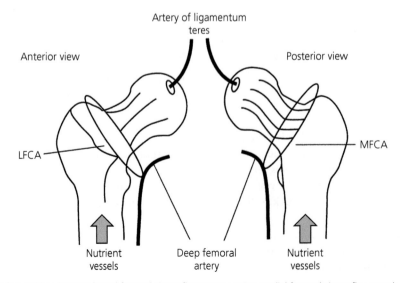

Figure 9.2 Blood supply to the femoral head (LFCA: lateral femoral circumflex artery; MFCA: medial femoral circumflex artery)

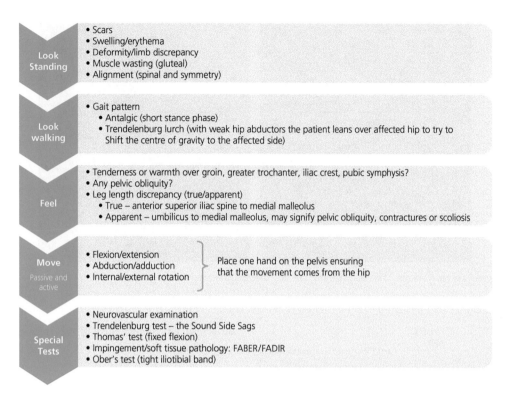

Figure 9.3 Hip examination

Table 9.2 Special tests for hip examination

Special tests
- Trendelenburg sign
  - Positive in patients with weak hip abductors (gluteus medius and minimus)
  - Whilst you support them, the patient is asked to stand on one leg at a time. If the patient's pelvis tilts on one side, this is a positive finding.
  - Remember: the sound side sags.
- Thomas's test
  - Used to assess if a hip flexion contracture is present
  - Whilst lying supine, the unaffected hip is flexed to bring the knee to the chest. This acts to stabilize the pelvis and obliterate lumbar lordosis. If the evaluated thigh lifts off the table, there is a flexion deformity present.
- Leg length measurements
  - True leg length – from anterior superior iliac spine to medial malleolus
  - Apparent leg length – umbilicus to medial malleolus
  - A true length discrepancy can arise due to conditions such as Perthes, slipped upper femoral epiphysis, developmental dysplasia of hip, avascular necrosis, or arthritis.
  - An apparent leg length discrepancy may arise from contractures, scoliosis or pelvic obliquity.

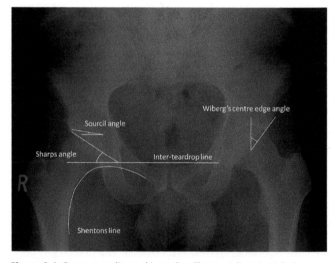

Figure 9.4 Common radiographic angles. Shenton's line. Acetabular angle (of Tonnis) or Sourcil angle normal value 0–10 degrees. Vertical centre edge angle (of Wiberg) normal value ≥25 degrees; Sharp's acetabular angle (between Sourcil's angle and pelvic tear drop) < 38 degrees, if higher than signifies dysplasia. Note small cam lesion of left hip

Table 9.3 General hip conditions according to age groups

15–45 years	45–60 years	>60 years
Developmental dysplasia	Osteoarthritis	
Leg length discrepancy	Avascular necrosis	
	Impingement	Post-THR

rarely undergo avascular necrosis or nonunion. As the surface area of contact is greater at the fracture site, they are more likely to achieve union. Surgical fixation is the treatment of choice, and this is often in the form a dynamic hip screw (DHS) or intramedullary nail (Figure 9.7). In DHS, the screw slides in its plate and allows the fracture to impact on itself as the patient bears weight, hence the "dynamic" nature of the screw. There are certain fracture configura-

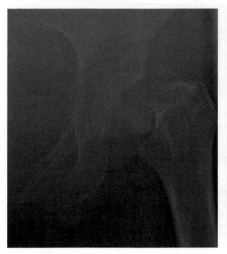
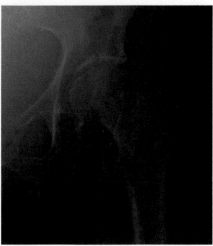

Figure 9.5 Plain radiographs of hip fractures: (L) intracapsular fracture, (R) extracapsular fracture

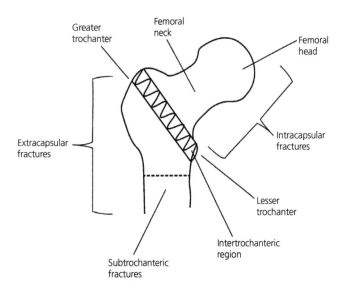

Figure 9.6 Hip fracture patterns

tions that are unstable (e.g. reverse oblique), and these may require fixation with an intramedullary nail.

Intracapsular neck of femur fractures

Garden's classification (I-IV) is commonly used to categorise intracapsular femoral neck fractures (Figure 9.8). These fractures may interrupt the blood supply to the femoral head and can result in avascular necrosis since the blood supply is important to allow the fracture to heal. Patients should be surgically managed if they are medically fit for anaesthesia such as general or spinal.

Surgical management depends on degree of fracture displacement, the patient's age, mentation, and the preinjury mobility (Figure 9.9).

Undisplaced

Undisplaced fractures can be managed with surgical fixation of the femoral neck (e.g. cannulated screws or dynamic hip screw). This is done with the assumption that the blood supply to the femoral

head is minimally interrupted, as the fracture is not displaced to allow healing.

Displaced in the young

Displaced fractures in the young may also be treated with surgical fixation in the hope that the vascular supply will be maintained after reduction and fixation of the fracture. If successful, the patient's fracture will unite and they may achieve a fully functional hip joint. However, if they develop AVN or nonunion, then a total hip replacement may be required to resolve these complications.

Displaced in the elderly

In the elderly, displaced fractures of the femoral neck are associated with higher rates of avascular necrosis (up to 30% in 18 months) and nonunion. For this reason, it is recommended that they undergo replacement arthroplasty where the femoral head can be replaced as a sole procedure (hemiarthroplasty, Figure 9.10) or as part of a total hip arthroplasty (acetabulum replaced, too, Figure 9.11). Total hip replacements should be reserved for those who have no cognitive impairment, were able to walk independently preinjury, and were fitter and younger patients, as they demand more of their hips.

Outline of hip fracture guidance

In order to standardise and improve the management of hip fractures in the United Kingdom, nationally approved guidelines have been recommended (Table 9.4).

Osteoarthritis of the hip

Overview

Osteoarthritis is the most common form of arthritis and can lead to disabling pain when affecting the hip joint. In the young adult, it can occur secondary to other causes such as Perthes disease, development dysplasia of the hip, or slipped upper femoral epiphysis. In older patients, it may arise secondary to trauma, AVN, or Paget's disease. It is referred to as primary osteoarthritis in cases

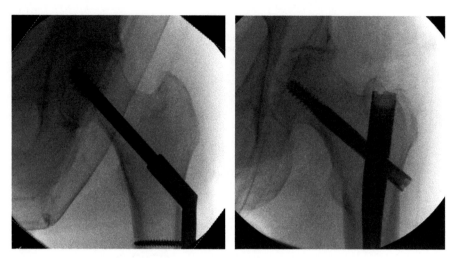

Figure 9.7 Radiographs of (L) dynamic hip screw, (R) intramedullary nail for treatment of extracapsular hip fracture

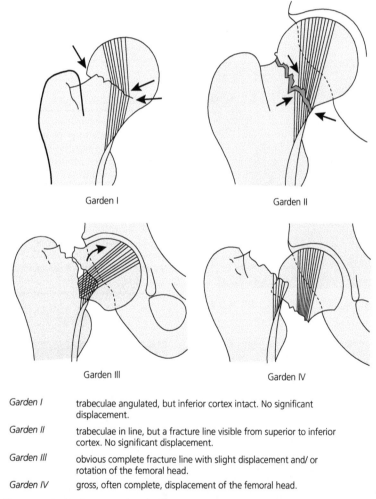

Garden I

Garden II

Garden III

Garden IV

Garden I	trabeculae angulated, but inferior cortex intact. No significant displacement.
Garden II	trabeculae in line, but a fracture line visible from superior to inferior cortex. No significant displacement.
Garden III	obvious complete fracture line with slight displacement and/ or rotation of the femoral head.
Garden IV	gross, often complete, displacement of the femoral head.

Figure 9.8 Garden classification of intracapsular hip fractures. This classification was used to describe intracapsular neck of femur fractures but more recently has been simplified to displaced or undisplaced. Classification is for historical reference

where no underlying cause can be found. It is thought that there is increased stress to the articular cartilage of the hip joint leading to damage and eventual loss of the cartilage, leading to exposure of the underlying bone.

Symptoms and signs

Patients often report a gradual onset of pain affecting their groin or anterior thigh. Often pain radiates to the knee, and can occasionally present as isolated knee pain. It may become worse after periods

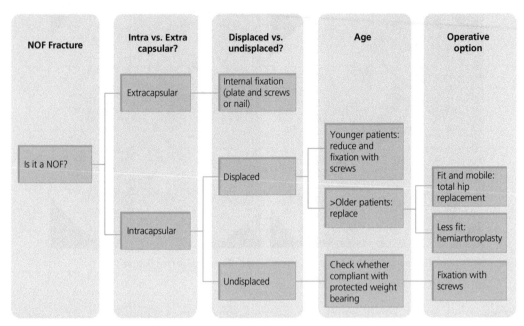

Figure 9.9 Management options for NOF fractures

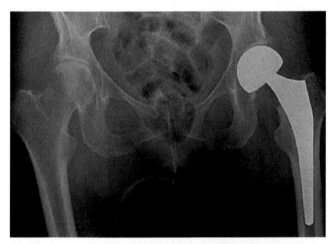

Figure 9.10 Radiograph of a cemented hemiarthroplasty for treatment of a displaced intracapsular hip fracture

Table 9.4 National NOF targets

- Time to surgery within 36 hours from arrival in Emergency Department
- Admitted under joint care of ortho-geriatric team
- Admitted using an assessment protocol agreed by geriatric medicine, orthopaedic surgery, and anaesthesia
- Assessed by a geriatrician in the perioperative period (defined as within 72 hours of admission)
- Post-operative geriatrician-directed care
- Multiprofessional rehabilitation team
- Fracture prevention assessments (falls and bone health)
- Pre- and post-op abbreviated mental test score (AMTS)

www.nice.org
CG124 Hip fracture: quick reference guide
22 June 2011

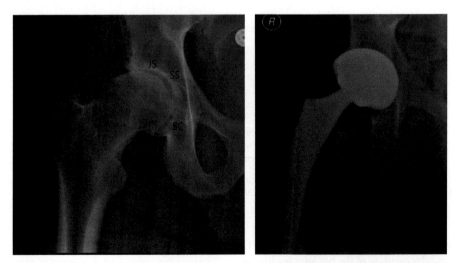

Figure 9.11 Radiographs of (L) osteoarthritis (OP - osteophyte; JS - loss of joint space; SS - subchondral sclerosis; SC - subchondral cyst) of the hip. (R) uncemented total hip replacement

of activity and is commonly associated with hip stiffness. They may walk with a painful limp and may use a walking stick to help them mobilise (helps offload the hip, reducing pain).

As the disease progresses, the range of movement at the hip joint declines. Internal rotation is the usually the first movement to be affected. In later stages of the disease there may be shortening of the affected leg, due to bone loss from the femoral head. Thomas's test may reveal a fixed flexion deformity of the hip and the Trendelenburg test may be positive, indicating weak abductors or secondary to pain.

Diagnostic Imaging

The characteristic radiographic signs of osteoarthritis are loss of joint space, osteophytes, subchondral bone cysts, and subchondral sclerosis (Figure 9.11).

Management

Nonoperative: In early osteoarthritis, exercise should be a core treatment, including local muscle strengthening and improving general aerobic fitness. This may be complemented with simple analgesics such as paracetamol, NSAIDs, or weak opioids.

Operative: In the latter stages of the condition, the combination of joint pain, loss of function, and impaired quality of life may lead to consideration for total hip replacement surgery.

Total hip replacement

A total hip replacement can be fixed with bone cement or by bone ingrowth onto the surface of the implant (Figure 9.11). The damaged femoral head is removed and a metal stem is implanted within the femur. A replacement ball made from ceramic or metal is then placed on the stem. The acetabulum is shaped, and then either a plastic socket or a metallic socket with a plastic or ceramic liner is cemented in. The two components constitute the new artificial hip joint.

Inflammatory arthritis of hip

Inflammatory arthritis describes the systemic conditions that are the result of an underlying immune-mediated pathology. These include rheumatoid arthritis, SLE and ankylosing spondylitis. In these conditions there is inflammation of the synovium of the hip joint. Patients may experience pain similar to that of osteoarthritis with pain in the groin, buttock, or thigh. They may walk with a painful limp and examination may demonstrate reduced range of movement of the hip. Laboratory studies will reveal raised inflammatory markers such as ESR and CRP. An immunological screen should be performed. Hip radiographs may show joint space narrowing, articular erosions, osteophytes, and diffuse osteopenia. Nonoperative management includes exercise and simple analgesia. Patients may be on disease-modifying anti-rheumatic drugs such as methotrexate or sulfasalazine that may help to slow the progression of the disease. Patients who are refractory to conservative measures may be considered for total hip replacement surgery.

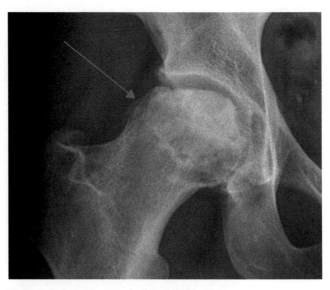

Figure 9.12 Avascular necrosis of the right hip

Avascular necrosis of hip

Avascular necrosis (AVN) of the hip is thought to arise due to a disruption to the blood supply to the femoral head. This leads to death of both cartilage and bone and to eventual collapse of the bone (Figure 9.12). Traumatic causes include intracapsular neck of femur fractures and hip dislocation. Nontraumatic causes include heavy alcohol intake, steroids, sickle cell disease, SLE, inflammatory bowel disease, and myeloproliferative disorders. Patients may present with a gradual onset of hip pain that may progress to severe pain with reduced range of movement. Radiographs may show flattening of the femoral head with subchondral bone cysts and sclerosis. Patients with early stages of the disease may gain benefit from bisphosphonate therapy. Surgical management includes a core decompression of the femoral head (for early stages), osteotomy, or total hip replacement (later stages).

Trochanteric bursitis

Trochanteric bursitis is a common condition characterised by inflammation of the bursa overlying the greater trochanter. It may occur as a result of overuse injury or trauma to the greater trochanter, but often no underlying cause can be found. Patients may complain of pain on the lateral aspect of the thigh and may have difficulty sleeping on the affected side. They often point to their greater trochanter as the site of pain, and passive adduction of the hip may exacerbate this. Ultrasound scan or MRI may reveal increased fluid within the trochanteric bursa. Nonoperative measures include NSAIDs and physiotherapy. Local infiltration of corticosteroid to the trochanteric bursa may act to reduce inflammation and provide pain relief. A bursectomy can be performed in patients who remain refractory to conservative measures. There may be radiation distally leading to ITB syndrome.

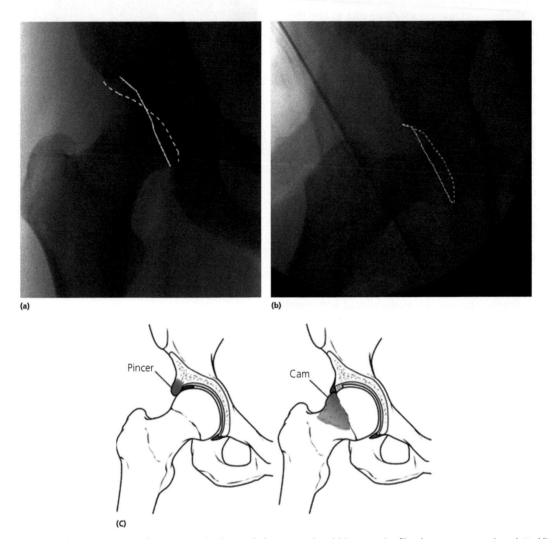

Figure 9.13 Femoro-acetabular impingement: The cross-over sign in acetabular retroversion. (a) Preoperative film shows cross-over sign, dotted line represents anterior rim of acetabulum. (b) This patient was treated successfully for a pincer lesion with acetabular rim resection and labral refixation. The anterior dotted line and posterior solid line meet at the edge, as they should in normal hips. (c) A schematic demonstrating pincer and cam lesions

Labral tear

Labral tears occur within the acetabular labrum of the hip joint. They are often the result of traumatic injuries to the hip and may occur in athletic individuals. Patients may only complain of hip pain during strenuous activity, and it is commonly associated with a "*clicking*" sensation in the hip. Examination may reveal pain and clicking on combined hip flexion, abduction, and internal rotation. An MR arthrogram may confirm the tear. Nonoperative measures include physiotherapy, NSAIDs, and corticosteroid injections. In patients in whom these measures fail, a hip arthroscopy can allow debridement or repair of the labral tear.

Femoroacetabular impingement

Femoroacetabular impingement is a condition that tends to affect young adults. There is an abnormal shape of the femoral neck (cam) or acetabulum (pincer), as in Figure 9.13. This leads to abnormal abutment of the femoral neck on the acetabulum during the extremes of hip motion, specifically flexion and internal rotation, with associated pain. It is now thought that this may be the cause of

the majority of cases of primary or idiopathic hip osteoarthritis. Examination may reveal reduced hip flexion, particularly with internal rotation. Radiographs may indicate loss of contour of the femoral head–neck junction and asphericity of the femoral head. MR arthrogram may also indicate if there are any associated labral tears and articular cartilage damage. Treatment includes refraining from exacerbating activities and physiotherapy. Surgical management includes arthroscopic or open resection of the deformity, which can provide symptomatic benefit.

Further reading

American Academemy of Ortopaedic Surgeons website, http://orthoinfo.aaos.org/main.cfm

British Orthopaedic Association Standards for Trauma (BOAST) 1 guideline: Patients sustaining a fragility hip fracture, https://www.boa.ac.uk/wp-content/uploads/2014/12/BOAST-1.pdf

NICE guidelines. Hip Fractures, https://www.boa.ac.uk/wp-content/uploads/2014/12/BOAST-1.pdf

Nice guidelines. Osteoarthritis, http://www.nice.org.uk/nicemedia/pdf/CG59NICEguideline.pdf

CHAPTER 10

The Knee

Nawfal Al-Hadithy[1] and Chinmay M. Gupte[1,2]

[1] Imperial College Healthcare NHS Trust, London, UK
[2] MSk Lab, Charing Cross Hospital, Imperial College London, London, UK

OVERVIEW

- Knee joint conditions can be divided into
  - traumatic (e.g. fracture)
  - sports injuries or repetitive strain
  - degenerative or inflammatory conditions (osteo- or rheumatoid arthritis)
- Osteoarthritis of the knee is one of the most common causes of reduced mobility in the developed world.
- Treatment of OA depends on symptoms including rest pain, night pain, disability and deformity. Treatment consists of conservative measures (e.g. walking aids, physiotherapy, analgesia, intra-articular injections) are relieving symptoms.
- Most common sport injuries include meniscal tears, cruciate ligament injuries and patella injuries. Operative treatment includes meniscal repair, resection, and ligament reconstruction (most commonly anterior cruciate ligament). Physiotherapy is also key in the management of these conditions.
- Surgical treatments of a degenerate knee consist of osteotomy and joint replacement. There is almost no role for arthroscopy for treatment of osteoarthritis.
- Patellofemoral disorders can result in anterior knee pain or patellar instability. Most can be managed with conservative measures such as physiotherapy, orthotics, or weight loss.

Anatomy and function

The knee is a synovial joint that comprises the tibiofemoral and patellofemoral joints. It is inherently unstable due to the incongruency of the bony surfaces; however, stability is maintained through a combination of the major ligaments in the knee, capsule, and muscles. The knee joint functions include:

- Transient load when standing
- Transmit muscle forces during movement, propulsion, and stair climbing
- Shock absorption when jumping

Tibiofemoral

The tibiofemoral joint transmits the body weight from the femur to the tibia and has a normal range of $-5°$ (hyperextension) to $150°$ (flexion). Additionally, the tibia externally rotates $5°$ as the knee fully extends, which is known as the *screw home mechanism*, allowing the knee to lock during standing to reduce fatigue on the quadriceps.

Ligaments

Knee ligaments (Figure 10.1 and Table 10.1) serve to stabilise the knee joint and can be divided into intra-articular (ACL/PCL) and extra-articular (MCL/LCL/PCL). These ligaments stabilise both translation and rotation of the knee in three different planes (x, y, z). Rupture of any of these ligaments can result in instability, that can be detected by appropriate clinical examination. Complete ruptures are commonly associated with tears to the medial and posterior capsule, and if the force is sufficient the ACL and medial meniscus may also be damaged (also known as O' Donahue's triad, Figure 10.2).

The knee anatomy is outlined in Figure 10.3. Within the tibiofemoral joint are the medial and lateral menisci, which are C-shaped fibro-elastic cartilage that have two main functions:

1 *Force transmission*: The increase in the congruity between the femur and tibia reduces stress contact forces and aids in shock absorption and transmits up to 80% of the load.
2 *Stability*: They deepen the tibial surface further, thus acting as choc blocks and contributing to anteroposterior stability.

Patellofemoral joint

The patellofemoral joint (PFJ) consists of the articulation between the patella and distal femur (femoral trochlea) and is part of the extensor mechanism. Its main function is to transmit the force generated from the quadriceps to the patella tendon and increase the lever arm of the extensor mechanism. The extensor mechanism consists of the quadriceps muscle, which attaches into the patella (quadriceps tendon), which attaches to the tibial tubercle via the patella tendon.

ABC of Orthopaedics and Trauma, First Edition. Edited by Kapil Sugand and Chinmay M. Gupte.
© 2018 John Wiley & Sons Ltd. Published 2018 by John Wiley & Sons Ltd.

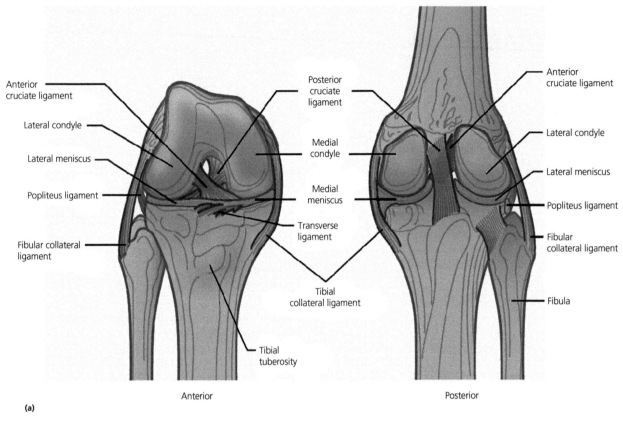

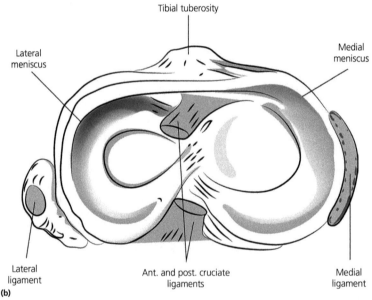

Figure 10.1 Knee anatomy: (a) Supporting structures of the anterior and posterior knee (b) Cross-section of the knee joint showing the menisci and cruciate ligaments

Table 10.1 Anatomy and functions of knee ligaments

Ligament	Anterior cruciate	Posterior cruciate	Medial collateral	Lateral collateral
Function	Prevents anterior translation of the tibia relative to the femur	Prevents posterior translation of the tibia relative to the femur	Prevents valgus angulation	Prevents varus angulation
Intra or extra articular?	Intra-articular	Intra-articular	Extra-articular	Extra-articular
Attachments	Mid-tibial plateau to lateral femoral condyle	Posterior tibia to medial femoral condyle	Medial femoral epicondyle to proximal medial tibia	Lateral femoral epicondyle to proximal fibula
Specific examinations	Anterior drawer Lachman's Pivot shift	Posterior drawer Posterior sag	Laxity and pain in response to valgus stress testing	Laxity and pain in response to varus stress testing

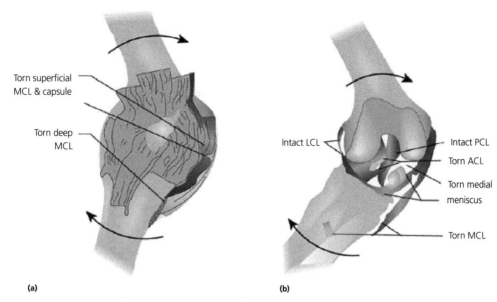

(a)　　　　　　　　　(b)

Figure 10.2 Unhappy triad of O'Donoghue: (a) Torn superficial and deep components of the MCL and ruptured medial capsule. (b) 'Unhappy triad of O'Donoghue: torn ACL, MCL, and medial meniscus (which could have occured at the time or subsequent to injury)

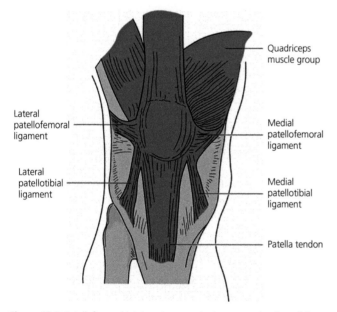

Figure 10.3 Patellofemoral joint anatomy and extensor mechanism of the knee

The patella has a tendency to deviate laterally and is restricted by the lateral femoral condyle, and the medial pull from the quadriceps (vastus medialis oblique) and the restraint of the medial patellofemoral ligament.

Blood supply

The knee joint is supplied by the anastomosis around it. The chief sources are:

1 Five geniculate branches of the popliteal artery
2 The descending geniculate branch of the femoral artery
3 The descending branch of the lateral circumflex femoral artery
4 Two recurrent branches of the anterior tibial artery
5 The circumflex fibular branch of the posterior tibial artery

Nerve supply

1 Femoral nerve through its branch to the vasti
2 Sciatic nerve through the geniculate branches of the tibial and common peroneal nerves
3 Obturator nerve through its posterior division

History and examination

A well-taken history should explore the patient's symptoms, mechanism of injury, treatments to date, and impact on their lifestyle. The latter includes functional limitations and pain especially at rest or night affecting their sleep. This will help direct the examination and subsequent investigations and treatment. It is extremely important to note that knee pain can be the initial presentation of hip or back pathologies. History should include pain, associated symptoms (locking giving way, swelling), history of injury, treatment already received, functional disability (walking distance, restrictions to play), other joints affected (rheumatology), and childhood problems (e.g. osteochondral defects, patella instability).

The examination should include the observations described in Figure 10.4.

Osteoarthritis

Background

Knee osteoarthritis is common and is due to progressive loss of articular cartilage. It is more common in females and older patients (>60 years). Risk factors include high BMI and trauma, including previous meniscal/ligament tears, abnormal alignment (varus/valgus), and hereditary tendency.

Symptoms

Patients often report a gradual onset of pain. A focus on the history should include functional activity such as walking distance, pattern of arthritis involvement (e.g. PFJ often is exacerbated by climbing

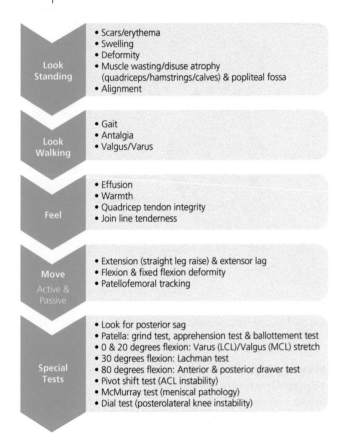

Look Standing
- Scars/erythema
- Swelling
- Deformity
- Muscle wasting/disuse atrophy (quadriceps/hamstrings/calves) & popliteal fossa
- Alignment

Look Walking
- Gait
- Antalgia
- Valgus/Varus

Feel
- Effusion
- Warmth
- Quadricep tendon integrity
- Join line tenderness

Move Active & Passive
- Extension (straight leg raise) & extensor lag
- Flexion & fixed flexion deformity
- Patellofemoral tracking

Special Tests
- Look for posterior sag
- Patella: grind test, apprehension test & ballottement test
- 0 & 20 degrees flexion: Varus (LCL)/Valgus (MCL) stretch
- 30 degrees flexion: Lachman test
- 80 degrees flexion: Anterior & posterior drawer test
- Pivot shift test (ACL instability)
- McMurray test (meniscal pathology)
- Dial test (posterolateral knee instability)

Figure 10.4 Examination steps

Table 10.2 Osteoarthritis – Relevant history/symptoms

Pain history	Location – does it radiate? (If pain is from the groin, it may be hip OA; if it is down to the foot, it may be referred from the lumbar spine.)
	Pain on stairs – PFJ arthritis
	Night pain – indicates severe disease, infection, or tumour
	Other joints affected – rheumatological cause
Function	Walking distance
	Locking and giving way – loose bodies / meniscal tears/ PFJ pathology
	Stiffness – pre-op ROM is best predictor for post-op ROM
Previous treatments	Previous treatments – physiotherapy / analgesia / injections/ arthroscopy
	If they had injections, did they help? If not, it may be referred pain from the hip or spine
Previous injuries	History of ACL tears / meniscal tears / arthroscopic surgery – risk factor for arthritis
	Patella dislocations is a risk factor for PFJ arthritis
Family history	Inflammatory arthritis / osteoarthritis

stairs and deep flexion), and severity of pain (pain at rest or at night) (Table 10.2). Patients may develop a limp and, as the arthritis progresses, the range of motion may decrease. Examination often reveals an effusion, malalignment (varus – medial compartment and valgus – lateral compartment), crepitations behind the patella, and tenderness at the tibiofemoral joint.

Imaging

Imaging usually consists of a weight-bearing AP, lateral (HBL), skyline (patellofemoral joint), and Schuss/Rosenberg view, which assesses for lateral compartment osteoarthritis (Figure 10.5). Loss of joint space and pain in a single compartment may represent isolated arthritis and affects management. History of knee symptoms (Table 10.3) that should be elicited include the following:

Treatment options
- *Nonoperative:* Nonsurgical treatments include weight loss, walking aids, and analgesia (i.e. paracetamol, NSAIDS or weak opioids). Physiotherapy and nonimpact exercises (cycling, cross trainer and swimming) are well tolerated even in late disease. Corticosteroid and hyaluronic acid injections have limited and short-lived benefits. Local anaesthetics are used as a diagnostic tool or with steroids in patients in whom surgical intervention is not being considered.
- *Operative:* In the later stages when conservative therapies have failed, realignment osteotomy or joint replacement (unicondylar/ unicompartmental or total) may be considered.

Total knee replacement (TKR)

More than 80,000 total knee replacements (TKR) are performed each year (Figure 10.6). Indications for TKR include severe symptoms, nonresolution with conservative measures, and increasing deformity.

Operative steps
A TKR is performed through a midline incision, and excising the affected distal femur and proximal tibia and replacing it with metal components, which are held in place with cement or through an interface that allows osseo-integration (e.g. hydroxyapetite). In between the metal components is a polyethylene tray. The ACL is always sacrificed and the PCL may need sacrificing, too. The technical aim of TKR is to implant components in optimal alignment with long-lasting fixation, thereby providing a well-balanced joint with good patellofemoral tracking with infection-free healing.

Complications
Complications (amongst others) include infections, early loosening, malalignment, patellofemoral maltracking, and general complications such as venous thromboembolic disease and neurovascular damage.

Outcomes
Outcomes after TKR are very good with 80 to 90% satisfaction, though not as successful as THR and patients can still have pain and sensitivity or stiffness. According to the National Joint Registry (NJR), the cumulative percentage probability of a TKR requiring revision at 10 years is just over 3%.

Unicompartmental knee replacement (UKR)

When there is arthritis affecting one compartment, it may be replaced in isolation. Most commonly, it is the medial compartment, followed by the PFJ and rarely the lateral compartment. This is done by removing the arthritic compartment and replacing it with metal and polyethylene. Advantages of unicompartmental/unicondylar knee replacements (UKR; Figure 10.7) include a preservation of nonarthritic bone and ACL, with some studies reporting better

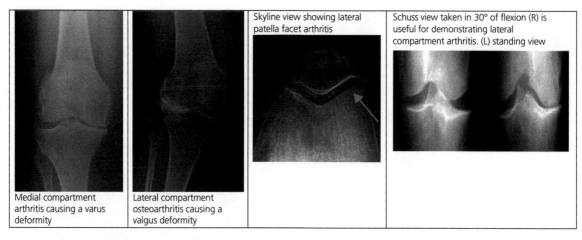

Skyline view showing lateral patella facet arthritis

Schuss view taken in 30° of flexion (R) is useful for demonstrating lateral compartment arthritis. (L) standing view

Medial compartment arthritis causing a varus deformity

Lateral compartment osteoarthritis causing a valgus deformity

Figure 10.5 Radiographic evidence of knee osteoarthritis

Table 10.3 Important issues to highlight in the history

- Pain: rest, night, activity-related
- Disability: e.g. giving way when pivoting or descending stairs
- Walking distance
- Associated symptoms: swelling, giving way, locking
- Deformity development: varus/valgus
- Limp

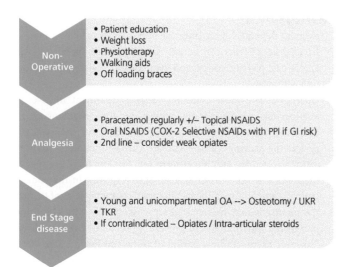

Non-Operative
- Patient education
- Weight loss
- Physiotherapy
- Walking aids
- Off loading braces

Analgesia
- Paracetamol regularly +/– Topical NSAIDS
- Oral NSAIDS (COX-2 Selective NSAIDs with PPI if GI risk)
- 2nd line – consider weak opiates

End Stage disease
- Young and unicompartmental OA --> Osteotomy / UKR
- TKR
- If contraindicated – Opiates / Intra-articular steroids

Figure 10.6 Management options of knee OA

function than TKR (e.g walking downhill). UKR is safer than TKR with a lower risk to life and deep infection. It is important to note that arthritis can progress in other compartments, necessitating revision surgery to a TKR down the line. The 10-year cumulative percentage probability for revision for UKR and PFJ is 12% and 19%, respectively. This is higher than TKR.

Management of osteoarthritis: overview

Management options can be divided into the following cascade in Figure 10.8. Arthroscopy is not usually indicated in arthritis except for mechanical symptoms of locking and giving way. Steroid injections may also be used as a diagnostic aid.

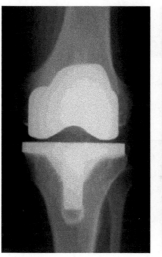
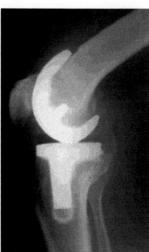

Figure 10.7 Plain radiograph of TKR

Sports injuries

Some of the common causes are highlighted in Figure 10.9. History and examination points are addressed in Table 10.4.

Meniscal tears

Background

The menisci commonly tear either acutely following significant injury in the younger active patient, or as part of a degenerative process in the elderly patient. The medial meniscus is more commonly injured than the lateral side, and both tear more commonly in anterior cruciate deficient knees.

Symptoms and signs

The main symptom is of pain localised to either the medial or lateral compartment. Locking can occur due to the meniscus interposing in the tibiofemoral joint in extension, and rarely fixed flexion deformities can occur in large flipped meniscal tears (bucket handle tears). Other causes of locking include loose bodies, ACL rupture, and patellofemoral pathology (*refer to Table 14.2.1*).

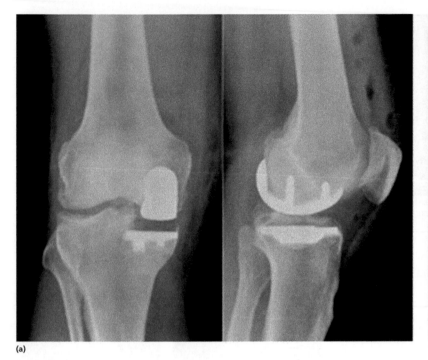
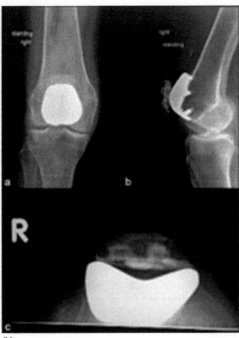

(a)   (b)

Figure 10.8 (a) Medial UKR (b) Patellofemoral joint replacement

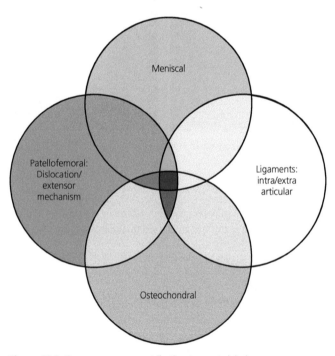

Figure 10.9 Common causes contributing to sports injuries

Imaging

Radiographs are often normal in the young patient, but calcification may be seen in the elderly patients (chondrocalcinosis). MRI is the gold standard imaging modality.

Management

Treatment depends on the duration and severity of symptoms:

- *Nonoperative:* Tears can initially be treated nonoperatively with analgesics, physiotherapy, and avoidance of twisting and squatting activities.
- *Operative:* The most common surgical treatment involves an arthroscopic meniscectomy, where the torn segment of the meniscus is excised. There is good evidence that meniscal surgery in the presence of a degenerate knee with established osteoarthritis provides only short-term relief unless there are specific mechanical symptoms of locking or giving way. In the younger patient, depending on the location and characteristics of the tear, the meniscus may be repaired arthroscopically with the aim of preserving function and of preventing secondary osteoarthritis. However there can be a period of restricted flexion and weight bearing post-operatively (up to 6 weeks) and a risk of retearing requiring meniscectomy. Table 10.5 summarises the main points of meniscal repairs.

ACL tears

ACL tears occur commonly in young, active patients participating in pivoting sports and usually involves a noncontact twisting injury when the foot is fixed to the floor. Patients may often feel a "pop" with an immediate haemarthrosis. Examination may reveal an effusion, and anteroposterior instability can be elicited via the Lachman's test (most sensitive), anterior drawer, or pivot shift test and should be compared with the unaffected knee (Table 10.6).

MRI scanning is the image of choice and is also useful at assessing other structures, including concomitant meniscal tears.

Table 10.4 Sports Injuries: History and Management

Sports injury	Relevant history/examination	Management
ACL tear	• Immediate swelling (haemarthrosis) • Ongoing instability, especially when pivoting • Examination: Lachman's / Anterior drawer test	• Conservative (physiotherapy and activity modification) or operative • Surgery more indicated in younger, more active patients intending to return to pivoting or contact sports
Other ligament injury (Collateral / PCL)	• Instability on descending stairs • Anterior knee pain • Ongoing instability PCL – Posterior sag and posterior drawer	• Usually can be managed nonoperatively with a brace. If ongoing instability and failure to heal, consider reconstruction
Acute meniscal tear	• Swelling (but less than ligament tear) occurring 6–24 hours after injury • Mechanical symptoms (locking/giving way)	• Meniscal repair / resection
Knee dislocation (tibiofemoral)	• High energy injury usually involving several ligaments • Acute orthopaedic emergency (10% popliteal artery injury)	• Vascular assessment for popliteal artery injury • Surgical reconstruction of affected ligaments
Patella dislocation	• Twisting or direct injury • Swelling and pain • Patella malposition • Unable to straight leg raise	• Reduce in a patella brace • Reconstruction of medial patellofemoral ligament or stabilisation procedures in recurrent cases

Table 10.5 Indications for meniscal repair

Indications for meniscal repair	Advantage of meniscal repair	Disadvantages of meniscal repair
• Tear characteristics: longitudinal tear, in vascular area, less than 3 months old • Younger/more active patients • No systemic disease (e.g. immunosuppression) • BMI <30 • Willingness to comply with post-operative rehabilitation regime	• Reduced risk of osteoarthritis compared with meniscectomy • Aids knee stabilising • Better post-operative function (e.g. sports)	• Risk of retearing requiring further procedure (meniscectomy) • Post-operative rehabilitation regimen: non–weight bearing for 6 weeks and avoid twisting or squatting for 3 months

Table 10.6 Special tests for knee examination

	Lachman's	Anterior Drawer	Pivot shift
Position of knee	Knee flexed to 30°	Knee flexed to 80–90°	Extension to flexion with valgus stress and internal rotation of the tibia
Positive finding	Excessive anterior translation Soft endpoint	Excessive anterior translation Soft endpoint	Whilst in extension, the lateral tibial plateau subluxes anteriorly due to the action of the iliotibial band. As the knee is flexed, a "clunk" will be felt as the tibiofemoral joint reduces

NB* Best performed when patient is relaxed

Treatment depends on age, activity level, and severity of instability. Patients should be referred for ACL rehabilitation to maintain ROM, increase the quadriceps and hamstring function, and restore proprioception. In younger patients who are more active and keen to perform twisting-type or contact sports, surgical intervention can be considered where a graft is used to reconstruct the ACL and fixed in place with implants and screws (Figure 10.10). Graft choice depends on patient factors and surgeon preferences, and can range from the patient's own hamstring, patellar tendon, quadriceps tendon to allograft.

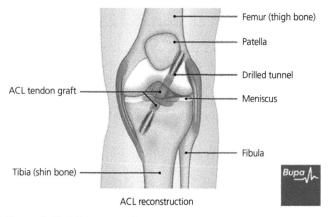

Figure 10.10 ACL reconstruction

Extensor mechanism rupture

Mechanism of injury

The extensor mechanism can fail due to a quadriceps rupture, patella fracture, or patella tendon rupture. Generally, the more proximal the injury to the extensor mechanism, the older the patient. Thus, quadriceps rupture is most commonly seen in men in their 40–70s and it is either due to eccentric loading of the extensor mechanism or direct trauma (patellar fractures). Patients may reveal that they had a sudden tearing sensation when they jumped or missed a step on stairs. Patellar tendon injuries are more common in younger patients (20–40 years), whilst quadriceps injuries are more common in middle-aged and older patients. Patella fracture can occur as a result of hyperflexion of the knee, yielding a transverse fracture, or direct trauma often resulting in a multifragmentary or stellate fracture.

Examination

Examination will reveal displacement of the patella (superiorly in patellar tendon rupture and antero-inferiorly in quadriceps rupture) and loss of active extension. When asked to perform a straight leg raise, an extensor lag will be seen.

Imaging

Radiographs will reveal displacement of the patella or a patella fracture. If the diagnosis is in doubt, an ultrasound or MRI may be performed.

Management

- *Nonoperative:* Partial tear of the quadriceps/patella tendon or undisplaced patella fractures with an intact extensor mechanism can be treated nonoperatively with immobilisation in full extension and progressive weight bearing and knee flexion in a hinge knee brace.
- *Operative:* Surgical intervention for quadriceps and patella tendon ruptures include open suture–based repairs. In displaced patella fractures, open reduction and internal fixation with tension band wires is often used. A multifragmentary fracture may require circumferential (cerclage) wires rather than tension band (*figure of 8*) wire.

Anterior knee pain

The causes of anterior knee pain are extensive and can be difficult to treat. Table 10.7 shows possible areas of pathology causing pain. Causes, according to age, include:

- *Adolescents:* Patellar instability, Osgood-Schlatter, patella chondropathy (chondromalacia patella)
- *Adults:* Patellar/Quadriceps tendinitis, bursitis, patellofemoral joint arthritis, fat pad impingement, iliotibial band syndrome

Patellar instability
Causes

Patellar instability can occur after acute trauma or may be due to generalised laxity and usually occurs in the second decade. It is often multifactorial (Figure 10.11) and may be due to hyperlaxity or

Table 10.7 Pathologies at different anatomical sites

Area	Pathology
Quadriceps	Tendinitis Rupture
Patella	Bipartite Chondropathy Lateral overload Instability Fracture
Patellar tendon	Proximal tendinitis Distal tendinitis Tendinosis Rupture
Iliotibial band	Tight Inflamed
Fat pad	Inflammation Avulsion
Plica	Medial/lateral/suprapatellar Inflammation
Pes anserinus	Tendinosis Bursitis
Bursas	Bursitis acute or chronic

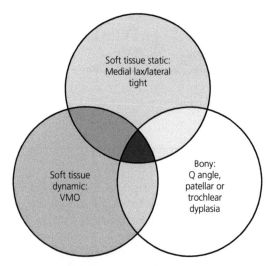

Figure 10.11 Causes contributing to patellar instability

weakness of the vastus medialis oblique muscles; however, it may also be due to a hypoplastic lateral femoral condyle, lateralised tibial tubercle, shallow trochlea groove, or rupture of the stabilising ligament (medial patellofemoral ligament).

Presentation

Patients may either present with dislocating patellas, or features of instability with apprehension on passive lateral patellar translation. A "J sign" may be seen where there is excessive patellar lateralisation in extension, which pops into the groove as the patella engages with the trochlea during flexion.

Management

- *Nonoperative:* Treatment is usually conservative with physiotherapy to increase gluteus and quadriceps strengthening.
- *Operative:* Surgical treatment is indicated in ongoing instability and treatment, depends on the aetiology of the instability, and is summarised in Table 10.8.

Osgood-Schlatter disease (OSD)

OSD is a traction apophysitis of the tibial tubercle and is most commonly seen in teenage overweight boys. Patients will reveal anterior knee pain exacerbated by kneeling, and an enlarged tender tibial tubercle may be found on examination. Pain may be provoked on resisted knee extension. A lateral radiograph will demonstrate fragmentation of the tibial tubercle (Figure 10.12). Conservative therapy is successful in over 90% of cases, and includes analgesics, activity modification, and quadriceps stretching.

Patella chondropathy

Patella chondropathy is a condition characterised by changes in the articular cartilage of the patella. It most commonly occurs in young females and its cause is unknown. Symptoms are similar to patellofemoral joint arthritis and include anterior knee pain and sensation of giving way worse on climbing/descending stairs and after periods of prolonged knee flexion (squatting/sitting).

Examination may be unremarkable in very mild cases. However, it may include crepitus, signs of patella maltracking, and pain on compression of the patella. MRI scan reveals high signal in the articular cartilage and underlying bone.

The mainstay of treatment is nonoperative and includes NSAIDS and physiotherapy with emphasis on gluteal and VMO strengthening. Surgical treatment has unreliable outcomes but aims to offload the lateral patella facet and can include a lateral release or shaving uneven chondral surfaces or flaps arthroscopically.

Patella/Quadriceps tendinitis

Patella/quadriceps tendinitis is an overuse condition most commonly affecting jumping athletes and is due to repetitive eccentric contractions of the extensor mechanism. Examination will reveal tenderness usually at the tendon-bone junction and pain on eccentric loading. Radiographs are usually normal; however, MRI will reveal thickening of the tendon with increased signal (Figure 10.13).

Treatment involves activity modification with abstinence of sporting activity until the symptoms have resolved and physiotherapy to stretch the extensor mechanism. Rarely, surgical debridement is required.

Prepatellar bursitis

Prepatellar bursitis is characterised as inflammation of the anterior knee and is common with excessive kneeling (plumbers/decorators). Examination reveals an isolated swelling anteriorly (Figure 10.14), with relatively preserved knee range of motion (cf septic arthritis). It may be warm, especially in infected cases, which should be treated with intravenous antibiotics. Treatment for aseptic bursitis includes compressive wrap and NSAIDS. Aspiration may be considered; however, recurrence is seen in more than 50% of cases. Rarely, surgical excision is indicated.

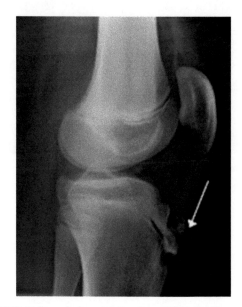

Figure 10.12 Radiograph demonstrating Osgood-Schlatter Disease

Table 10.8 Surgical management of patella instability

Cause of instability	Medial patellofemoral ligament rupture	Tibial tubercle malposition	Shallow femoral trochlea
Explanation	The MPFL attaches from the patella and medial femoral epicondyle and is the primary stabiliser to lateral displacement of the patella	If the tibial tubercle is malpositioned, the patella will have a tendency to subluxate laterally	If trochlea is flat or shallow, patella will tend to glide laterally
Surgical treatment	MPFL reconstruction with gracilis/ semitendinosis graft	Tibial tubercle realignment osteotomy	Trochleoplasty to deepen trochlea

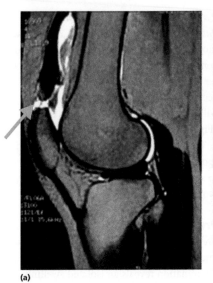
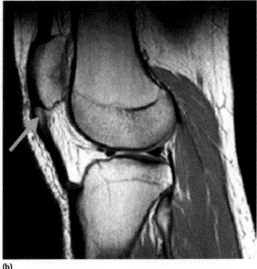

(a)   (b)

Figure 10.13 (a) Sagittal T2 MRI – revealing increased uptake in the distal quadriceps tendon (b) Sagittal T1 MRI – revealing increased uptake in the proximal patellar tendon

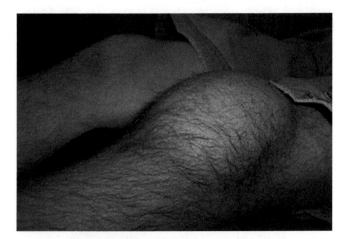

Figure 10.14 Prepatellar bursitis

Further reading

Moseley, J.B., O'Malley, K., Petersen, N.J., et al. (2002, July). A controlled trial of arthroscopic surgery for osteoarthritis of the knee. *New England Journal of Medicine* 347 (2): 81–88.

Sihvonen, R., Paavola, M., Malmivaara, A., et al. (2013, December). Arthroscopic partial meniscectomy versus sham surgery for a degenerative meniscal tear. Finnish Degenerative Meniscal Lesion Study (FIDELITY) Group. *New England Journal of Medicine* 369 (26): 2515–2524.

Skou, S.T., Roos, E.M., Laursen, M.B., et al. (2015, October). A randomized, controlled trial of total knee replacement. *New England Journal of Medicine* 373 (17): 1597–1606.

van Adrichem, RA1, Nemeth, B1, Algra, A1, et al. (2017 February). Thromboprophylaxis after knee arthroscopy and lower-leg casting. *New England Journal of Medicine* 376 (6): 515–525.

CHAPTER 11

Foot and Ankle

Nadeem Mushtaq[1], Ali Abbasian[2], Kapil Sugand[3,4], and Chinmay M. Gupte[3,5]

[1] Imperial College Healthcare NHS Trust, London, UK
[2] Guy's & St. Thomas' Hospital, London, UK
[3] MSk Lab, Charing Cross Hospital, Imperial College London, London, UK
[4] North West London Rotation, London, UK
[5] Imperial College Healthcare NHS Trust, London, UK

OVERVIEW

- Foot and ankle pathology is common in the population and can be divided into acute traumatic conditions and chronic conditions such as malalignment, arthritides, and diabetic foot.
- Foot and ankle pathology can be a manifestation of systemic disease.
- Radiographs should always be taken weight-bearing to ascertain the joint under stress.
- Nonsurgical treatment includes corrective orthotics, plaster casting, and physiotherapy.

Anatomy

Basic bony anatomy of the foot and ankle is outlined in Figure 11.1.

Pain

Foot and ankle pain is a common presentation often seen in both general practice and urgent care centres in the emergency department. Patients range from children to the elderly, with varying pathologies from trauma to systemic illnesses. Pain can be divided into the following causes, as seen in Table 11.1.

Hallux valgus (bunion)

Hallux valgus is a deformity of the forefoot at the level of the first metatarsophalangeal (MTP) joint. There is medial deviation of the first metatarsal and lateral deviation of the hallux. It is a common condition, with a prevalence of around 20% in adults aged 18–65 years and 35% in elderly people aged over 65 years. Prevalence increases with age and is twice as common in females.

Aetiology

Causes are thought to be a genetic predisposition with an imbalance of intrinsic and extrinsic forces on the joint. Instability in the MTPJ or TMT joint, combined with tight footwear, results in the classical deformity, which over time becomes fixed and painful.

Medical conditions may also predispose to developing the condition (Table 11.2).

Presentation

Presentation is usually due to pain:

1. Pain over the bunion (adventitious bursa pain)
2. Joint pain (capsule stretching, joint subluxation, arthritic changes)
3. Lesser toe pain (transfer metatarsalgia – overloading of the lesser toes due to a malfunctioning great toe, with resultant hammer toe deformity) primarily affecting the second and third rays
4. Sesamoid pain (due to their subluxation out of cristae)

Examination

The examination should assess the following, as all can affect treatment:

- Degree of hallux valgus whilst standing (weight-bearing; Figure 11.2 showing IM [intermetatarsal] angle and HV [hallux valgus] angle)
- Pronation of toe and resulting medial callus (Figure 11.2)
- Passive ROM of first MTPJ – restricted dorsiflexion in corrected position is unlikely to improve after surgery
- Pain and stiffness in the first MTPJ with a palpable dorsal osteophyte (hallux rigidus)
- Associated transfer pathology such as lesser toe deformities, metatarsalgia, planter callosities, or tarsometatarsal OA
- Shape of the arch: Cavus or plano-valgus foot
- First TMTJ instability – defined as elevation of first MT above level of second MT with dorsal pressure

Treatment

- *Nonoperative*: Nonsurgical treatments involve wide, high-boxed shoes to accommodate the primary and secondary deformities. Orthotics may be required if there in associated hypermobility or pes planus.
- *Operative*: Surgery mainly involves a distal soft tissue release and a metatarsal osteotomy (various types exist such as chevron, scarf, proximal). Occasionally, a first TMTJ arthrodesis has to be performed to address hypermobility of the joint and the hallux valgus is addressed simultaneously. If there is an associated

---

ABC of Orthopaedics and Trauma, First Edition. Edited by Kapil Sugand and Chinmay M. Gupte.
© 2018 John Wiley & Sons Ltd. Published 2018 by John Wiley & Sons Ltd.

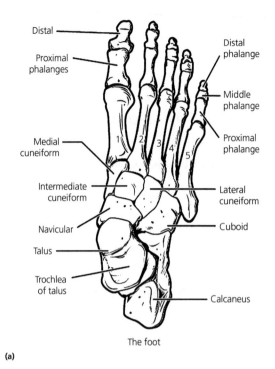

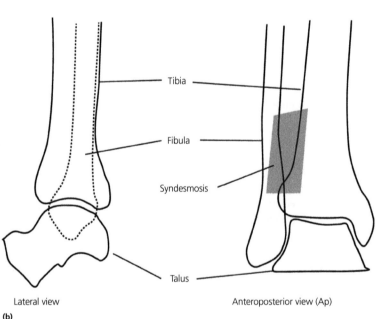

Figure 11.1 Anatomy of (a) foot and (b) ankle

Table 11.1 Some causes of pain in foot and ankle

Ankle	Foot		
	Fore-	Mid-	Hind-
Trauma, fractures, joint dislocation, sprains, tendinitis, arthritis, ulcers, flat foot, medial and lateral plantar nerve irritation			
	Paronychia, metatarsalgia, Morton's neuroma, gout, bunion, tarsal tunnel syndrome	Lisfranc injury, avascular necrosis (e.g. Kohler's disease), tarsal tunnel syndrome	Plantar fasciitis, Achilles tendinitis, bone spur

hallux valgus interphalangeus (valgus deviation of the proximal phalanx), then an Akin (medial closing wedge) osteotomy of proximal phalanx is also performed (Figure 11.2).

Hallux rigidus

Hallux rigidus is stiffness of the first MTPJ. It is a result of degenerative arthritis, which may be primary or secondary.

Table 11.2 Medical conditions predisposing to hallux valgus

Gout
Rheumatoid arthritis
Psoriatic arthropathy
Joint hypermobility in connective tissue disorders (e.g. Ehlers-Danlos and Marfan's syndromes)
Ligamentous laxity (e.g. in Down syndrome)
Multiple sclerosis
Charcot-Marie-Tooth disease
Cerebral palsy

Presentation and examination

Activities that require dorsiflexion will be affected, such as wearing high heels, sprinting, or lunging. Patients complain of pain at toe-off (part of stance phase of the gait cycle). Dorsiflexion is affected more than plantar flexion and is associated with pain. The radiographs demonstrate a loss of joint space and a dorsal osteophyte (Figure 11.3).

Treatment

- *Nonoperative*: Management begins with stiff insole (Morton's extension) to limit the range of movement in the first MTPJ and activity modification. A steroid injection has only a temporary benefit.
- *Operative*: Cheilectomy is a useful procedure to remove bony spurs to increase the range of motion and help with pain on dorsal impingement. For severe disease, a first MTPJ fusion is the surgery of choice. Various artificial joint replacements are available but they have so far provided unreliable results.

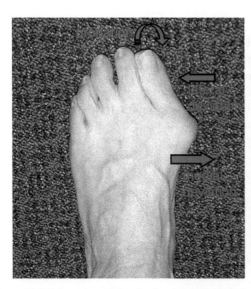
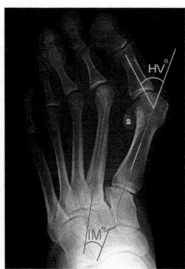
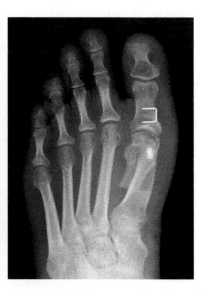

Figure 11.2 Hallux valgus: deformity showing medial deviation of the first MT and lateral deviation and pronation of the hallux. The preoperative radiograph shows an inter-metatarsal (IM) angle greater than the normal 9° and the hallux valgus is greater than 15°. The sesamoids are subluxed. The postoperative radiographs show a scarf and akin osteotomy with improvement of angles

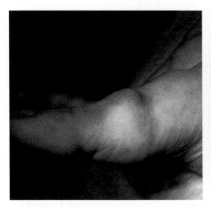
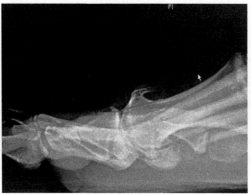
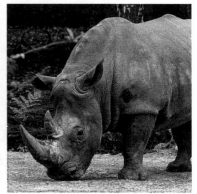

Figure 11.3 Hallux rigidus: a clinical photograph with corresponding radiograph showing the classical dorsal osteophyte that grows like a rhinoceros' horn

Metatarsalgia

Metatarsalgia is a general term for pain under the ball of the foot (metatarsal heads) and is a common symptom in the foot and ankle surgical practice.

Aetiology

Numerous causes include genetic, acquired, and iatrogenic, but the underlying mechanism is uneven weight distribution that can ultimately result in forefoot overload. Overload may result in callus formation, as seen in Figure 11.4. Patients with long metatarsals or with high arches (pes cavus) are predisposed to this condition. A metatarsal may be made relatively longer after surgery to its neighbouring metatarsal – an iatrogenic cause of metatarsalgia.

Presentation

The patient may complain of the sensation of "walking on a marble or stone."

Treatment

- *Nonoperative*: Treatment consists of orthotics to elevate and offload the affected metatarsal heads.
- *Operative*: If conservative measures fail, then a shortening (+/–elevating) MT osteotomy can be performed (i.e. Weil's osteotomy).

Morton's neuroma

A benign neuroma of an intermetatarsal plantar nerve, Morton's neuroma results from repetitive trauma and ischaemia to the plantar digital nerve at the distal edge of the transverse intermetatarsal ligament. Neuromas are most common in the third intermetatarsal space, followed by the second webspace, and finally the fourth webspace (Figure 11.5). The third plantar digital nerve is formed from both the medial and lateral planter nerves and so has an increased tendency to undergo tethering and traction.

Aetiology

The aetiology is variable, and any factor that increases the pressure on the nerve can cause the neuroma: tight shoes, repetitive hyperextension of MTPJ by running, tight gastrocnemius, or space-occupying lesions – ganglion, cyst, and synovitis.

Presentation, examination, and investigations

A Morton's neuroma will cause pain in between the metatarsal heads and not on the metatarsal head as in metatarsalgia. There may be associated parenthesis and a palpable click on metatarsal compression (Mulder click). This is generally overdiagnosed. All causes of forefoot overload and metatarsalgia should be carefully excluded before a neuroma is diagnosed. In one study, over half of those with asymptomatic feet had a neuroma on ultrasound. Hence, USS or MRI can help with the diagnosis.

Treatment

- *Nonoperative*: Treatment consists of shoe modification, orthotics to release pressure from the webspace, neuromodulators such as gabapentin, and ultrasound-guided steroid injection. Steroid injections have only a temporary effect, regardless of the size of the neuroma, and by 12 months, the symptoms have reoccurred in all patients.

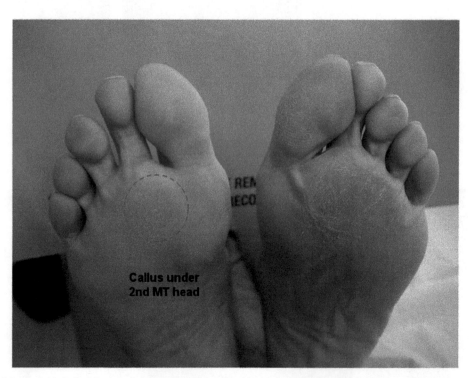

Figure 11.4 Metatarsalgia: hard skin (callus) forms underneath the metatarsal heads due to uneven weight distribution as the patient overloads his metatarsal heads

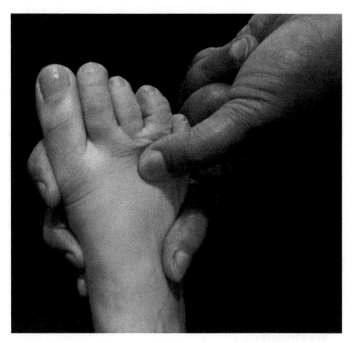 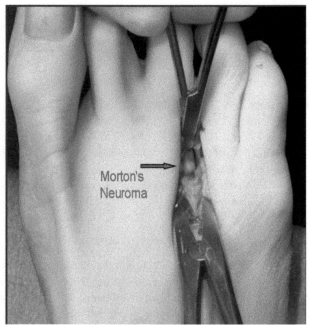

Figure 11.5 Morton's Neuroma: a demonstration of a Mulder's click for a neuroma in the third web space – squeeze the metatarsal heads together whilst pinching the webspace between index finger and thumb. The neuroma is visible at time of surgery

- *Operative*: Surgery involves releasing the transverse intermetatarsal ligament and/or neurectomy. If the nerve is excised, then permanent sensory loss is expected and the patient should be warned of this.

Claw, hammer, and mallet toe deformities

These are sagittal-plane deformities involving the lesser toes. They occur through various aetiologies, but claw toes are more common in neurological conditions and these should be sought in the examination. A claw toe has an MTPJ hyperextension, a hammer toe has a PIPJ flexion deformity, and a mallet toe has a DIPJ flexion deformity. Treatment depends on whether the deformities are flexible or fixed. For flexible deformities, options include nonoperative therapy, such as a high box shoe, or soft tissue procedures (e.g. tendon transfers). For fixed deformities, a bony procedure such as arthrodesis is preferable.

Plantar fasciitis

This is the most common cause of heel pain and results from inflammation and microtears in the plantar fascia (sole; Figure 11.6). Its aetiology is not fully understood, but it is associated with certain types of foot shape (e.g. pes planus or cavus). A heel spur is found in 50% of patients (usually in people in their thirties and forties). Otherwise, there may be tensile overload of the attachments to the fascia. Causes consist of primary (idiopathic), trauma, prolonged standing, and obesity.

Presentation and examination

Unilateral heel pain is worsened by full weight-bearing, especially after prolonged rest, or startup pain (pain on movement after resting for a while, especially on waking up). The heel spur is not the cause of the inflammation, and treatment should not be addressed

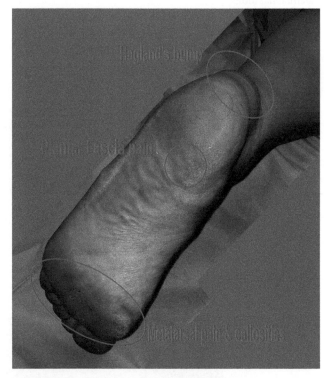

Figure 11.6 Plantar fasciitis: a clinical photograph of a patient with a tight gastrocnemius muscle. Presenting with a Haglund's bump, retro-calcaneal bursa, plantar fasciitis and metatarsalgia with metatarsal callosities

towards it. The condition is associated with a tight gastrocnemius muscle, and pain is increased on toe dorsiflexion (windlass test). Tenderness may be elicited by palpating the site of fascial insertion at the medial calcaneal tuberosity and is increased with dorsiflexion of toes, which tenses the plantar fascia.

Investigation

Diagnosis is usually clinical, and imaging is mainly used to exclude other causes of pain. USS or MRI scans are the first choice of investigations, but a bone scan can also show increased uptake at the origin of the fascia.

Treatment

- *Nonoperative*: The treatment involves physiotherapy to stretch out the calf muscles and wearing night splints to keep the gastrocnemius stretched. NSAIDs and steroids also play a significant role. Shockwave therapy is still controversial.
- *Operative*: A gastrocnemius or plantar fascia release can be considered as a last resort.

Acquired adult flat foot (plano-valgus)

The acquired flat foot is a painful loss of the medial arch height. It is one of the most common problems involving the foot and ankle, affecting 10% of the population (mainly females). As the disease progresses, the hindfoot drifts into valgus and the forefoot supinates to compensate. As the talo-navicular joint subluxes, the forefoot abducts at the talo-navicular joint.

This pathology should be differentiated from the two forms of congenital flat foot:

- *Mobile and pain free,* which are usually physiological and seen more predominantly in the African-Caribbean population
- *Rigid,* which is associated with coalition, previous trauma, or Charcot (neuropathic) deformity

The most common cause is tibialis posterior tendon dysfunction (from inflammation, degeneration or rupture) that can be precipitated by many causes (degenerative, tight gastroc-soleus, inflammatory arthritis, midfoot arthritis, fracture mal-unions, diabetes mellitus, and obesity).

Presentation and examination

There is complaint of pain and sometimes swelling at the medial aspect of the ankle extending distally into the foot. With disease progression, there is pain on the lateral aspect from calcaneo-fibular impingement. After observing gait, watch the patient from behind to assess the extent of valgus deformity of hindfoot (Figure 11.7). Look for "too many toes sign" due to forefoot abduction (normally only fifth and half of fourth toes are seen), as well as "single leg heel rise" test, which usually disappears with disease progression. Test the strength of heel inversion. Only half of radiographs are diagnostic showing arthritic changes and abnormal angulation, whereas MRI can identify the posterior tibialis tendon accurately. The dysfunction can be classified into four broad groups (Table 11.3).

Treatment

- *Nonoperative*: Treatment is based on the stage of the disease but essentially, if the hindfoot is still mobile and only has minimal degenerative changes, then a joint-preserving procedure should be recommended, as it can achieve around 95% of pain relief and functional improvement. Supportive management with rest, analgesia, and orthoses are also effective.
- *Operative*: For severe stages, joint sacrificing surgery is preferred. It allows the correction of the deformity and addresses any

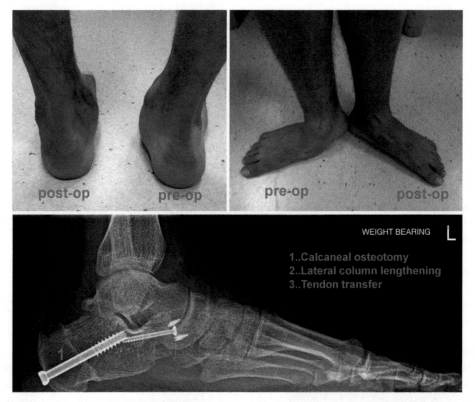

Figure 11.7 Flatfoot deformity: This patient had bilateral symptomatic plano-valgus. The left side has been operated on and he is awaiting surgery on the right. The surgery involved a calcaneal osteotomy to change the vector force of the tendo-Achilles, a lateral column lengthening to recreate the medial arch, a gastrocnemius lengthening, and a tendon transfer to compensate for the weak tibialis posterior (FDL was used)

Table 11.3 Myerson's modification of Johnson & Strom's classification for Tibialis Posterior dysfunction

Stage	Stage description	Symptoms	Treatment
1	Tenosynovitis without deformity	Pain and swelling along Tendon – power intact. There is no deformity.	Orthotics
2	Ruptured tendon and flexible flat foot	Arch collapse, mobile hindfoot. Single-leg heel raise is not possible. Hindfoot is still passively mobile.	Tendon augmentation, lateral column lengthening, calcaneal osteotomy
3	Rigid hindfoot valgus	Hindfoot no longer moves.	Selective/triple fusion
4	Ankle valgus	Ankle arthritic changes occur.	As above and then treat ankle separately

degenerative changes in the joints. Classically triple fusion is the operation of choice, with a 60% success rate, but subsequent degeneration of the ankle joint occurs in half of the cases. Other options include calcaneal osteotomy, tendon repair, or transfer (e.g. FDL).

Cavus Foot (cavo-varus)

A foot with a higher than normal medial arch is known as a cavus foot. It is commonly seen in neuropathic patients (hereditary sensory motor neuropathy, spinal cord abnormalities, and polio), but it does also occur in non-neuropathic feet. Thus, examination of the cavus foot must include a thorough assessment of the spinal cord. The trigger for cavus can be either forefoot driven (abnormally plantar flexed first ray) or hindfoot driven (varus heal), but with time both will coexist. Patients present with clawing of toes, recurrent ankle sprains, peroneal tendonitis, lateral foot overload with stress fractures, and metatarsalgia. The gastrocnemius becomes tight and the patients also develop plantar fasciitis.

Treatment

- *Nonoperative*: Treatment starts with orthotics – the principle is to allow the first MT head to planter flex more and so return the hindfoot into valgus, not to fill up the medial arch, as this will only push the hindfoot into more varus. The gastrocnemius has to be stretched though a physiotherapy program.
- *Operative*: For failed nonoperative treatment, one can consider selected tendon transfers and osteotomies along with a gastrocnemius release. For fixed deformities, arthrodesis is considered.

Ankle arthritis

Arthritis, as elsewhere in the body, can be inflammatory, degenerative, and posttraumatic. More than 85% of patients with RA have painful feet or ankles during the course of the disease.

Primary ankle arthritis is much less common than hip and knee arthritis, and most patients will get arthritis secondary to previous trauma. The ankle joint is such a congruent joint that any malalignment postfracture or significant chondral damage will progress to end-stage arthritis within two decades. Symptoms will include pain (especially on weight-bearing), swelling causing deformity, giving way and typical radiographic signs (AP, lateral, weight-bearing, and mortise view for ankles).

Treatment

- *Nonoperative*: Treatment starts with physiotherapy, analgesia, rocker-bottom shoes, and ankle brace. A steroid injection may give some temporary relief.

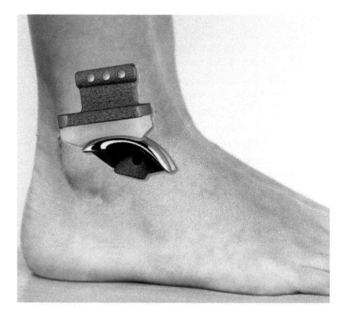

Figure 11.8 Ankle replacement: This is a third-generation ankle replacement. It is anatomically shaped, unconstrained, and cementless. Results suggest a 90% 10-year survival rate

- *Operative*: With more advanced cases, the osteophytes will cause pain, and soft tissue and bony impingement at the front (and occasionally back) of the ankle. This can be treated with arthroscopic or open cheilectomy and debridement. If the ankle joint is severely involved then the only alternatives are arthroplasty or arthrodesis. Arthrodesis can be performed either arthroscopically or through open approach. Ankle arthroplasty (Figure 11.8) has previously demonstrated poor long-term results, but now third-generation ankle replacements results show 90% survivorship at 10 years. Early treatment strategy in patients with RA includes synovectomy.

Foot arthritis

Arthritis of the other hindfoot and midfoot joints produces pain and deformity. There is no successful replacement for these joints, and if nonoperative measures fail, then arthrodesis is the only option that allows the deformity to be corrected and also provides good pain relief. The patient has to be counselled about the risk of nonunion and necessity of further surgery, especially if they are smokers. There is also a significant risk to the adjacent joints developing arthritis because they have to compensate for the fused joint.

Achilles tendon disease

Types and examination

Achilles tendon disease can be divided into acute or chronic. Acute pathology usually presents as a complete or a partial tear of the tendon. Chronic pathology presents as inflammation of the tendon at either its insertion into the calcanium (insertional tendonitis) or, more commonly, around 4–5 cm above the insertion (noninsertional tendonitis).

Acute

In acute cases, patients will complain of feeling a sudden "pop" after the sensation of being kicked, cut, or shot at the heel. Visibly, there is a swelling, bruising, haematoma collection, and loss of continuity of the tendon with a palpable gap (Figure 11.9). Some trigger activities include playing racquet sports (badminton, squash, and tennis) and sprinting, where there is sudden stretching of the tendon. Patients will be unable to bear weight due to pain. They have an inability to plantar flex the ankle against gravity (beware of a false negative because of an intact plantaris). The resting tone will be decreased (Figure 11.9) and Simmond's test will be positive – with the patient lying prone and the feet hanging off the edge of the bed, squeezing the calf will not produce plantar flexion.

Treatment options could be conservative, using rigid equinus casting or functional bracing, or operative. Research is pointing to there being no difference in rupture rates between operative and nonoperatively managed Achilles tendon rupture if both groups commence early movement in a functional brace. There may be a slight advantage in operating to improve the push-off power important in sprinters, for instance.

Chronic

In chronic cases, patients usually present with pain along the tendon at the back of the leg, which worsens with repetitive stress, intense activity, and overuse. Presence of a bone spur at the tendon attachment may also be a pain generator. It is important to exclude

sinister causes, especially deep vein thrombosis. Chronic background inflammation leads to tendinitis (pain, swelling, and thickening), which increases the risk of tearing (Figure 11.9). Treatment options include physiotherapy, steroid injections (increased risk of rupture with multiple injections), shockwave, or surgical decompression (+/– grafting/tendon transfer).

Investigations

Plain radiography imaging can demonstrate calcification or hardening of the Achilles tendon in its mid-substance or at its insertion (Haglund's bump).

Ultrasound is very useful in acute tears because the ankle can be moved to evaluate the gap between the torn tendon ends, and if the gap remains large, then surgery should be considered.

MRI imaging is more relevant for chronic pathology. It demonstrates tendonitis well and any inter-substance tears.

Ankle fractures and dislocation

Ankle fractures are a common injury presenting to the emergency department and sometimes to general practice as a late presentation if the pain is initially manageable. Dislocations may be due to unstable fractures or ligamentous injury. Patients sustain these types of injuries after falling, tripping, and playing a sport. Fracture patterns depend on the mechanism of injury involving supination vs. pronation and external rotation vs. ab/adduction.

Depending on the mechanism of injury, direction and severity of the injury, and joint integrity, there is a predictable pattern and chronology of injury with respect to the anterior and posterior tibiofibular ligaments, all three (medial, lateral and posterior) malleoli, site of fibular fracture (according to Weber classification, Figure 11.10), and the deltoid ligament. A talar shift over 2 mm

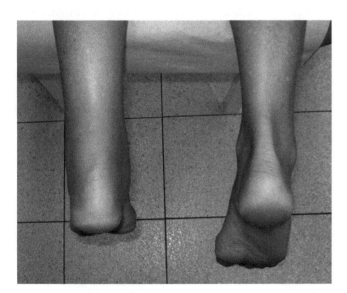

Figure 11.9 Clinical photograph showing absence of outline of the left Achilles tendon

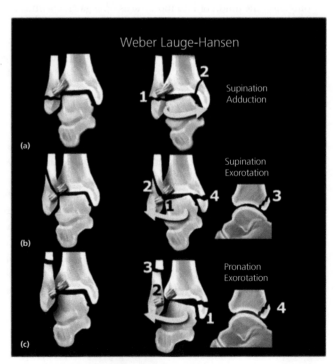

Figure 11.10 Weber and Lauge-Hansen classifications for ankle fractures

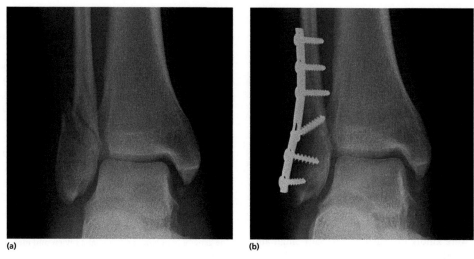

(a)   (b)

Figure 11.11 Plain radiographs showing (a) Weber B and medial malleoli avulsion fracture with talar shift and (b) ORIF with plate and screws

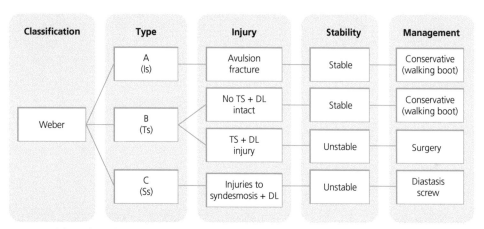

Key: Is – infrasyndesmotic, Ts – transyndesmotic, Ss – suprasyndesmotic, TS – talar shift, DL – deltoid ligament

Figure 11.12 Management options of Weber fracture classification

(Figure 11.11a) is likely to result in an unstable joint and will require ORIF (Figure 11.11b). Otherwise, if the shift is minimal, then a walking cast or boot is adequate.

Management

Management options have been outlined in Figure 11.12. Open fractures in the elderly with comorbidities like peripheral vascular disease or lymphoedema are at a high risk of fracture fixation failure. A pilon fracture (intra-articular fracture of distal tibial plafond) may become unstable and lead to dislocation in which the mantra "span (ExFix as temporary fixation), scan (CT), and plan (for definitive treatment)" is applicable.

Ankle dislocations do not need to be imaged before being reduced. The joint needs to be reduced as soon as the clinical diagnosis has been made. Waiting too long may lead to skin blistering and necrosis on either malleoli, requiring skin cover by the plastics team later down the line. Rarely, the surgeon will use a hindfoot nail to fix an ankle fracture whereby the subtalar joint is sacrificed to achieve a solid fixation of the ankle. However, this will lead to ankle and subtalar arthritis if the nail is removed, as the joints are not

formally fused during the procedure. In severe fractures, one may consider fusing the ankle joint as a primary procedure, but one should then avoid fusing the subtalar joint. Thus, a screw or plate fixation should be used instead of a nail.

Calcaneal fractures

Calcaneal fractures are common and tend to occur in a specific demographic. Typically, the patient will be a young male labourer (e.g. roofer, builder, painter) who falls from a height and lands on his heels. The presentation will be a painful, swollen, and bruised hindfoot with the inability to bear weight. It is imperative to rule out associated injuries that are less obvious. Ensure to exclude bilateral calcaneal or vertebral fractures and be vigilant for compartment syndrome in the foot (10% incidence each).

Early management is symptomatic and conservative because premature surgical intervention leads to a high rate of complications. Poor prognosis and operative risks include being an active smoker, being obese, and having peripheral vascular disease or osteoporosis. The patient will have to be admitted for bed rest, have the foot elevated onto a Braun splint, while in a backslab for several days, and have strong analgesia. There is usually intra-articular (75% of cases) involvement on radiological imaging: plain radiographs and CT are required to delineate the severity of the injury. Wrinkling of skin is a good indicator that the swelling is resolving.

Treatment options include nonoperative management with 6 weeks avoiding bearing weight (no cast), followed by 6 weeks weight-bearing in a boot. Operative management involves fixation of the fracture through minimal invasive techniques or open surgery. In severe pathology, a primary subtalar fusion should be considered.

Acknowledgements

Some of the figures were kindly provided by Mr. Sam Singh and Miss Sandhya Lamichhane.

Further reading

Asplund, C.A., and Best, T.M. (2013). Achilles tendon disorders. *BMJ* Mar 12: 346: f1262.

Gulati, V., et al. (2015). Management of Achilles tendon injury: A current concepts systematic review. *World Journal of Orthopedics* 6 (4): 380–386.

Horisberger, M., Valderrabano, V., and Hintermann, B. (2009). Posttraumatic ankle osteoarthritis after ankle-related fractures. *Journal of Orthopaedic Trauma* 23 (1): 60–67.

Mann, J.A., Mann, R.A., and Horton, E. (2011, May). STAR™ Ankle: Long-term results. *Foot and Ankle International* 32: 473–484.

Mann, R., and Reynolds, C. (1983). Interdigital neuroma—a critical clinical analysis. *Foot Ankle* 3: 238–243.

Riskowski, J., Dufour, A.B., and Hannan, M.T. (2011). Arthritis, foot pain and shoe wear. *Current Opinion in Rheumatology* 23 (2): 148–155.

Sheree, N., Smith, M., and Vicenzino, B. (2010). Prevalence of hallux valgus in the general population: a systematic review and meta-analysis. *Journal of Foot and Ankle Research* 3: 21.

CHAPTER 12

Spine

Syed Aftab and Robert Lee

Royal National Orthopaedic Hospital, Stanmore, UK

OVERVIEW

- Back pain is a common presentation and can be caused by pathology within the disc, bone, nerve root, or cord.
- Always be on the lookout for red flags to exclude cauda equina syndrome in acute back pain and tumours in chronic back pain.
- Much of back pain can be managed nonoperatively in the community with physiotherapy, lifestyle adaptations, and analgesia.
- Investigations include plain films, MRI, CT, and blood tests if infection or tumour is suspected.
- Spinal trauma can lead to long-lasting disability, and appropriate management is crucial to preserve quality of life and functionality.

Introduction

Back pain and/or nerve root compression and injury are among the most common reasons for presentation to the emergency department as well as to general practitioner. While the majority might not lead to permanent disability or be life threatening, it is important to identify those patients at risk. Even if back problems do not cause paralysis or loss of function, the pain and discomfort can be extremely severe and the burden on society is great.

Anatomy

The spine (Figure 12.1) is made up of 7 cervical vertebrae, 12 thoracic vertebrae, and 5 lumbar vertebrae. There are also 5 sacral vertebrae (fused together) and the coccyx. Each vertebrae is made up of a body anteriorly, the lamina, spinous process posteriorly, and contains a vertebral foramen that contains the spinal cord. These posterior elements are connected to the body by the pedicle. Facet joints connect each vertebra to the level above and below. Thoracic vertebrae also articulate with ribs. The space between the vertebrae is occupied by the intervertebral disc, which is composed of a tough outer annulus and a soft inner nucleus pulposus. Soft tissue structures like ligaments along with the bony architecture provide stability to the construct.

The spinal cord begins at the foramen magnum and passes through the vertebral foramen. It ends at the level of L1/L2 as the conus medullaris. The cauda equina begins here and ends at S2. The cord gives off nerve roots that exit at the neural foraminae. Dermatomes are areas on the surface of the skin that are control by specific nerve roots from the spinal cord (Figure 12.2). Myotomes correspond to muscles that are controlled by specific nerve roots from the spinal cord (Table 12.1). Reflexes are outlined in Table 12.2.

History

History of spinal symptoms to ask about include the following:

- Pain: neck vs. back, over spinal processes, paraspinal muscles, limb pain (at what level), worse pain on sitting/squatting/being still worse vs. standing/walking (neurogenic vs. vascular claudication for spinal stenosis)
- Imbalance
- Limb weakness
- Sensory changes: numbness, pins and needles
- Restriction of spinal movements and stiffness
- Functional limitations e.g. walking
- Disability: bladder, bowel, erectile dysfunction
- Deformity (and its onset)
- Associated symptoms: fever, weight loss, fatigue and night sweats

Examination

The examination should include observations as shown in Figure 12.3.

Structural spinal pathology

Some common degenerative structural changes of the spine can be seen in Figure 12.4.

Slipped disc and discogenic back pain

Cause

One of the most common causes of back pain is a slipped disc due to herniation of the nucleus pulposus (Figure 12.5). This is caused by traumatic or degenerative changes to the disc: loss of water content, tearing of the annulus fibrosus, and herniation of the nuclear

---

ABC of Orthopaedics and Trauma, First Edition. Edited by Kapil Sugand and Chinmay M. Gupte.
© 2018 John Wiley & Sons Ltd. Published 2018 by John Wiley & Sons Ltd.

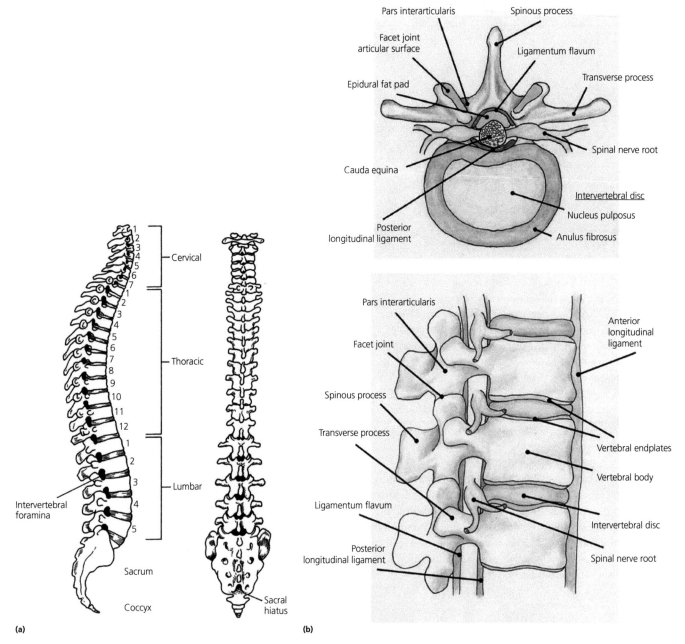

Figure 12.1 Anatomy of spine (a) entire column (b) single-level cross section of the lumbar vertebra

material. Discs can bulge or protrude into the canal without a tear of the annulus. Depending on the location, the cord, cauda equine, which all lead to myelopathy, or nerve roots can be affected leading to back pain, radiation, and distal neurological dysfunction, collectively known as radiculopathy. The most common disc affected is the L4/5 disc, closely followed by the L5/S1 disc.

Presentation
Patients often present with a combination of severe back pain and muscle spasms (loss of lumbar lordosis on plain lateral X-ray), radiation (e.g. sciatica), and neurological dysfunction (such as foot drop). There may be a precipitating injury, such as a fall or an episode of heavy lifting.

Examination
Clinical examination may reveal localised pain in and near the area of the pathology. Neurological findings will vary, depending on the nature and location of lesion. A loss of knee or ankle reflexes along with weakness may be observed. Straight leg raise and bow stringing are often possible.

Imaging
In a nontrauma situation, plain radiographs usually do not reveal anything other than a loss of lumbar lordosis. There may be other signs of degeneration such as loss of disc height or osteophytes. MRI scans may be used to confirm the diagnosis or rule out any other suspected pathology.

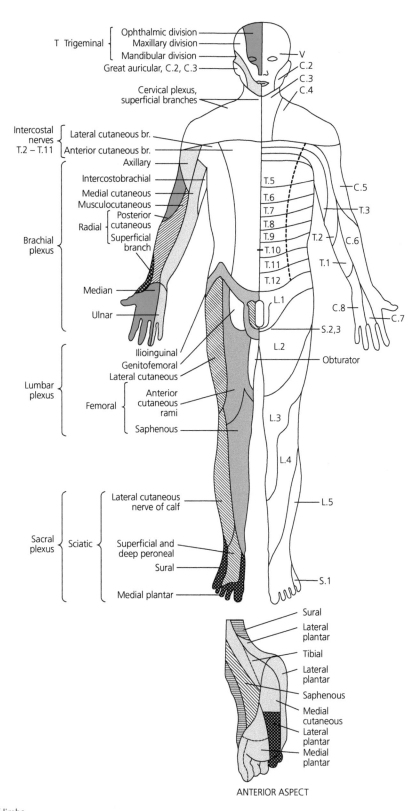

Figure 12.2 Dermatomes of limbs

Management

- *Nonoperative:* Mainstay of management is with analgesics, mobilisation, and reassurance (large majority of patients will experience resolution of symptoms within 12 weeks). If pain is severe, nerve root blocks or caudal epidural injections may be considered. Bed rest is not recommended due to risks of immobility (such as DVT) and muscle wasting. Physical therapy, swimming, pilates, and yoga to improve core stability are extremely useful measures to expedite recovery and prevent recurrence.

Table 12.1 Myotomes of limbs

Movement	Nerve root segments
Upper limb	
Shoulder girdle elevation	C3/4
Shoulder flexion / abduction	C5
Elbow flexion	C5/6
Elbow extension	C7/8
Wrist flexion / extension	C6/7
Finger flexion / extension	C7/8
Finger abduction / adduction	T1
Lower limb	
Hip flexion	L2/3
Hip extension	L4/5
Hip adduction	L2/3
Hip abduction	L4/5
Knee extension	L3/4
Knee flexion	L5/S1
Ankle dorsiflexion	L4/5
Hallux extension	L5
Ankle plantarflexion	S1/2

Table 12.2 Limb reflexes

Reflex	Nerve segments
Upper limb	
Biceps jerk	C5/6
Triceps jerk	C7/8
Brachioradialis jerk	C6/7
Lower limb	
Knee jerk	L3/4
Ankle jerk	S1/S2

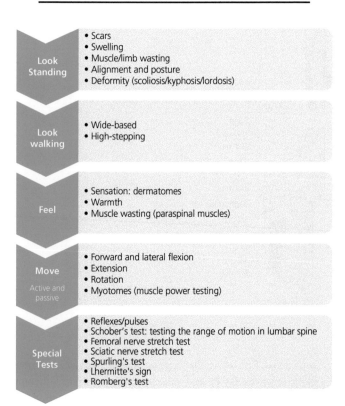

Look Standing
- Scars
- Swelling
- Muscle/limb wasting
- Alignment and posture
- Deformity (scoliosis/kyphosis/lordosis)

Look walking
- Wide-based
- High-stepping

Feel
- Sensation: dermatomes
- Warmth
- Muscle wasting (paraspinal muscles)

Move *Active and passive*
- Forward and lateral flexion
- Extension
- Rotation
- Myotomes (muscle power testing)

Special Tests
- Reflexes/pulses
- Schober's test: testing the range of motion in lumbar spine
- Femoral nerve stretch test
- Sciatic nerve stretch test
- Spurling's test
- Lhermitte's sign
- Romberg's test

Figure 12.3 Spinal examination

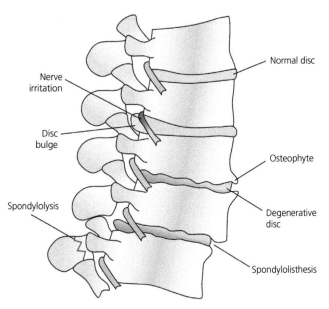

Figure 12.4 Schematic diagram of the spine showing a normal vertebral unit with examples of structural abnormalities

- *Operative:* In severe cases or where there is significant neurological compromise (such as foot drop from L5/S1 compromise), a surgical decompression (laminectomy and discectomy) may be useful.

Disc degeneration

This can also lead to back pain without radiation. Often, this pain is worse when sitting or leaning forward (i.e. neurogenic claudication). Nonsurgical management is along the lines described above. Surgical management may also include a fusion of the affected vertebrae, but the results for fusion for back pain alone are poor.

Sciatica

Cause

Sciatica is one of the most common causes of severe lower back pain. The sciatic nerve lies in the posterior thigh and branches into the tibial, common fibular, superficial fibular, deep fibular, sural, medial, and lateral plantar nerves, thus making it the largest nerve in the body. Sciatica results from compression or irritation of the nerve roots (L3–S4) or the sciatic nerve itself. Causes include slipped disc, spinal stenosis, pregnancy or centripetal obesity, and trauma.

Presentation

Symptoms include lumbar pain, weakness, and numbness to the buttock and legs along sciatic nerve distribution.

Examination

Diagnosis is mainly from history and clinical examination. Other signs to look out for include Lasague's sign and foot drop.

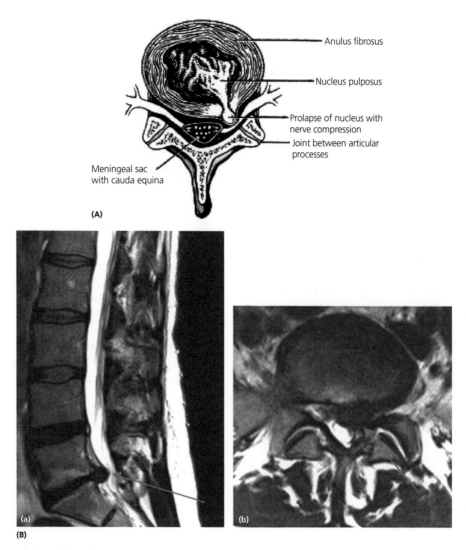

Figure 12.5 (A) Schematic of slipped disc and (B) Disc protrusion (a) Sagittal T2 weighted (T2w) image of the lumbar spine. (b) Axial T2w images show an L5/S1 left paracentral disc protrusion impinging on the left S1 nerve root. Note the degenerative vertebral endplate changes, loss of disc height and disc dehydration at this level

Investigations

MRI is not relied upon as much as clinical symptoms and signs. Imaging is reserved for patients displaying "red flag" symptoms to rule out cauda equina (Figure 12.6; see Chapter 14.7) and for cases not responding to conservative management after 2 months. Nerve conduction tests may also be considered.

Management

Management is initially nonoperative with weight loss, strong analgesia, and aggressive physiotherapy before resorting to surgical decompression in refractory cases.

Spinal narrowing (stenosis)

Cause

Stenosis of the spinal canal or neural foramen (Figure 12.7) can cause referred pain.

Presentation

Patients often complain of symptoms that are worse when upright and relieved in a flexed position such as when pushing a supermarket cart or a baby pram or riding a bicycle. This is also known as *neurogenic claudication* and must be differentiated from vascular claudication. In vascular claudication, leg pain will be worse with usage and Buerger test positive (elevating the leg above the level of the hip for 30 seconds brings on similar pain).

Management

MRI scanning will confirm the diagnosis. The three most common pathologies include disc prolapse, facet joint hypertrophy (from arthropathy), and hypertrophy from ligamentum flavum (from degenerative disease). Treatment is again with analgesics, physical therapy, and reassurance. Caudal epidural injections or nerve root blocks may be a useful temporising measure. Surgical management with decompression is indicated when quality of life is unacceptably impaired.

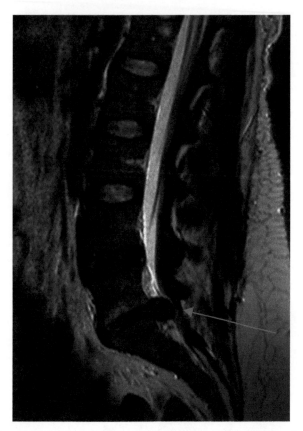

Figure 12.6 Cauda equina compression. Sagittal T2-weighted MRI showing a large L5/S1 disc protrusion causing compression of the thecal sac and cauda equina

Facet joint arthropathy

Cause

Wear of the facet joints also often leads to back pain. Due to its close proximity to the neural foramen, nerve root compression and referred pain is common concurrently. Facet joint cysts can also occur, which may cause neural compression.

Presentation

It is rare that a patient presents with only one pathology. Facet joint arthropathy, disc degeneration, referred pain, and back pain may all coexist.

Differentials

It is also important to consider other causes of back pain. These include abdominal or thoracic aortic aneurysms, metastatic disease (e.g. prostate or breast), spinal infections, or rheumatological conditions such as ankylosing spondylitis.

Management

Here an attempt at percutaneous aspiration of the cyst may be successful, but in cases of recurrence of symptoms or failure to decompress the cyst, surgical decompression is necessary.

Spondylosis, spondylolysis, and spondylolisthesis

Cause

- Spondylosis refers to generalised degenerative (arthritic) spinal (e.g. intervertebral disc) disease (Figure 12.8).

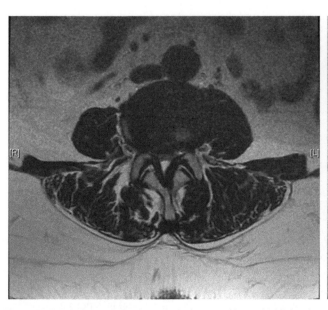
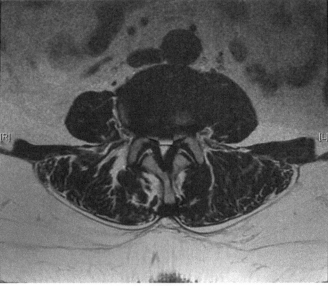

Figure 12.7 Spinal stenosis (lumbar spine). The second image highlights the vertebral canal available for the cauda equina (blue). The areas for the transiting nerve roots (or lateral recesses) are coloured red. In a normal spine, both the blue and the red areas would be much larger, giving much more space for the neurological structures

- Spondylolysis refers to a defect in the pars intra-articularis (part of vertebra located between the inferior and superior articular processes of the facet joint).

- Spondylolisthesis occurs when one vertebral segment slips forward or backward on the level below as a result of the ensuing instability (Figure 12.9).

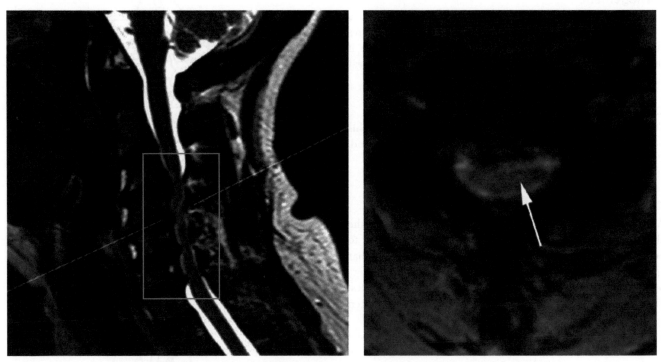

Figure 12.8 Cervical myelopathy from spondylosis. Sagittal MRI images showing spinal cord compression by a horizontal osteophyte at the C5–C6 (arrow) and C6–C7 levels. At those levels the spinal cord is abnormally hyperintense in these T2-weighted images

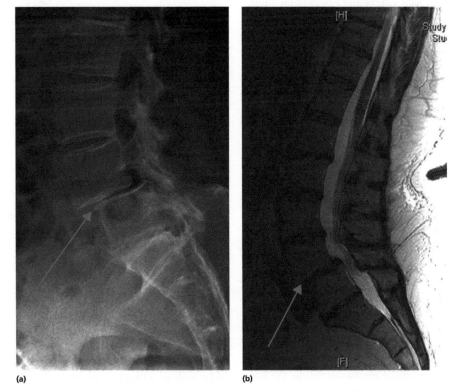

(a)　　　　　　　　　　　　(b)

Figure 12.9 Degenerative listhesis. Lateral radiograph (a) shows grade 1 (25%) slip of L4 on L5; (b) the sagittal T2W MRI shows reduction in the calibre of the spinal canal as a result of the degenerative listhesis (c.f. in lytic listhesis the canal is increased in diameter)

Presentation

Depending on the level and how capacious the canal is, patients may complain of back pain and referred pain.

Management

It is often visible on plain lateral standing films. In the absence of a progression with well-controlled symptoms, conservative measures such as analgesia and physical therapy are sufficient. However if there is progression, surgical stabilisation of the affected segment (often L5/S1) is indicated.

Congenital

Some individuals may be born with a congenital pars defect. This often leads to back pain in the teenage years or early adulthood. Treatment is often with surgical stabilisation and fusion.

Low mechanical back pain

Also known as lumbago, this refers to pain in the back in the absence of any clear radiological findings. It is often thought to be as a result lumbar segmental instability such that the lumbar spine is unable to withstand physiological loads without abnormal spinal motion causing pain. Management is with analgesics, physical therapy, and reassurance. Surgical treatment is not often appropriate.

Deformity

Scoliosis refers to a S-shaped curved spine (Figure 12.10). It is a three-dimensional deformity with a curve and a twist of the spine. There are many causes, but the most common is an idiopathic scoliosis affecting adolescents (female predominance). Neuromuscular conditions such as cerebral palsy or Duchenne's muscular dystrophy can also lead to scoliosis as well as severe spinal degeneration. The majority will not require management other than reassurance, but in some cases the deformity rapidly progresses and can cause pain, functional limitation, cardio-respiratory compromise and is unsightly. Management often starts with bracing and progresses to surgical correction and fusion when indicated. Kyphosis (from the Greek for hump) refers to a hunched forward spine. It can be congenital (e.g. Scheuermann kyphosis) or acquired (e.g. as a result of osteoporotic vertebral body collapse in the elderly or ankylosing spondylitis).

Tumours of the spine

Tumours in the spine can be primary or secondary (i.e. metastatic disease, Table 12.3). Metastases can occur outside or inside the spinal canal. If inside the canal, it can spread to the dura or the spinal cord itself. Common malignancies that metastasise to the spine include breast, lung, thyroid, kidney, and prostate. Patients can present with a history of malignancy elsewhere and associated back pain and radiation. Sometimes spinal metastases will be the first presentation of a primary malignancy elsewhere. X-rays may show metastatic disease in terms of lytic or blastic lesions, but MRI and

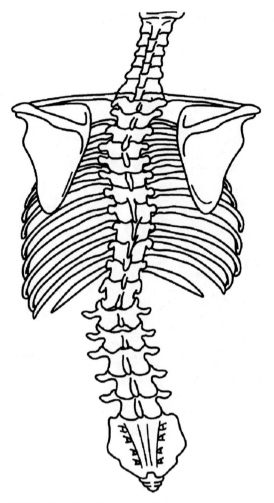

Figure 12.10 Scoliosis: the spine curves and rotates

Table 12.3 Sources of metastatic spread to spine

1 Breast
2 Prostate
3 Lung
4 Thyroid
5 Kidney
6 Multiple myeloma

CT scans reveal the pathology in more detail and help to stage the patient. Chemo-radiotherapy may be useful. In some cases, surgical treatment for debulking and decompression for symptomatic treatment or occasionally with curative intent is possible.

Infections of the spine

Infections can affect the discs (discitis, Figure 12.11a), bones (osteomyelitis, Figure 12.11b), or in the structures surrounding the spine. Patients can present with back pain or referred pain with or without the hallmarks of sepsis. Tuberculosis in the spine (Pott's disease) is its most common extra-pulmonary location. Radiographs may show destructive lesions. Treatment

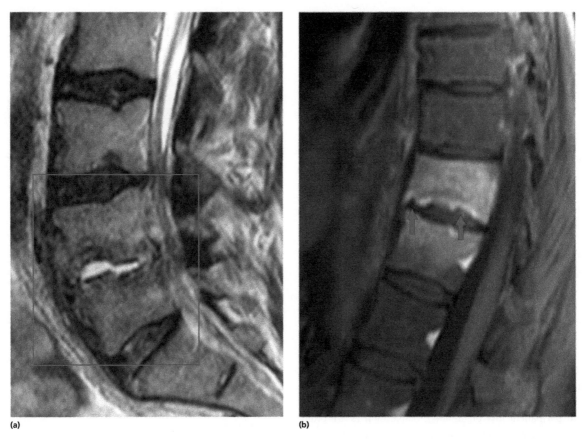

(a)　　　　　　　　　　　　　(b)

Figure 12.11 (a) Sagittal T2W MRI showing loss of disc height and ↑ disc signal at the L4–5 level (b) Sagittal T1W MRI showing eroded, ragged end-plates (arrows) in a patient with thoracic osteomyelitis. Blood cultures revealed Staph. aureus

is with long-term (months) antibiotics and surgical clearance if necessary.

Spinal trauma

Background

One person is paralysed by spinal cord injury every 8 hours. There are approximately 40,000 people living with paralysis as a result spinal cord injury in the United Kingdom. The initial management of an individual with spinal injury may mean the difference between life and death if not permanent paralysis and functional recovery.

Cause

The mechanisms of injury are primarily road traffic accidents, falls, penetrative trauma, assault, and sports (e.g. rugby).

Presentation

An injury to the cord at C1/2 is often fatal. C3/4/5 injury may be compatible with life, depending on its effects on the phrenic nerve. A spinal cord injury may be complete (AIS A) or incomplete (AIS B, C, or D). Some cord injuries may expect varying degrees of functional recovery. Long-term effects of cord injury include muscle wasting, pressure sores, and chest and urinary sepsis.

Resuscitation

The immediate management of a person with suspected spinal cord injury follows ATLS principles with airway, breathing, and circulation. Life-threatening injuries are treated and the spine is subsequently immobilised using a spinal board and C-spine rigid collar. Intravenous access is gained and fluid resuscitation started.

Examination

Once the patient is stabilised, a full neurological examination and secondary survey is required. An assessment of the spine is incomplete without a per-rectum examination, looking for loss of tone, sensation, and voluntary contraction. All documentation should be made on the ASIA chart for validated scoring and to assist with monitoring.

Initial management

Once completed, intravenous steroid therapy may be considered according to the protocols of the local spinal cord injury referral centre.

Complication

A patient with a cord injury may develop neurogenic shock characterised by hypotension and bradycardia along with a flaccid paralysis. This is different from hypovolaemic shock (tachycardia) and is a result of disruption to sympathetic outflow and loss of peripheral vascular resistance.

Imaging

Investigations often include plain radiographs, but not all injuries are easily visible with this modality. CT scans are used in the acute setting to identify and characterise bony injuries. If there is loss of neurological function, MRI scans are used to assess the cord and surrounding soft tissue structures.

Fractures

Background

Most spinal injuries will not involve cord injury. The bony and ligamentous structures can be damaged. There are varying patterns of injury, depending on the anatomical location and mechanism of injury.

Classification

The Denis three-column theory (Figure 12.12) suggests that compromise of at least two columns lead to structural instability. A CT is usually reserved for CT traumagrams in major or polytrauma. Otherwise, plain radiographs or MRI may be used, depending on complexity, comorbidities, and presence of neurological deficit.

Management

Management depends on how unstable the injury is deemed to be. An unstable injury managed inappropriately may lead to cord injury and permanent loss of function. Stable injuries are often treated without any immobilisation or fixation. A brace may be used to prevent deformity while healing is taking place (e.g. in an osteoporotic vertebral body wedge fracture). In cases where there is instability and risk of damage to neural structures a stabilisation procedure would often be performed. This may be nonsurgical (such as use of a hard collar, or halo-jacket) or surgical. For the unfortunate individuals in whom there has been permanent loss of neurological function due to spinal cord injury, management is supportive and requires input from a dedicated multidisciplinary spinal injury unit.

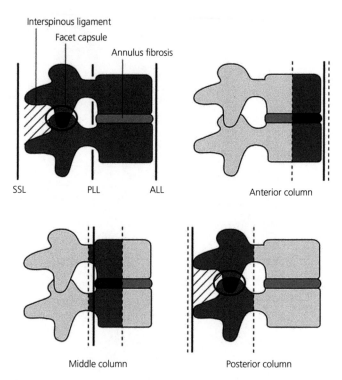

Figure 12.12 The three anatomical columns: SLL, supraspinatus ligament; PLL, posterior longitudinal ligament; ALL, anterior longitudinal ligament

Further reading

Jacobs, W.C., van Tulder, M., Arts, M., et al. (2011). Surgery versus conservative management of sciatica due to a lumbar herniated disc: a systematic review. *European Spine Journal* 20 (4): 513–522.

Manchikanti, L., Helm, S., Singh, V., et al. (2009). ASIPP. An algorithmic approach for clinical management of chronic spinal pain. *Pain Physician*. 12 (4): E225–264.

Yue, J.K., Upadhyayula, P., Chan, A.K., et al. (2015, November). A review and update on the current and emerging clinical trials for the acute management of cervical spine and spinal cord injuries – Part III. *Journal of Neurosurgical Sciences* 24.

CHAPTER 13

Paediatric Orthopaedics

Bassel El-Osta[1], Alex Shearman[2], and Neel Mohan[1]

[1] St. George's Hospital, London, UK
[2] North West London Rotation, London, UK

OVERVIEW

- Children's bones are unique in that they have growth plates (physes), are more flexible (therefore can bend rather than break), have a characteristic blood supply (especially around the metaphysis), and have thick periosteum surrounding the cortex.

- Injuries around the growth plate can be classified using the Salter-Harris classification.

- Nonaccidental injury should be suspected in any child, or where the clinical history does not match the pattern of injury.

- It is vital to build a rapport with the paediatric patients and their parents.

- Beware of referred pain that may be the only symptom of proximal joint pathology.

Anatomy of a paediatric bone

Paediatric long bones consist of a shaft (diaphysis), metaphysis, physis (growth plate), and epiphysis (part of the joint). An apophysis is a normal bony outgrowth (site of tendon and ligament attachments) that initially arises from a separate ossification centre before fusing with age. Figure 13.1 shows a paediatric femur.

Injuries during childbirth

A fracture of an otherwise healthy bone (i.e. not a pathological fracture through diseased bone like in *osteogenesis imperfecta*) may be sustained during complex deliveries, particularly in those associated with the use of forceps and difficult extraction, such as in shoulder dystocia (where the infant's shoulder is trapped behind the mother's pubic bone). Fractures tend to involve the clavicle or humerus; excess traction may lead to brachial plexus injuries (i.e. obstetric Erb's palsy [upper brachial plexus paralysis] seen in Figure 13.2a or Klumpke's palsy [lower brachial plexus paralysis] seen in Figure 13.2b). A thorough examination must therefore be carried out after a complicated delivery. Clavicle fractures may be missed, as it is difficult to assess active range of shoulder motion in

a newborn. Humeral, or more rarely, femoral shaft fractures may be suspected if the child is distressed when being held or changing nappies or clothes.

Management

Management is normally nonoperative, consisting of appropriate splintage. Most heal within 2–4 weeks. This is due to the strong periosteum around bone in children and a rich vascular supply. Radiologically, the healing process becomes evident by the formation of abundant callus around the fracture. Even if the bones heal with some angulation, they usually remodel, and within a few months the radiograph will likely become completely normal.

Fractures during childhood

Introduction

Fractures in children are common. According to Landin (1997), the percentage of children sustaining at least one fracture from 0 to 16 years of age is 42% in boys and 27% in girls. A fracture of immature bone may be incomplete, while the encircling periosteum remains in continuity. These are called greenstick or buckle fractures and are usually stable. Another common type of a stable fracture pattern is a Toddler's fracture, which is a spiral fracture of the tibia in a child of 2 or 3 years. Fractures may occur through the growth plate (physis) of growing bone. Physeal injuries account for up to a third of all childhood fractures, but associated growth disturbance is uncommon and happens in less than 10% of these injuries.

Classification

Salter and Harris classified these injuries in 1963, which is still widely in use today (Table 13.1). In their original paper, they described five types of injury (Figure 13.3).

The risk of growth disturbance increases with the type of fracture. The most common injury is type 2, which represents around 75–80% of all physeal injuries, types 1 and 3 together around 10% and Type 4 occurs in 5–10%; type 5 is uncommon.

ABC of Orthopaedics and Trauma, First Edition. Edited by Kapil Sugand and Chinmay M. Gupte.
© 2018 John Wiley & Sons Ltd. Published 2018 by John Wiley & Sons Ltd.

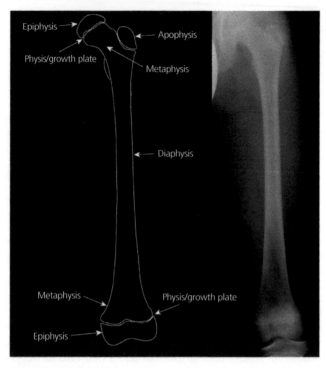

Figure 13.1 Paediatric bone anatomy

Clinical assessment of paediatric fractures

Sometimes it can be difficult to detect if a child has a fracture, particularly if the mechanism of injury was not witnessed by the accompanying adult, as sometimes happens in a playground. Some reliable signs to watch out for include limping, swelling, and bruising, marked tenderness (particularly in one area), and an inability or unwillingness to move the limb.

Management

Fractures in general may be treated conservatively or operatively, however most fractures in children can be treated conservatively. Some fracture patterns may need to be manipulated if widely displaced, if the limb is visually deformed or in displaced Salter Harris fractures. Fractures that are unstable, or rotationally deformed, may require internal fixation.

Nonaccidental injury (NAI)

It is the responsibility of the healthcare team to screen all paediatric patients for safeguarding issues and to ensure that the mechanism of injury is congruent with the history from the patients and their parents. Otherwise, there have been many cases of child abuse that have led to avoidable deaths. Be on the look out for red flags outlined in Table 13.2 and unusual injuries in Table 13.3.

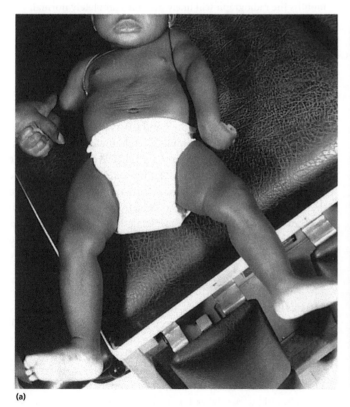

(a)

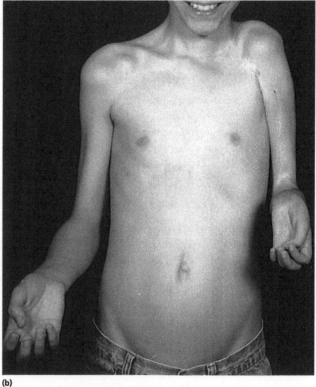

(b)

Figure 13.2 Brachial plexus paralysis: (a) Erb's Palsy due to an upper brachial plexus lesion on the left involving the C5, 6, and 7 roots. The arm hangs at the side internally rotated at the shoulder, with elbow extended and pronation of the forearm producing the so-called "waiter's tip" posture (courtesy of Rolf Birch FRCS); and (b) Klumpke-type paralysis due to lower brachial plexus avulsion earlier in childhood. A marked disturbance of subsequent growth especially affects the clavicle, scapula, and humerus. Horner syndrome was present. Nerve transfer operations have restored some hand grasp. Nonetheless, the residual weakness is characteristic orthopaedic with paralysis of wrist flexion and a claw hand (courtesy of Rolfe Birch FRCS)

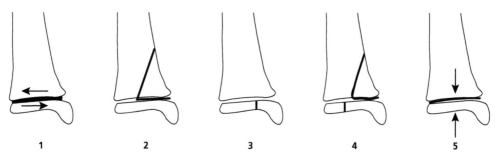

Figure 13.3 Salter-Harris classification of paediatric fractures

Table 13.1 Salter and Harris injury classification

Class	Definition
1	Fracture through the hypertrophic zone of the growth plate
2	Fracture through the growth plate with a metaphyseal fragment
3	Fracture through the growth plate with an epiphyseal fragment
4	Fracture through the growth plate with both metaphyseal and epiphyseal fragments
5	Crush injury or compression fracture of the growth plate

Box 13.1 **Mnemonic for Salter Harris fractures (SALTER):**

S: Slipped physis
A: Above (into metaphysis)
L: Low (into epiphysis)
TE: Through Everything (metaphysis, physis and epiphysis)
R: Rammed/crushed physis

Table 13.2 Red flags for suspecting NAI

Delayed presentation or multiple attendances to the Emergency Paediatric Department	History or evidence of Munchausen syndrome by proxy
Inconsistent history from patient or parents not matching injury	Unusual injuries (caused by twisting motion or direct blow)
Unwitnessed trauma	Neglect, poor hygiene, and dentition
Signs of domestic abuse or violence	Multiple injuries
Malnutrition	Children with learning difficulties, delay in development, or chronic illness

Table 13.3 Injuries suggestive of NAI

Multiple/cluster of bruising, especially in a shape of a hand or instrument and in a nonambulatory child	Leg, rib, or skull fractures (from twisting, squeezing, and hitting)
Burns	Recurrent fractures not down to metabolic bone disease

Ensure whether the paediatric patient is already known to social services or to the child protection registry. If suspicious of NAI then discuss with your consultant, the ED consultant, and the lead paediatric consultant and specialist paediatric nurse in charge of safeguarding issues.

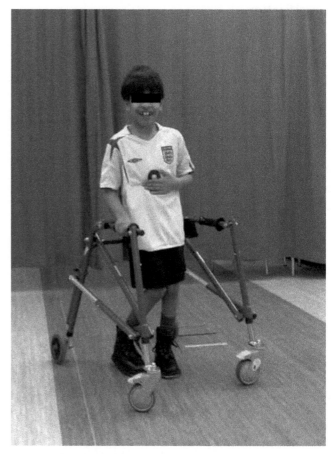

Figure 13.4 Cerebral palsy

Cerebral palsy (CP)

Introduction

Cerebral palsy (CP, Figure 13.4) describes a nonprogressive neuromuscular disorder that is caused by an injury to an immaturely developed brain. It is the most common cause of physical disability in children, and has an estimated incidence of between 1 and 3 out of 1000 live births.

Aetiology

The cause of injury is often unknown; contributing factors include prematurity, head injury, intrauterine problems, perinatal infection (e.g. meningitis) or anoxia.

Presentation

The cerebral lesion leads to upper motor neurone impairment of the musculoskeletal system, leading to a heterogeneous syndrome of muscular hypotonia and spasticity. Initially the musculoskeletal system is normal but progressive spasticity around joints will lead to fixed contractures, bony deformities and joint subluxation, with associated gait disorders and reduced function. Whilst the cerebral injury is considered nonprogressive, the effect on the muscles and joints is progressive. Assessment of these patients is aimed at identifying and preventing deterioration of these deformities.

Classification

This may be considered to be physiological, anatomical, or functional.

Physiological refers to a classification of the neurological presentation:
- Spastic (60%): hypertonic, hyperreflexia, contractures leading to slow and restricted movements
- Dystonic (20%): slow and writhing involuntary movements with choreiform athetosis. Involvement of basal ganglia where severity is related with emotional stress.
- Ataxic (10%): weakness, malcoordination, and tremor due to cerebellar involvement
- Hypotonic
- Mixed

Anatomical refers to the distribution of involvement and is related to the site of cerebral injury:
- Hemiplegia where one side (upper and lower limb) is involved
- Diplegia where the lower limbs are affected more than the upper limbs
- Tetra-/quadri-plegia where the whole body is involved, associated with low IQ and increased mortality

Functional classification considers the ability of the child to walk and the need for aids. This is most commonly associated with the Gross Motor and Functional Classification System (GMFCS, Table 13.4).

Management

A multidisciplinary approach to the management of these patients is essential. Identifying patients with deteriorating function using objective measures such as the GMFCS will help in the early years. In general treatment options considered are outlined in Table 13.5.

Table 13.4 Gross motor and functional classification system

GMFCS	Mobility	Limitation
1	Walks without restrictions	Limited in advanced gross motor skills
2	Walks without assistive devices	Limited in walking outdoors and in the community
3	Walks with assistive mobility devices	
4	Self-mobility with limitations	Transported or use powered mobility outdoors or in the community
5	Self-mobility is severely limited even with the use of assistive technology	

Table 13.5 Management options for cerebral palsy

Issue	Management
Spasticity	• Botulinum toxin injections are used, which act at the neuromuscular junction to inhibit muscular contraction, so preserving joint laxity. • Baclofen, which acts on GABA receptors, can also help. This is either delivered systemically or locally through a pump. • Dorsal rhizotomy (selective surgical sensory neurectomy) may be effective in ambulatory patients with spastic diplegia.
Orthotics	To support weak muscle and aid gait, such as ankle-foot orthoses (AFOs).
Soft tissue rebalancing	Tendon lengthening or transfer procedures in addition to localised tenotomy (e.g. adductor tenotomy at the hip).
Bony procedures	These include corrective osteotomies, fusion and salvage procedures. Surgery should treat the limb as a whole and aim to prevent deterioration of function.

Spina Bifida

Background

Spina bifida (Figure 13.5) is a congenital neural tube defect leading to incomplete formation of the vertebral arch, with or without protrusion of a meningeal sac (meningocoele) through the defect. This sac may contain neural elements in which case it is termed a myelomeningocoele. Myelomeningocoele accounts for approximately 75% of all spina bifida and has an estimated incidence of 1 in 800. This may be decreasing with intrauterine diagnosis and folic acid supplementation.

Presentation

Aside from the obvious meningocoele, clinical features include a neurological deficit, relating to the level at which the cord is involved (for example, patients with lesions above the level of L4 will have no quadriceps function and therefore will be unable to ambulate). In patients without meningocoele (spina bifida occulta), the skin normally covers the defect but there may be an associated tuft of hair or dimpling at the sacrum. Associated conditions include hydrocephalus, scoliosis, and syringomyelia as well as bladder and bowel dysfunction. Fractures are common and often difficult to diagnose.

Management

Fractures are normally treated with splintage and heal readily. Treatment is multidisciplinary and involves orthopaedic, paediatric, urologic, and neurosurgical input. Initial repair of the defect is followed by close observation of developmental milestones. Orthoses are used to aid ambulation. Surgery aims to rebalance muscles and correct deformity.

Metabolic Bone Disease

Rickets
Background

A metabolic disorder of bone in which a deficiency of available calcium and/or phosphate ions leads to altered development and mineralisation of bone. This leads to short stature, pain, and limb deformities as well as fracture (Figure 13.6).

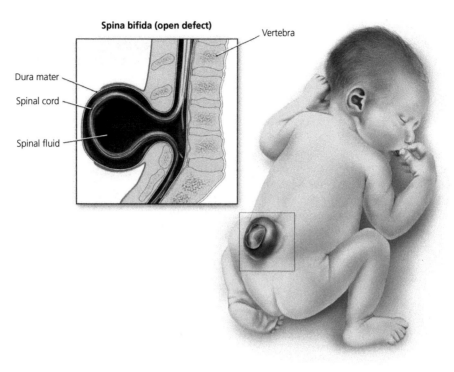

Figure 13.5 Types of spina bifida

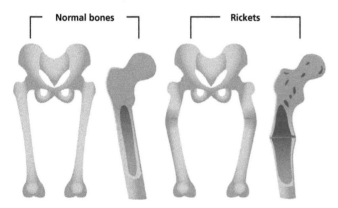

Figure 13.6 Rickets

Aetiology

Causes include dietary insufficiency as well as lack of exposure to sunlight. There are some associated disorders (malabsorption, X-linked hypophosphataemia).

Assessment

Clinical assessment includes full history and examination, particularly examining for varus deformities of the limbs, ligamentous laxity, and thoracic kyphosis (cat-back).

Investigations

Radiographs may demonstrate these deformities as well as widening or blunting of the physis, Looser zones, and enlarged costal cartilages (rachitic rosary). Serological tests should include calcium, phosphate, ALP, PTH, and vitamin D Levels.

Management

Treatment is with phosphate and vitamin D, as well as addressing any nutritional deficiencies.

Osteogenesis Imperfecta (OI)
Background

This is a genetic disorder of type I collagen formation leading to increased bone fragility and subsequent fracture. Incidence is estimated at 1:20,000 live births.

Presentation

Clinical features include bone fragility (often presenting as atypical fractures), scoliosis, tooth defects, hearing problems, blue sclerae, and ligamentous laxity.

Subtypes

Sillence classified osteogenesis imperfecta in 1979 into four types based on differing phenotypes. Subsequent research and histological examination has led to further subtypes being described.

Genetics

Inheritance is most commonly autosomal dominant (80–85%), meaning that affected individuals have a 50% likelihood of having a child with OI. In a smaller proportion of patients, OI is inherited in a recessive fashion, or is a result of mosaicism.

Management

There is no cure for OI. Treatment aims to prevent fractures and deformity. Bisphosphonates have been shown to reduce fracture rates. Bracing of long bones may help prevent deformities.

Corrective osteotomies with intramedullary rods may be necessary in severe deformity. Severe scoliosis may require surgical correction.

Bone dysplasias

Achondroplasia
Background
Dysplasia describes abnormal development. Applied to bone, this leads to shortening of the affected areas (i.e. dwarfism). Dwarfism may be proportionate (symmetric decrease in trunk and limb size) or disproportionate (either short trunk or short limbs relative to the other). Pathogenesis is due to disruption in the proliferative zone of the physis, so it is considered a disorder of the growth plate. Disproportionate bone formation in the limbs leads to shortening.

Genetics
Achondroplasia describes a genetic disorder of disproportionate dwarfism, due to a mutation of the fibroblast growth factor receptor 3 (FGFR3) gene. Inheritance is autosomal dominant.

Presentation
Clinical features include short stature (Figure 13.7), frontal bossing, and button nose. *Trident hands* (Figure 13.7) describe an apparent separation between the middle and ring fingers. Patients with achondroplasia also present with spinal problems consisting of thoracolumbar kyphosis, excessive lumbar stenosis (which may cause peripheral neurological compromise) and excessive lordosis.

Management
Management involves addressing any spinal problems such as decompression and fusion for stenosis. Deformities such as tibia vara can be corrected with osteotomy or hemiepiphysiodesis.

Paediatric Hip Disorders

Developmental dysplasia of hip (DDH)
Background
DDH is an abnormal development or dislocation of the hip secondary to capsular laxity and associated mechanical factors. It was previously known as congenital hip dysplasia (CHD), before it was accepted that this condition can develop post-partum.

Risk factors
These include breech positioning, family history, female gender, firstborn child, and oligohydramnios.

Examination
Prognosis is best if picked up early and the role of screening is pivotal. In the neonate (up to 6 weeks), Barlow's and Ortolani's tests are conducted. Ortolani tests whether the hip is dislocated by abducting and gently elevating the affected hip (Figure 13.8).

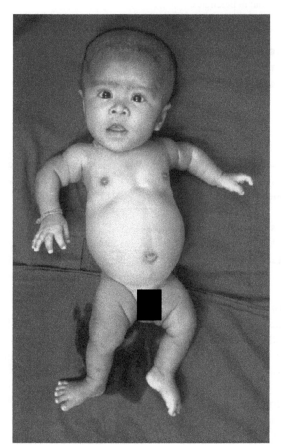

(a)

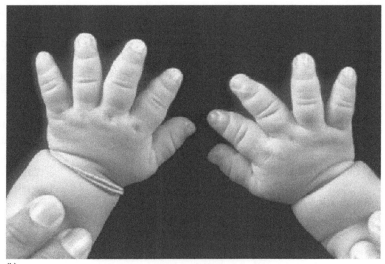

(b)

Figure 13.7 Achondroplasia

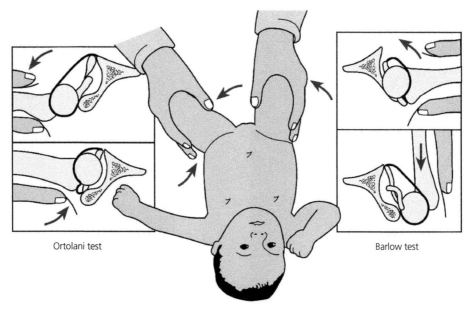

Ortolani test

Barlow test

Figure 13.8 Barlow and Ortolani tests for DDH

A palpable "clunk" as the hip is reduced is considered positive. Barlow's test involves pressure and depression of the adducted hip. The test is positive if the hip is felt to sublux or dislocate. On the basis of these findings, the hip may be considered: *dislocated* (Ortolani+), *dislocatable* (Barlow++), or *subluxatable* (Barlow+). Beyond 6 weeks, the hip becomes stiffer and these clinical tests are less useful. Other signs include restricted abduction compared to the contralateral side (although this is not useful in cases of bilateral dislocation), Galeazzi sign (apparently shortened femur), and asymmetric gluteal folds.

Imaging
Ultrasound is ideal, as the femoral head does not ossify before 6 months and radiographs are difficult to interpret.

Treatment
Treatment is based on the age at presentation:
- <6 months: a Pavlik harness (Figure 13.9a) is designed to hold the hips in a reduced position. Reduction of the hips must be confirmed after application.
- 6–18 months: the patient may be suitable for a closed reduction in theatre. An arthrogram is performed intraoperatively, and adductor tenotomy is performed to help maintain reduction. The reduction is held in a hip spica cast (Figure 13.9b) and post-operative CT is performed to confirm reduction.
- 18–36 months: it is less likely that closed reduction will be successful and open reduction is therefore preferred. After 3 years, corrective osteotomies can reshape the hip.

Perthes disease
Background
Legg-Calvé-Perthes disease (Figure 13.10), more commonly known just as Perthes disease, is defined as a noninflammatory aseptic avascular osteonecrosis of the proximal femoral epiphysis (i.e. femoral head).

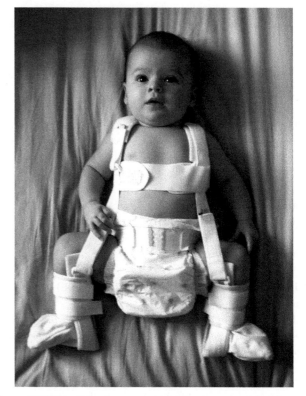

Figure 13.9(a) Pavlik harness

Demographics
With an incidence of 1:1,200, 10% will have both hips affected. Males are four to five times more likely to be affected than females. This disease typically affects children aged 4–8 years.

Presentation and examination
Patients typically present with a painless limp but may occasionally complain of anterior thigh or groin pain. Sometimes, referred knee pain may be present. Examination may reveal limited hip

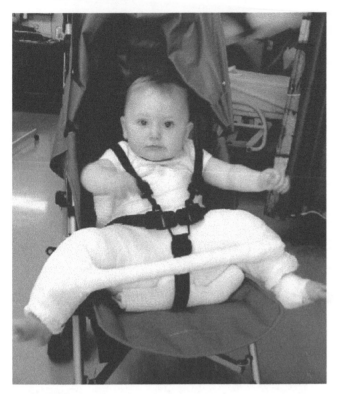

Figure 13.9(b) Hip spica

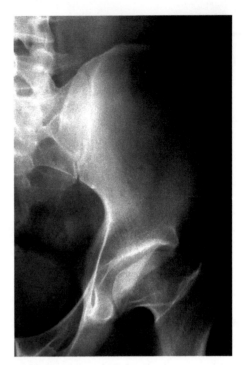

Figure 13.10 Radiograph showing Perthes disease

movements, particularly internal rotation and abduction, and altered gait.

Imaging

Radiographs in the early stages show a smaller ossified nucleus in the femoral head, which is denser and may be flattened and lateralised. There are also segmental collapses and lucencies.

Management

Prognosis is related to maintaining femoral head sphericity. Treatment is primarily nonsurgical, but corrective osteotomy may be considered in severe cases.

Slipped capital femoral epiphysis (SCFE)
Background

SCFE (Figure 13.11) is defined as a *"disorder of the proximal femoral epiphysis caused by weakness of the perichondral ring and slippage through the hypertrophic zone of the growth plate."*

Demographics

The incidence is 1 in 100,000, but early diagnosis is critical. It typically affects overweight adolescent males where 25% of cases are bilateral. It is important to exclude associated endocrinological disorders (hypothyroidism, growth hormone deficiency) in the young.

Presentation and examination

Presentation is normally with a limp, hip or thigh pain, but ipsilateral referred knee pain may be the only symptom. Consequently, any child presenting with knee pain should undergo hip examination.

Table 13.6 Classifications of SCFE

Classification	Description
Loder	Stable vs. unstable (unable to walk even when on crutches)
Radiological	Grade 1 = < 1/3 slippage
	Grade 2 = 1/3 – ½ slippage
	Grade 3 = > ½ slippage
Temporal	Acute vs. chronic vs. acute-on-chronic

Patients have decreased internal rotation and demonstrate obligate external rotation when the hip is flexed.

Imaging

Plain radiography confirms the diagnosis. Lateral imaging is helpful but frog-leg lateral views should be avoided in unstable slips to avoid further damage.

Classifications

Prognosis is related to the ability to bear weight, which indicates the stability of the hip according several classifications (Table 13.6).

Treatment

The treatment of choice is in-situ pinning of the slip. Aggressive reduction methods are not used. Corrective surgery may be necessary at a later stage. Although controversial, prophylactic fixation of the contralateral hip should be considered at the time of surgery, as a significant number of these cases are bilateral.

Transient synovitis

Transient synovitis is a common cause of painful hip in childhood. Diagnosis remains one of exclusion. It is essential to ensure that septic arthritis and osteomyelitis are excluded and where diagnostic doubt remains further investigation like ultrasound +/- MRI should be considered. Clinical features are of antalgic gait, limp, reduced range of motion, and muscle contraction.

Kocher described four criteria to help distinguish between septic arthritis and transient synovitis.
1 Leukocytosis with WCC > 12 × 10⁹
2 Pyrexia with temperature > 38.5 °C
3 Erythrocyte sedimentation rate (ESR) > 40 mm/hr
4 Non–weight-bearing on the affected limb

If none of these criteria are met, there is a 0.2% likelihood of septic arthritis. Where all four of these criteria are met, there is a 99.6% likelihood of septic arthritis. Septic arthritis (Chapter 19) is a surgical emergency, and if left alone it will lead to cartilage destruction. Aggressive management, urgent exploration, and washout are required in septic arthritis. However, treatment of transient synovitis is with NSAIDs, rest, and observation. Symptoms should settle within 48–72 hours.

Paediatric knee disorders

Genu valgum/varum

Genu varum describes a deformity of the knee where the tibia is angulated towards the midline with reference to the femur. It may be physiological under the age of 2 years. Abnormal varus is associated with Blount's disease (growth disorder of tibia resembling bowleg), OI, osteochondromas, or trauma. Treatment is based on age and may vary from bracing in the early stages through to corrective osteotomies in latter years. Genu valgum is also known as *knock-knees*. Again, this may be physiological in the ages 2–6 years. Pathological causes include infection, osteochondromas, or trauma. Surgical correction is normally required.

Osgood-Schlatter disease

This is a traction apophysitis at the tibial tubercle, seen in growing children. It has a characteristic radiographic appearance (Figure 13.12). Patients will present with pain and swelling, with localised tenderness at the tibial tubercle. This condition is usually self-limiting and treatment consists of rest from sports, topical ice therapy, and NSAIDs.

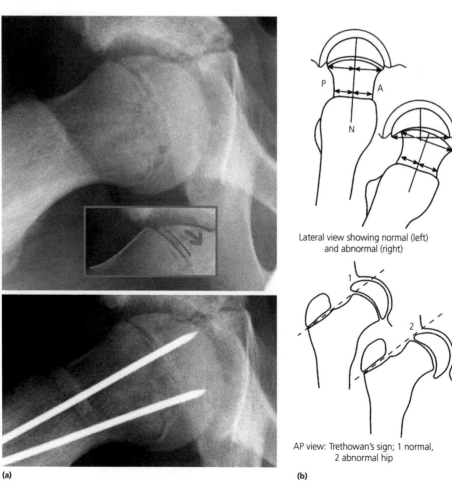

(a)   **(b)**

Lateral view showing normal (left) and abnormal (right)

AP view: Trethowan's sign; 1 normal, 2 abnormal hip

Figure 13.11 Slipped capital femoral epiphysis (a) radiograph and (b) measurements

Paediatric knee injuries

These can be divided into congenital or acquired.

Congenital

The most common congenital paediatric condition is the discoid lateral meniscus. The lateral meniscus can be of an abnormal shape or have abnormal connections. This can lead to a clunking sensa-

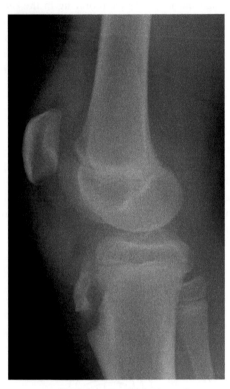

Figure 13.12 Radiograph showing Osgood–Schlatter disease

tion, a lack of extension or lateral pain. The meniscus is also suscepible to tearing. Asymptomatic discoid lateral meniscus should be managed conservatively. However discoid lateral meniscus with history of locking or a tear may require either reshaping with arthroscopic treatment, resection or repair depending on the type of tear.

Paediatric acquired knee conditions is divided into the following:

1 *Bony* (e.g. osteochondritis dissecans [OCD]). OCD is a condition which is poorly understood but related to repetitive high impact activities and sporty young individuals. Occasionally there may be a history of direct trauma. Most OCD lesions can be managed conservatively with activity modification and physiotherapy. Impact activity should be stopped for 6-12 months depending on symptoms. However some lesions can be unstable on MRI scan and if associated with appropriate symptoms, this may require either fixation of the lesion or removal of lose body of the detached lesion.

2 *Meniscal injuries.* Meniscal injuries should be treated if symptomatic for more than six weeks with arthroscopic repair if possible. If the meniscus is displaced in a bucket handle tear fashion, it should ideally be reduced and repaired. Occasionally the meniscus can be too damaged for this and may require removal which can predispose to early degenerative change.

3 *Cruciate ligament injury.* The most common being ACL rupture either in the mid-substance or avulsion at the tibial bony insertion (tibial spine fracture). Paediatric mid-substance ACL ruptures are best managed with early reconstruction. Reconstruction methods are controversial and may involve either reduced trauma to the physeal growth plates or extra-physeal reconstruction.

4 *Patellafemoral dislocation/instability.* This has many causes, including abnormal bony anatomy (eg shallow femoral trochlea),

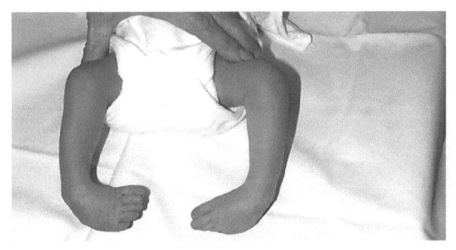

Figure 13.13 Clubfoot pathology

abnormal patellar alignment, medial patellofemoral ligament injury or hyperlaxity. First time patella dislocation should be managed with bracing and physiotherapy. Repeated dislocations require investigation of the possible causes. If conservative measures fail, operative options include medial patellofemoral ligament reconstruction or reshaping of the femoral trochlea if this is particularly dysplastic.

Paediatric tibial spine fractures

These can be either displaced or undisplaced. Undisplaced fractures should be managed conservatively with a period in a plaster followed by bracing in resisted flexion.

Foot and ankle disorders

Congenital talipes equinovarus (clubfoot)

Clubfoot (Figure 13.13) describes a congenital deformity of the hindfoot and midfoot. Specifically, it is an adducted and supinated forefoot combined with hindfoot varus and equinus. This is relatively common, affecting 1:1000 live births. Males are predominantly affected (3:1). Normally idiopathic, though there are some genetic associations. Previously, this condition was treated surgically with tendon lengthening and releases to alter the biomechanics of the foot. The widespread adoption of the *Ponseti technique* of deformity correction has revolutionised the management of this condition, and surgery is now only reserved for refractory cases. The Ponseti method is a technique of serial casting in which the three-dimensional deformity is corrected in a sequential manner, commonly remembered using the mnemonic CAVE (Table 13.7).

Metatarsus adductus

This condition is a true varus deformity of the forefoot, caused by adduction at the tarsometatarsal joint. It typically affects 1:1000 live births. It is important to recognise in neonates, as it is

Table 13.7 CAVE deformities for clubfoot

Mnemonic	Description	Site	Tight and tense...
C	Cavus	Midfoot	Intrinsics, FHL, and FDL
A	Adductus	Forefoot	Tibialis posterior
V	Varus	Hindfoot	Achilles tendon and tibialis posterior
E	Equinus		Achilles tendon

associated with DDH in 10–15% of cases. Clinical assessment focuses on whether the deformity is correctable. In the majority of cases (85%), this condition will resolve without intervention. Serial casting may be necessary in fixed deformity. Surgery is reserved only for refractory cases.

Further reading

Brown, J.H., and DeLuca, S.A. (1992). Growth plate injuries: Salter-Harris classification. *American Family Physician* October 46 (4): 1180–1184.

Forlino, A., and Marini, J.C. (2015). Osteogenesis imperfecta. *Lancet.* November 2. pii: S0140-6736(15)00728-X.

Kerr, Graham, H., and Selber, P. (2003, March). Musculoskeletal aspects of cerebral palsy. *Journal of Bone and Joint Surgery (Br.)* 85 (2): 157–166.

Kocher, M.S., Zurakowski, D., and Kasser, J.R. (1999). Differentiating between septic arthritis and transient synovitis of the hip in children: an evidence-based clinical prediction algorithm. *J Bone Joint Surg Am.* 81 (12): 1662–70.

Landin, L.A. (1997, April). Epidemiology of children's fractures. *Journal of Pediatric Orthopedics,* part B 6 (2): 79–83.

Morris, C. (2009). Current and future uses of the Gross Motor Function Classification System: the need to take account of other factors to explain functional outcomes. *Developmental Medicine & Child Neurology* 51 (12): 1003.

Salter, R., and Harris, W. (1963). Injuries involving the epiphyseal plate. *Journal of Bone and Joint Surgery (Am.)* 45: 587–622.

Sillence, D.O., Senn, A., and Danks, D.M. (1979). Genetic heterogeneity in osteogenesis imperfecta. *Journal of Medical Genetics* 16 (2): 101–116.

Wall, E.J., and May, M.M. (2012, June). Growth plate fractures of the distal femur. *Journal of Pediatric Orthopaedics* 32 Suppl 1: S40–46.

Orthopaedic Emergencies
14.1 Emergency: Dislocated Hip

Simond Jagernauth and Joshua KL Lee

The Royal London Hospital, Barts Health NHS Trust, London, UK

OVERVIEW

- A native traumatic hip dislocation is a rare orthopaedic emergency that requires a high-energy mechanism of injury (usually a dashboard injury).
- Total hip replacements can also dislocate with low-energy mechanisms, such as certain movements or fall from standing height.
- Most hip dislocations are posterior that can lead to sciatic nerve dysfunction.
- Dislocated hips ought to be reduced within 6 hours to reduce the risk of neurovascular compromise, avascular necrosis, and recurrence, while increasing the likelihood of successful closed reduction.

Introduction

A dislocated hip is a rare injury, where the femoral head is forced out of the acetabulum and is an orthopaedic emergency. The hip joint is inherently very stable due to the bony anatomy and soft tissue constraints; it therefore requires a high-energy injury to dislocate it.

Mechanism of injury

The hip dislocates posteriorly in the majority of cases (90%). A *dashboard injury* is the classic mechanism; sitting with the hip flexed, an axial load is transmitted through the femur when the knee impacts with the dashboard, forcing the femoral head posteriorly out of the acetabulum. Falling from a height or industrial accidents are other injuries with sufficient force to dislocate a hip.

Examination

This injury is extremely painful. The patient is unable to bear weight. The hip adopts a classical position of slight flexion, adduction, and internal rotation (Figure 14.1.1).

It is important to perform a thorough neurovascular examination of the lower limbs, as a sciatic nerve injury is present in 10–20% of cases.

Imaging

A radiograph (Figures 14.1.2 and 14.1.3) will readily identify a dislocation and any associated fractures. A CT scan is often obtained as part of a trauma protocol and can more accurately define any fractures.

Management

Due to the high energy required to sustain this injury, the patient should be treated as a major trauma and initial management as per Advanced Trauma Life Support (ATLS). In 95% of hip dislocations, there are also associated injuries. The hip should ideally be relocated within 6 hours, as there is an increased risk of avascular necrosis and sciatic nerve injury the longer the hip is left out of joint. The hip can be reduced closed in the majority of cases; there is some controversy as to whether this should be done in the emergency department or in the operating theatre. With the patient sedated or anaesthetised lying supine, the knee is flexed to relax the hamstrings and the hip brought to 90° flexion, longitudinal traction is then applied to the femur and the femoral head is manipulated back into the acetabulum. If the hip does not go back into joint, one must proceed to a surgical relocation of the hip. A CT scan should be obtained after the reduction to check for any associated fractures and possible retained bone fragments in the hip joint. These may require further surgical management.

COMPLICATIONS

- Sciatic nerve injury: 8–20%
- Avascular necrosis: 5–40%
- Posttraumatic arthritis: 20% for simple dislocation, much increased if there is an associated acetabular fracture
- Recurrent dislocation: 2%

ABC of Orthopaedics and Trauma, First Edition. Edited by Kapil Sugand and Chinmay M. Gupte.
© 2018 John Wiley & Sons Ltd. Published 2018 by John Wiley & Sons Ltd.

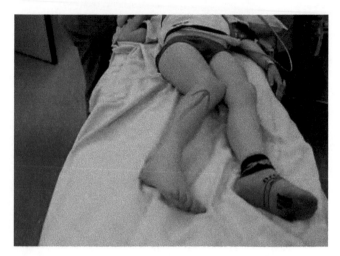

Figure 14.1.1 Classic position of lower limb in posterior dislocation of the hip. Slight flexion, adduction, and internal rotation

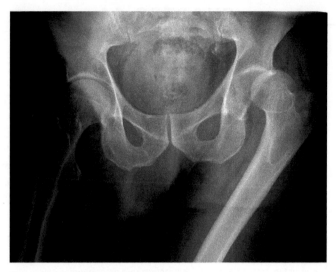

Figure 14.1.2 Left hip joint dislocation

Further reading

Mandell, J.C., Marshall, R.A., Weaver, M.J et al. (2017, November–December). Traumatic hip dislocation: What the orthopedic surgeon wants to know. *Radiographics* 37 (7): 2181–2201.

Massoud, E.I.E. (2018, March). Neglected traumatic hip dislocation: Influence of the increased intracapsular pressure. *World Journal of Orthopedics* 9 (3): 35–40.

Moreta, J., Foruria, X., Sánchez, A., et al. (2017, November–December). Prognostic factors after a traumatic hip dislocation. A long-term retrospective study. *Revista Espanola de Cirugia Ortopedia Y Traumatologia* 61 (6): 367–374.

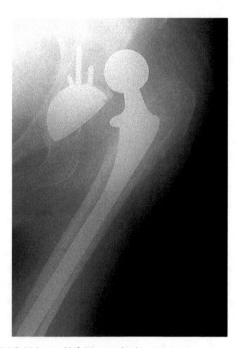

Figure 14.1.3 Dislocated left hip prosthesis

Emergency: Locked Knee and Dislocation

Sohail Yousaf[1], Mubeen Nazar[2], and Chinmay M. Gupte[3,4]

[1] Ashford and St. Peter's Hospitals, Surrey, UK
[2] Epsom and St. Helier University Hospitals NHS trust, London, UK
[3] MSk Lab, Charing Cross Hospital, Imperial College London, London, UK
[4] Imperial College Healthcare NHS Trust, London, UK

OVERVIEW

- True locked knee is the inability to fully extend the knee actively or passively.
  - Causes are either mechanical (meniscus, ligament, loose bodies) or nonmechanical (exaggerated pain, neurological, hysterical).
- If mechanical cause, arthroscopy should be done within a fortnight.
- Ideal choice of imaging is MRI.
- Knee dislocations may be transient but can lead to neurovascular compromise, compartment syndrome, and chronic disability if not diagnosed or managed early and correctly.
- Knee joint dislocations need to be reduced urgently and held in a brace or spanned with external fixators, and reconstructed expeditiously.
- If vascular injury after knee dislocation is suspected, then open reduction and direct visual examination of the vasculature are required.

Locked knee

Background

The knee is the most frequently injured joint in the body during sports. The term *locked knee* is applied to describe the inability of the patients to fully straighten their knee actively or passively. The symptoms of locking may occur immediately after injury or, more commonly, after the initial severe phase has resolved. An MRI scan is highly sensitive for diagnosis, and arthroscopic intervention is often required. The acutely locked knee is a common problem affecting active individuals, and often results in a significant lifestyle disruption and time off work due to pain and restricted function.

Pathophysiology

Locked knee implies an intra-articular disorder blocking full extension, resulting in a knee held in flexion, which is painful on attempting full extension. Most of the injuries are related to high stresses during twisting and turning motions, such as during football, skiing, and rugby. Causes can be divided into mechanical vs. nonmechanical, as seen in Table 14.2.1.

Meniscal injuries

The menisci have an important role in controlling complex rolling and gliding motions of knee joint. The meniscal injuries are usually produced by the twisting strains in relatively flexed knees, as in kicking a football. The meniscus may get separated from the capsule or may be torn. If the separated fragment remains attached front and back, the lesion is called a *bucket handle tear* (Figure 14.2.1) that typically cause locking due to displacement of torn portion towards the centre of the joint, and can become wedged between femur and tibia (Figure 14.2.2). The medial meniscus is more commonly injured than lateral, as it is less mobile due to its attachment to the joint capsule. Locking may start after a few days of injury and is associated with complaints of "giving way." Giving way can be caused by a mechanical block, instability from associated ligamentous injury, and is often followed by pain and swelling.

Presentation

A twisting injury during sports is a typical mechanism of injury. Patients may describe hearing a "pop." The symptoms of locking may occur immediately and are often associated with severe pain over the side of the joint. The swelling may appear some hours later or on the following day. It is important to determine whether the patient is able to continue playing sport or bearing weight immediately after the injury. If this is not possible, it implies a more severe injury, perhaps of the ligaments or bones.

Examination

The knee joint may be held in slight flexion, and there may be an effusion. There is joint-line tenderness on palpation. The range of motion is restricted and limited in extension, but full flexion can be possible. The symptoms can be intermittent, and in some chronic cases, patients are able to unlock the knee by twisting or bending the knee. Meniscal provocation tests such as McMurray's, Apley's grind, and Thessaly tests may not be appropriate due to acute pain.

ABC of Orthopaedics and Trauma, First Edition. Edited by Kapil Sugand and Chinmay M. Gupte.
© 2018 John Wiley & Sons Ltd. Published 2018 by John Wiley & Sons Ltd.

Table 14.2.1 Mechanical vs. nonmechanical causes of locked knee

	Mechanical		Non-mechanical
Soft tissues	**Loose bodies**	**Chondral and osteochondral fragments**	Due to pain after soft tissue or bony injury that is too severe to allow knee motion
Meniscus (bucket handle tear)	Detached osteophytes	Anterior tibial spine fracture	Neurological
Ruptured ACL	Synovial chondromatosis	Patella dislocation	Hysterical
		Osteochondritis dissecans (OCD)	Exaggerated pain

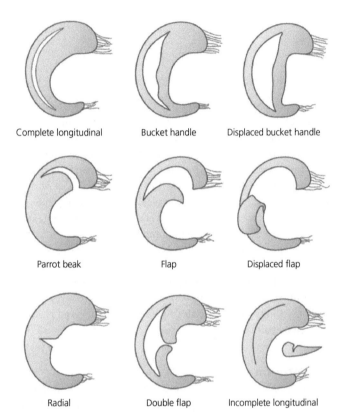

Complete longitudinal   Bucket handle   Displaced bucket handle

Parrot beak   Flap   Displaced flap

Radial   Double flap   Incomplete longitudinal

Figure 14.2.1 Meniscal tear patterns

Symptoms of acute meniscal injury

- Pain – often localised to medial or lateral joint line
- Swelling
- Locking or catching
- Giving way
- Restricted range of motion

Loose bodies

Loose bodies that move freely in the joint cavity are predisposed to being trapped between the articular surfaces, causing intermittent joint locking, limitation of motion, pain, and intra-articular effusion. Loose bodies in patients over 60 years of age are commonly derived from degenerative joint disease in the form of osteophytes. In paediatric patients, loose bodies can be from osteochondritis dissecans. Synovial osteo-chondromatosis is an uncommon condition resulting in multiple intra-articular loose bodies. Loose bodies can be removed arthroscopically.

Chondral or osteochondral fragments

Chondral or osteochondral fragments after an acute injury can also produce locking. One of the most common mechanisms is an acute patella dislocation causing a chondral fragment avulsion during dislocation or relocation. A fracture displacement involving the tibial spine may also cause a block in extension of the knee joint. The acute haemarthrosis is often a clue to the bony injury.

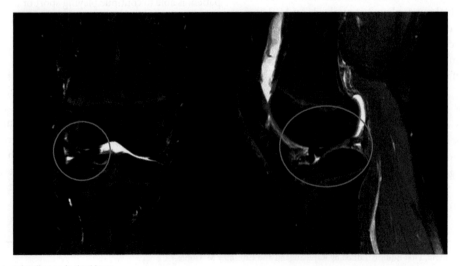

Figure 14.2.2 Meniscal tear leading to locked knee

Nonmechanical locking

Patients can also have a locked knee when they have severe pain with any knee motion. One further cause of locking is a perceived mechanical phenomenon due to patellofemoral chondral wear, degeneration, or maltracking. While this is not true, mechanical locking the patient perceives the sensation of locking, particularly after standing from a seated position after a long period or when squatting. It may be difficult for a patient to determine whether or not there is a physical block to their knee motion or if pain is the issue. A thorough physical examination can usually separate these problems from one another.

Investigation

A plain radiograph of the knee can diagnose fractures or loose bodies but is of little value for diagnosing soft tissue injuries. MRI scan is a noninvasive and reliable investigation that can detect meniscal injuries as well as associated ligamentous or osteochondral injuries responsible for locking of the knee. MRI scans are used for preoperative planning of soft tissue injuries such as meniscal pathology, and plain radiographs may be sufficient for preoperative planning in joint replacement.

Treatment

- *Nonoperative*: Treatment consists of analgesia, ice, compression, and a cricket pad splint (Figure 14.2.3). Physical therapy is required in the majority of cases. In cases of true locking, gentle passive manipulation can rarely overcome the mechanical block. Patients can also be treated with protected weight-bearing in a splint and quadriceps exercises for weeks.
- *Operative*: Treatment depends on pathology: a bucket handle meniscal tear should be treated by repair ideally or alternatively by resection of the torn segment. Arthroscopic examination and intervention is the mainstay treatment for a locked knee not responding to conservative treatment. Arthroscopic meniscal repair with a suture is reserved for young patients who have a peripheral tear with a capacity to heal in vascularised (red) zone of the meniscus (Table 14.2.2). Complications include failure to heal the tear, knee stiffness, and potential damage to articular surface. Tears in other peripheral zones (white-white) are treated with excision of torn meniscus (partial or sub-total meniscectomy) due to being more avascular and are likely to heal poorly if at all. ACL stump can be debrided, followed by delayed ACL reconstruction. Osteochondritis dissecans can be fixed back or removed.

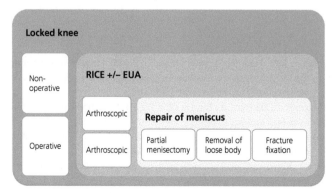

Figure 14.2.3 Treatment protocol for locked knee

Table 14.2.2 Vascular zones of the meniscus

Zone	Location	Status
Red-red	Peripheral third	Vascular
Red-white	Middle third	Avascular (in adult but vascular in child)
White-white	Central third	Avascular

Rehabilitation and follow-up

Procedures are performed as a day case and hospital stay is minimal. Patients undergoing repair of menisci usually require protected weight bearing for 4-6 weeks before being followed up in an outpatient clinic. However, patients requiring partial meniscectomy are advised physiotherapy and mobilisation as they are able immediately after surgery.

Knee dislocations

Definition

A knee dislocation is a complete disruption of the integrity of the tibiofemoral articulation resulting in a multiligament knee injury (Figure 14.2.4).

Epidemiology

It is a relatively uncommon but potentially limb-threatening injury associated with a high-energy injury mechanism. Road traffic accidents involving a dashboard injury and fall from a height are the most common presentations, and are occasionally associated with sports injuries (i.e. skiing or rugby). The majority of knee dislocations (relation of tibia to femur) are antero-posterior but can be medial or lateral (or combined). Ligamentous injuries vary, depending on the direction of dislocation. They can include ACL, PCL, PLC (posterolateral corner: e.g. LCL, popliteus, biceps femoris, iliotibial tract and lateral head of gastrocnemius), MCL, LCL or a combination.

Clinical examination

Initial assessment should be carried out according to ATLS principles. The deformity may not be obvious due to haemarthrosis, or signs of dislocation may be subtle, as most of the dislocation spontaneously reduce. The clue could be from anterior skin abrasions or bruising within the popliteal fossa. Complete neurovascular examination is mandatory. There is a significant incidence of associated vascular injury and nerve damage (common peroneal nerve). CT angiogram should be considered. Multi-ligament instability is present as a rule along with capsular damage and may lead to a compartment syndrome (Chapter 14.6).

Imaging

Plain radiographs may only demonstrate a small corner fracture of lateral tibial plateau (Segond fracture), or avulsion fracture of tibial spine or fibula. MRI scan, along with CT/MR angiogram, is usually performed to assess the extent of soft tissue damage (ACL, PCL, menisci, collateral ligaments, osteochondral fractures, and vascular injury).

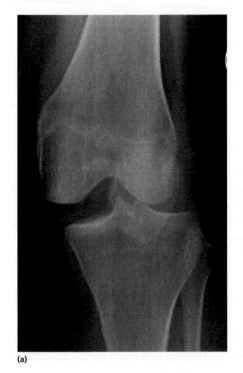

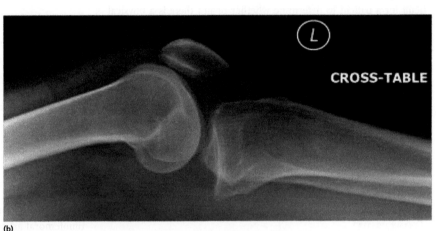

(a)   (b)

Figure 14.2.4 Radiograph showing a left dislocated knee (a) AP view and (b) lateral view

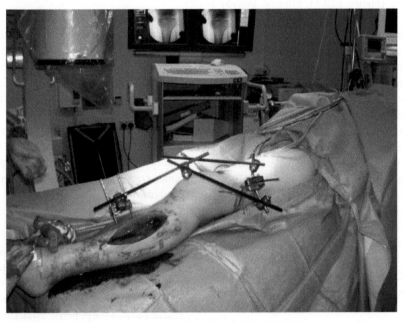

Figure 14.2.5 Fasciotomy for compartment syndrome and ExFix for knee dislocation

Management

Urgent reduction under general anaesthesia is required before the knee being assessed for stability. If stable, a POP or brace can be applied. If unstable, external fixators (temporary stabilisation) are usually the first line of treatment. In cases of absent pulses, open reduction and exploration for vascular injury is indicated (Figure 14.2.5). All ligaments can be reconstructed at the same sitting or in stages, depending on duration of procedure.

Acknowledgements

We thank Dr. Muhammad Ismail Khalid Yousaf from Shaikh Zayed Al Nahyan Hospital (Lahore) for his assistance.

Further reading

Holzer, L.A., Leithner, A., and Holzer, G. (2013). Surgery versus physical therapy for meniscal tear and osteoarthritis. *New England Journal of Medicine* 369(7): 677.

Macmull, S., Skinner, J.A., Bentley, G., et al. (2010). Treating articular cartilage injuries of the knee in young people. *BMJ* 340: c998.

Maffulli, N., Longo, U.G., Campi, S., et al. (2010). Meniscal tears. *Open Access Journal of Sports Medicine* 1: 45–54. eCollection.

Teh, J., Kambouroglou, G., and Newton, J. (2012). Investigation of acute knee injury. *BMJ* 344: e3167.

Emergency: Acute Shoulder Dislocation

Andrew Sankey and Peter Reilly

Chelsea and Westminster Hospital, London, UK

OVERVIEW

- Traumatic shoulder (i.e. glenohumeral) dislocations require a high-energy mechanism of injury and may be associated with fractures which may complicate reduction.
- Most dislocations are anterior, but posterior dislocations are easy to miss.
- Shoulder dislocations may be associated with Bankart or Hill-Sachs defects as well as axillary nerve dysfunction.
- There are numerous closed reduction techniques, the most popular being Kocher's.
- Risk of recurrent dislocation is inversely proportional with the age of the patient.

Anterior dislocation

An anterior dislocation is associated with a fall onto an abducted arm, and is easily identified on plain radiographs (Figure 14.3.1). The antero-inferior labrum becomes detached from the glenoid (Bankart lesion) and the posterior aspect of the humeral head engages on the anterior glenoid, creating an impression fracture (Hill-Sachs defect).

Reduction

If there is an associated fracture, relocation should be performed with caution so as not to further displace the fracture (Figure 14.3.2). Many techniques of reduction have been described. For example, Kocher's method of relocation is performed only after administration of adequate analgesia: longitudinal traction and counter traction are applied with the elbow flexed, followed by adduction across the chest and then internal rotation once the joint reduces. Post-op check radiographs confirms the reduction.

Posterior dislocation

Posterior dislocations are far less frequent and are all too commonly missed (up to 60%). There is an association with electric shocks and epilepsy. The patient will be in acute pain and will be

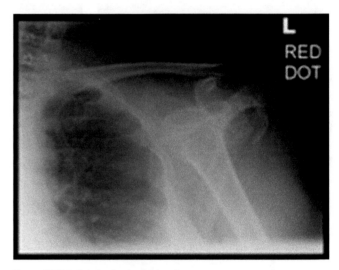

Figure 14.3.1 Anterior fracture dislocation

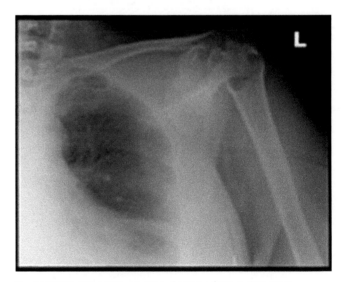

Figure 14.3.2 Attempted reduction of anterior fracture dislocation

ABC of Orthopaedics and Trauma, First Edition. Edited by Kapil Sugand and Chinmay M. Gupte.
© 2018 John Wiley & Sons Ltd. Published 2018 by John Wiley & Sons Ltd.

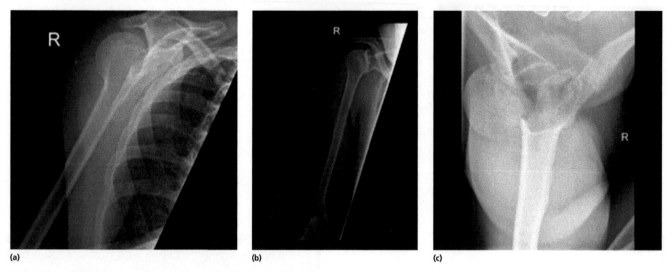

Figure 14.3.3 Radiographs showing (a) 'Y' view of posterior dislocation, (b) Light bulb sign and (c) Axial view of posterior fracture dislocation

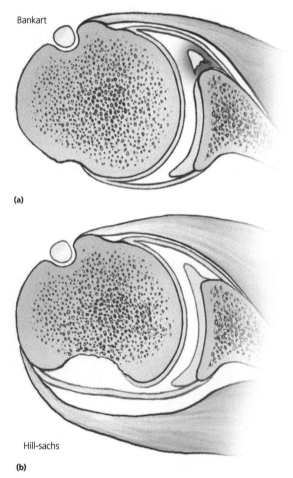

Figure 14.3.4 (a) Bankart and (b) Hill-Sachs defects

holding the arm in fixed internal rotation. Adequate plain radiographs are essential, including a GHJ view orthogonal to the glenoid and a modified axial. Lateral scapula Y views may be difficult to interpret (Figure 14.3.3a). As the arm is held in internal rotation, the humeral head has a "light bulb" appearance on the AP or GHJ view (Figure 14.3.3b). A missed dislocation may be picked up only when the patient secondarily sustains a fracture (Figure 14.3.3c).

Analogous to an anterior dislocation, there is a posterior Bankart and reverse Hill-Sachs defect (Figure 14.3.4). Relocation manoeuvres involve internal rotation to disengage the head, lateral traction and counter-traction, and an anterior force is applied to the posterior aspect of the humeral head. Once the head disengages, external rotation should be applied.

Treatment

The upper limb is then rested in a sling for several weeks, followed by physiotherapy to strengthen the surrounding musculature. In recurrent dislocations, glenohumeral instability, and chronic pain, surgical intervention may be required, including for Bankart and Hill-Sachs lesions. Operative options range from soft tissue repair, arthroscopy vs. open technique, and hemiarthroplasty vs. total shoulder arthroplasty.

Further reading

Brownson, P., Donaldson, O., Fox, M., et al. (2015). BESS/BOA Patient Care Pathways: Traumatic anterior shoulder instability. *Shoulder & Elbow* 7 (3): 214–226.

Emergency: Supracondylar Fractures of Distal Humerus in Children

Alex Shearman[1], Bassel El-Osta[2], and Neel Mohan[2]

[1] North West London rotation, London, UK
[2] St. George's Hospital, London, UK

OVERVIEW

- Common injury in children aged 5–7 years old, usually after a fall from a moderate height (trampoline, monkey-bars etc.).
- The fall is usually on a hyper-extended elbow leading to extra-articular fracture with posterior displacement of the distal fragment.
- Look out for injuries to adjacent neurovascular structures and always document your findings.
- Immediate and accurate assessment is essential to prevent chronic complications.

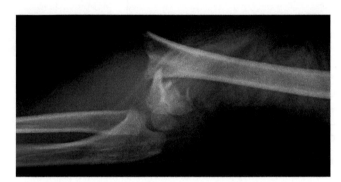

Figure 14.4.1 Gartland 3 extension type supracondylar fracture

Introduction

A supracondylar fracture is an extra-articular fracture of the distal humerus. This diagnosis incorporates a spectrum of injury, from undisplaced fractures that need nothing more than plaster immobilisation to severely displaced fractures requiring emergency exploration and stabilisation. Accurate and timely assessment of these injuries is crucial to ensuring a good outcome (Figure 14.4.1).

Relevant anatomy

The elbow is a complex hinge composed of the humero-ulnar, radio-capitellar, and proximal radio-ulnar joints (Figure 14.4.2). The brachial artery lies antero-medial to the distal humerus. The median nerve, derived from the medial and lateral cords of the brachial plexus, courses with the brachial artery before passing between the two heads of pronator teres and gives off the anterior interosseous nerve (AIN). These structures are at risk in supracondylar fractures with apex-anterior angulation (extension-type). The radial nerve passes from the lateral aspect of the distal humerus anterior to the lateral epicondyle. The ulnar nerve derives from the medial cord and passes on the medial side, underneath the medial epicondyle of the elbow. It is particularly important when considering surgical fixation.

Clinical assessment

History

Supracondylar fractures are most common in children aged 5–7 years. Males are more commonly affected. Classically children will present with a painful swelling and clinical deformity following a fall onto an extended arm.

Examination

Ensure that this is an isolated injury by using a systematic approach to examine the patient (e.g. *ATLS*® principles), particularly in cases involving high energy or where the history is unclear.

Move on to examine the upper extremity. This is often difficult in a distressed patient. Swelling can be significant, and meaningful examination of the elbow is therefore difficult.

The priorities are to examine (and document) the following:

- *Neurovascular status of the limb distal to the injury.* Examine both radial and ulnar pulses. Look at the hand for pallor and assess the perfusion by measuring the capillary refill time in the fingers. Use a saturation probe if there is any doubt. Examination of the nerves can be easily tested by asking the patient to make an 'OK' sign (anterior interosseous [AIN]/median nerve); 'thumbs up' sign (posterior interosseous/radial nerve); and spread out/cross

ABC of Orthopaedics and Trauma, First Edition. Edited by Kapil Sugand and Chinmay M. Gupte.
© 2018 John Wiley & Sons Ltd. Published 2018 by John Wiley & Sons Ltd.

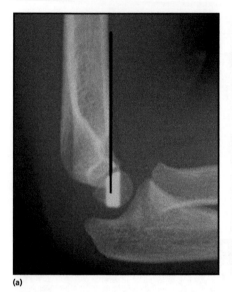
(a)

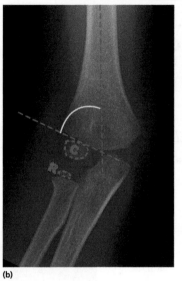
(b)

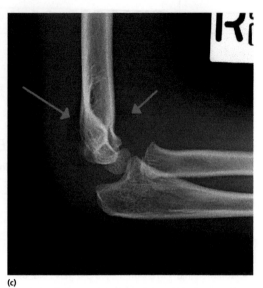
(c)

Figure 14.4.2 (a) anterior humeral line, (b) Baumann angle and (c) anterior and posterior fat pads

Table 14.4.1 Modified Gartland classification of supracondylar fractures

Classification	Description
1	Undisplaced
2 (a)	Angulated in extension/flexion with intact periosteal hinge WITHOUT rotational displacement on AP view
2 (b)	Angulated in extension/flexion with intact periosteal hinge WITH rotational displacement on AP view
3	Off-ended, complete separation of fracture ends

their fingers for the 'lucky' sign (ulnar nerve). Sensory neurological examination involves assessment of light touch sensation in the autonomous regions of the hand. The AIN does not have a sensory component.

- *Muscular compartments.* Compartment syndrome must be excluded. Significant swelling and tense forearm compartments should raise suspicion. Passive flexion and extension of the digits should be assessed for disproportionate severity of pain.
- *Soft tissues around the elbow.* Assess the soft tissues for signs of open injury. Record the sites and size of swelling and bruising. Specifically, look in the antecubital fossa for signs of puckering, which may indicate soft tissue involvement at the fracture site and therefore may predict a difficult reduction.

Imaging

This normally consists of radiographs only. AP and lateral views are obtained to identify and classify the injury (Figure 14.4.1).

Supracondylar fractures can be subdivided into flexion-type (5%) and extension-type (95%). The Gartland Classification (Table 14.4.1) has become a popular method of classifying these injuries and is relatively straightforward.

Radiographic indices to aid diagnosis in less displaced fractures include:
1 Anterior humeral line is a line drawn on the lateral view from the anterior cortex of the humeral diaphysis distally. It will normally intersect the capitellum (Figure 14.4.2a).

2 Baumann's angle is between the axis of the humerus and the growth plate of the capitellum. This normally measures about 60–80° (Figure 14.4.2b).
3 Presence of a posterior fat-pad and exaggerated anterior fat-pad (sail) sign on lateral radiograph may aid diagnosis in undisplaced fractures. An anterior fat-pad is usually normal (Figure 14.4.2c).

Management

Undisplaced (type 1) and angulated fractures without rotation (type 2a) can normally be managed successfully with above elbow immobilisation. A plaster backslab is applied with the elbow at 90° flexion. Check and document neurovascular status and take repeat radiographs after applying the plaster.

Angulated fractures with rotation (type 2b) and off-ended fractures (type 3) will normally require manipulation and open or percutaneous fixation. These fractures should be managed urgently because reduction becomes progressively more difficult as swelling increases.

Two golden rules of supracondylar fractures:
1 A pulseless, white hand associated with a supracondylar fracture should immediately go to theatre.
2 A compartment syndrome should immediately go to theatre.

In a small number of cases, the hand is clearly perfused but pulses cannot be felt – the *pink, pulseless hand.* These patients should be operated on urgently. If there is any doubt as to the perfusion of the limb (increasing pain, development of neurological dysfunction), then these should be taken to theatre immediately. Use of continuous pulse oximetry can help to monitor any reduction in perfusion.

If vascular involvement is suspected, a vascular surgeon must be involved early on. Whilst the brachial artery is often compressed or tethered by the fracture/soft tissue and blood flow can be restored by closed means, there are instances when exploration of the antecubital fossa may be indicated. Vascular repair is sometimes necessary.

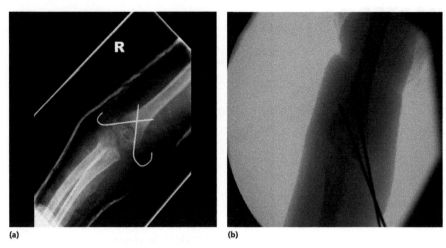

Figure 14.4.3 Examples of different wiring techniques: (a) crossed and (b) divergent K-wires

Technique of closed reduction

Reduction should be done in theatre with the patient under anaesthetic and with real-time fluoroscopy.

Deformities are corrected sequentially:
1 In-line traction is applied gently with appropriate counter traction (either directly or using a sheet) *to restore length.*
2 With traction still applied, any valgus/varus and rotation is corrected to *restore AP alignment.*
3 The elbow is *flexed* with pressure from the thumb over the posterior aspect of the olecranon process.
4 The reduction is *locked* by pronating the forearm.

Reduction can sometimes be blocked by soft tissue interposition. If this is the case, it may be necessary to open the fracture site and retrieve this. Following successful reduction the skeleton needs to be stabilised. This is normally achieved through open or percutaneous wire fixation. This is performed either by passing K-wires in a crossed fashion from each epicondyle across the fracture site (Figure 14.4.3) or divergent wires from the lateral epicondyle across the fracture site. There is a risk of ulnar nerve injury when passing a wire medially, and it is therefore good practice to make a mini-incision on the medial side and identify the nerve prior to passing the wire.

In the case of compartment syndrome fasciotomy should be performed. The patient is then placed in an above-elbow plaster and neurovascular observations are made at regular intervals postoperatively.

Further reading

British Orthopaedic Association. (2015). British Orthopaedic Association Standards for Trauma (BOAST 11): Supracondylar fractures of the humerus in children. www.boa.ac.uk/wp-content/uploads/2015/01/BOAST-11.pdf

Carson, S., Woolridge, D.P., Colletti, J., et al. (2006). Pediatric upper extremity injuries. *Pediatric Clinics of North America* 53 (1): 41–67.

Gartland, J.J. (1959). Management of supracondylar fractures of the humerus in children. *Surgery, Gynecology, and Obstetrics* 109: 145–154.

Roberts, S.B., Middleton, P., and Rangan, A. (2012). Interventions for treating supracondylar fractures of the humerus in children. *Cochrane Database of Systematic Reviews* 10: CD010131.

Wilkins, K.E. (1984). Fractures and dislocations of the elbow region. In Rockwood, C.A., Wilkins, K.E., King, R.E., eds. *Fractures in Children*, 3rd ed. JB Lippincott Co. 363–575.

Williamson, D.M., Coates, C.J., Miller, R.K., et al. (1992). Normal characteristics of the Baumann (humerocapitellar) angle: an aid in assessment of supracondylar fractures. *Journal of Pediatric Orthopedics* 12 (5): 636–639.

CHAPTER 14.5

Emergency: Septic Arthritis

James Donaldson and Jonathan Miles

Royal National Orthopaedic Hospital, Stanmore, UK

Introduction

Septic arthritis is defined as inflammation of the synovial membrane with purulent effusion into the joint capsule and is caused by bacteria within the joint space. The use of antibiotics has virtually eliminated mortality, but permanent joint damage may result if it is not treated within 24–48 hours. There are approximately 20,000 cases per year in the United Kingdom, with *S. aureus* being the commonest cause (approximately 70%).

Aetiology

Sources of infection include:
- Direct inoculation from a penetrating wound, surgery or aspiration
- Spread from adjacent infection or abscess
- Haematogenous spread from a distant site

Predisposing factors include rheumatoid arthritis, immuno-compromise, advanced age, chronic debilitating conditions, and intravenous drug abuse.

The joints commonly affected are labelled in Figure 14.5.1.

Pathology

The normal joint does have protective components with some phagocytic and bactericidal activity. However, a synovial joint is highly vascular and has no basement membrane to act as a barrier to microbes. In addition, previously damaged joints may demonstrate neovascularisation and have increased adhesion factors, making them more susceptible to infection. The organism crosses the synovial membrane and the acute inflammatory cascade is initialised. As pus appears in the joint, destructive enzymes within the exudate begin to erode the articular cartilage. In the early stages, this process is reversible. Within the next 24–48 hours, marked synovial proliferation, infiltration by mononuclear cells, and granulation tissue develop and permanent damage may ensue.

Microbiology

Figure 14.5.2 outlines the common pathogens causing septic arthritis.

Clinical features

The classical presentation is of an acutely hot and swollen joint with systemic signs of infection. It may differ according to the age of the patient. In the newborn, the emphasis is on septicaemia rather than joint pain; in children and adults, the typical features often include:
- Severe pain, which is worse with any degree of movement
- Fever, malaise, and systemic signs of sepsis
- A red, hot, and swollen joint with an effusion

Kocher criteria apply to children with painful joint (Table 14.5.1). In the immunocompromised, a high index of suspicion is needed, as there may be few systemic symptoms and signs.

Investigations

- White cell count is raised, CRP and ESR.
- Blood cultures may be positive.
- Radiographs may help in excluding other causes.
- Ultrasound is useful and an aspiration can be performed at the same time, especially for deeper joints like the hip.
- Synovial fluid examination is the gold standard:
  ○ A white cell count greater than 50,000 per mL is usually suggestive of infection.

Differential diagnoses

- Acute osteomyelitis. The two may coexist in young children – the treatment is the same.
- Trauma: synovitis or haemarthrosis.
- Irritable joint (the child will be systemically well).
- Crystal monoarthropathy.
- Haemophiliac bleed.

Management

Treatment may be started as soon as an aspirate is taken. The principles are similar to acute osteomyelitis.
- Supportive treatment with IV fluids, analgesia, and splintage
- Surgical drainage and washout is standard in the United Kingdom. This is usually an open procedure. A further washout may be needed if symptoms do not settle within 24–48 hours

ABC of Orthopaedics and Trauma, First Edition. Edited by Kapil Sugand and Chinmay M. Gupte.
© 2018 John Wiley & Sons Ltd. Published 2018 by John Wiley & Sons Ltd.

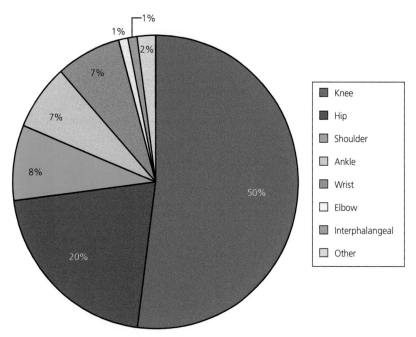

Figure 14.5.1 Common sites of septic arthritis

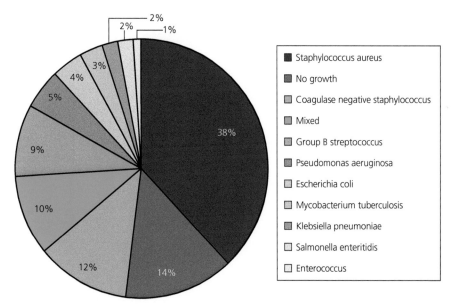

Figure 14.5.2 Common pathogens causing septic arthritis

Table 14.5.1 The Kocher criteria for a child with a painful hip include

- raised ESR (>40 mm/hr)
- raised white cell count (>12,000 cells/µL)
- inability to bear weight
- pyrexia (>38.5 °C)

4 of the criteria are 99% sensitive for septic arthritis; 3 are 93% sensitive; 2 are 40% sensitive; and 1 is 3% sensitive. Recent research has also included CRP.

- Antibiotics: Initially, best-guess broad-spectrum intravenous antibiotics are started, and are changed when microbiological sensitivities are known. Intravenous antibiotics may be converted to oral antibiotics once signs of sepsis have resolved and then continued for 6 weeks. The timescale is controversial and may be shorter or longer, depending on the response.

Prognosis

- 30% of adults with septic arthritis are left with reduced ROM or chronic pain post infection.
- Bone destruction and dislocation (especially the hip) may occur.
- Cartilage destruction may lead to ankylosis or secondary osteoarthritis.
- Growth disturbance and deformity occur in children.
- Predictors of poor outcome include:
  ○ Age >60 years
  ○ Infection of hip or shoulder joint

- ◦ Underlying rheumatoid arthritis
- ◦ Positive findings on synovial fluid cultures 7 days after starting antibiotics
- ◦ Delay in treatment

Further reading

Bulstrode, C., Wilson-MacDonald, J., Eastwood, D.M., et al. (eds.) (2011). *Oxford Textbook of Trauma and Orthopaedics*, 2nd ed. Oxford University Press.

Green, D.P. (2001). *Rockwood and Green's Fractures in Adults*. Lippincott Williams & Wilkins.

Osmon, D.R., Berbari, E.F., Berendt, A.R. et al. (2013) Diagnosis and management of prosthetic joint infection: Clinical practice guidelines by the Infectious Diseases Society of America. *Clinical Infectious Diseases* 56 (1): 1–10.

Solomon, L., Warwick, D., and Nayagam, S. (2001). *Apley's System of Orthopaedics and Fractures*. Hodder Publishing.

CHAPTER 14.6

Compartment Syndrome

Ahsan Sheeraz

Barts Health NHS Trust, London, UK

OVERVIEW

- Compartment syndrome is an orthopaedic emergency that can threaten the viability of a limb and is largely due to crush injury.
- The diagnosis is clinical, but compartment pressures can be measured to exclude the diagnosis.
- The mainstay treatment for acute cases is surgical with a fasciotomy of all limb compartments.
- Compartment syndrome can occur in both closed and open long-bone fractures.
- Management guidelines have been included in British Orthopaedic Association Standards for Trauma (BOAST) guideline 4.

Introduction

Compartment syndrome is a potentially limb-threatening complication that occurs due to increased pressure in any osseofascial compartment. Each compartment is bound by bone or fascia and contains muscles, nerves, and blood vessels. While it can occur in any compartment, it is most common in the leg.

Definition

Compartment syndrome is defined as an increase in pressure in an osseofascial compartment that leads to a compromise in blood supply to that part of the limb.

Pathophysiology

If not diagnosed promptly, the increased pressure within the compartment will lead to necrosis of the muscles due to ischaemia and loss of function of the nerve contained within the compartment. There is a vicious cycle (Figure 14.6.1) that continues to increase the pressure. The injury (open or closed fracture, tight cast, crush injury, rhabdomyolysis etc.) sets off the inflammatory cascade

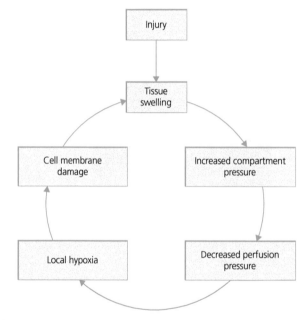

Figure 14.6.1 Vicious circle: Pathophysiology of compartment syndrome

that leads to swelling followed by increased compartmental pressure, then reduced venous return and decreased perfusion pressure, and tissue hypoxia from compression of arteries leading to necrosis, which then perpetuates further inflammation and tissue swelling.

Diagnosis

The diagnosis is clinical, with the patient complaining of severe pain on passive movement, refractory to strong analgesia (e.g. morphine), tense musculature, and paraesthesia. Late complications include paralysis and pallor with loss of distal pulses. If clinical diagnosis cannot be made, as would be the case in an unconscious patient, then devices (arterial lines and epidural catheters) can

---

ABC of Orthopaedics and Trauma, First Edition. Edited by Kapil Sugand and Chinmay M. Gupte.
© 2018 John Wiley & Sons Ltd. Published 2018 by John Wiley & Sons Ltd.

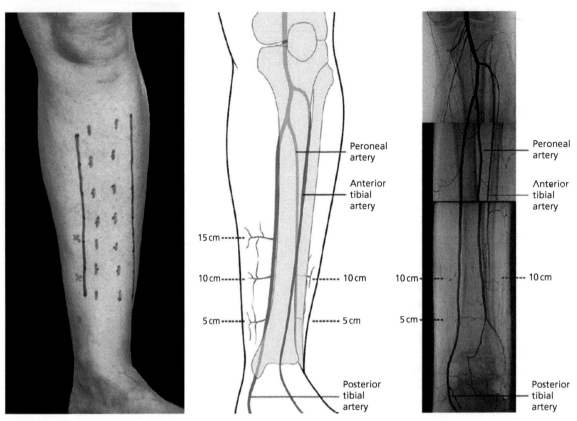

Figure 14.6.2 Sites of fasciotomy incisions in the leg and its compartments

be utilised on the bedside to measure the pressures within the compartment to confirm the diagnosis.

> Quantitative diagnosis can be made by the following:
> **i** If intracompartmental pressure (normally <10 mmHg) exceeds 30 mmHg, or there is a 20 mmHg pressure difference for over 4 hours
> **ii** Differential (delta) pressure measurement is more accurate (i.e. diastolic blood pressure – intracompartmental pressures) falls below 30 mmHg
> **iii** Threshold pressures are lower and are approximately 15–20 mmHg for the hand

Treatment

Once the diagnosis has been made, then patient needs to be taken to theatre immediately and the compartments decompressed with the help of fasciotomies (Figure 5.14). This involves cutting open the skin, fat, and the facial layers to allow all the collected blood to escape out, releasing the pressure off the neurovascular bundle within the compartment. The British Orthopaedic Society (BOA) has issued guidelines (BOAST 4) on management of compartment syndrome and where to make the fasciotomy incisions (Figure 14.6.2 and Figure 5.14).

Further reading

British Orthopaedic Association (2009). British Orthopaedic Association Standards for Trauma guideline 4. The management of severe open lower limb fractures. Available at www.boa.ac.uk/wp-content/uploads/2014/12/BOAST-4.pdf

von Keudell, A.G., Weaver, M.J., Appelton, P.T., et al. (2015). Diagnosis and treatment of acute extremity compartment syndrome. *Lancet* 386 (10000): 1299–1310.

CHAPTER 14.7

Emergency: Cauda Equina Syndrome

Syed Aftab and Robert Lee

Royal National Orthopaedic Hospital, Stanmore, UK

OVERVIEW

- Cauda equine syndrome is a constellation of symptoms including uni/bilateral leg pain, saddle anaesthesia, urinary/bowel/erectile dysfunction, and lower-limb weakness.
- Look out for "red flags" to confirm the clinical diagnosis before obtaining radiological evidence with a MRI.
- Causes include disc retropulsion (commonest), trauma, malignancy, or infection.
- Critical window of opportunity for surgical decompression is within 48 hours before prognosis becomes poor, leading to paralysis, bowel and bladder incontinence, and sexual dysfunction.
- Patients presenting with red flags need to be referred to the local spinal unit with access to MRI and an on-call spinal team led by orthopaedic or neurosurgeons.

Back pain is one of the most common presentations to the primary care physician and emergency department. The economic burden of back pain in terms of its management and lost days in employment is vast. A logical approach is necessary for effective management. Furthermore, while the majority of back pain can be treated with simple analgesics and physiotherapy, it is important to identify those individuals who may benefit from surgery or in whom surgery may be required as an emergency measure to prevent permanent functional impairment.

An assessment of back pain begins with history and examination. Mode of onset (acute, traumatic, or gradual), duration of symptoms, and associated symptoms are all important. It is important to assess whether the pain is isolated to the back (mechanical back pain) or radiates distally (sciatica). A neurological examination along with a digital rectal examination is also necessary.

Red flags are features in history and examination that would suggest that urgent specialist assessment is required for potential spinal cord or cauda equina compromise. Cauda equina syndrome occurs when there is compression to the neural structures in the cauda equina. Herniated nucleus pulposus is the most common cause, but other causes include trauma, malignancy, metastatic disease, or infection. This is a surgical emergency that ought to be confirmed by urgent MRI (Figure 12.6). Without urgent decompressive surgery, there is a high risk of permanent loss of bowel and bladder continence and paralysis of lower limbs, rendering a patient wheelchair bound. Return of bladder/bowel, motor, and sexual function is better if surgery is undertaken within 24 hours of presentation, but the outcome is much poorer if intervention is delayed beyond 48 hours.

Red flags

- Urinary retention
- Bowel or bladder incontinence
- Saddle paraesthesia or anaesthesia
- Loss of anal tone
- Motor weakness (such as foot drop)
- Fever
- History of malignancy or unexplained weight loss

Other features in the history – such as severe intractable pain, intravenous drug use, immunosuppression, or steroid use – may be relevant.

The duration of onset and nature of symptoms would guide whether an emergency referral is required. For symptoms that are acute in onset with any of these red flags, emergent referral is necessary to the local spinal team. Symptoms that have been ongoing for months or years are unlikely to require emergent attention.

ABC of Orthopaedics and Trauma, First Edition. Edited by Kapil Sugand and Chinmay M. Gupte.
© 2018 John Wiley & Sons Ltd. Published 2018 by John Wiley & Sons Ltd.

Further reading

Ahn, U.M., Ahn, N.U., Buchowski, J.M., et al. (2000, June 15). Cauda equina syndrome secondary to lumbar disc herniation: a meta-analysis of surgical outcomes. *Spine* (Philadelphia, Pa, 1976). 25 (12): 1515–1522.

Heyes, G., Jones, M., Verzin, E., et al. (2018, February). Influence of timing of surgery on Cauda equina syndrome: Outcomes at a national spinal centre. *Journal of Orthopaedics* 15 (1): 210–215.

Hussain, M.M., Razak, A.A., Hassan, S.S. et al. (2018, April). Time to implement a national referral pathway for suspected cauda equina syndrome: review and outcome of 250 referrals. *British Journal of Neurosurgery* 2: 1–5.

Srikandarajah, N., Wilby, M., Clark, S. et al. (2018 February). Outcomes reported after surgery for cauda equina syndrome: A systematic literature review. *Spine* (Philadelphia, Pa, 1976).

CHAPTER 15

Orthopaedic Procedures

Simon Mordecai[1] and Jacqueline Waterman[2]

[1] North West London Rotation, London, UK
[2] Hillingdon Hospital, London, UK

OVERVIEW

- A safe stepwise approach should be followed for all orthopaedic procedures.
- For joint injections, aseptic technique must be followed to avoid introducing infection.
- Palpate and mark bony landmarks before injecting or aspirating joints.
- Plan all surgical approaches carefully.
- Beware of the surrounding anatomy and the nerves and blood vessels that may enter a surgical field.

Joint injection and aspiration

Joint aspiration is a commonly performed procedure in orthopaedics providing an important diagnostic tool for evaluating red, hot, painful, swollen joints. It can also be used therapeutically to relieve pain caused by a tense effusion. Joint injections usually steroids or local anaesthetic are used to relive pain and inflammation in joints. Caution should be taken on patients with coagulopathy or on anticoagulant treatment. The risk of bleeding should be weighed against the potential benefit of the injection or aspiration. Joint injections/aspirations should not be performed through cellulitic skin owing to the risk of seeding the infection. In patients with joint prosthesis, the procedure should be performed in a sterile environment to minimise the risk of infecting the metalwork. Complications are outlined in Table 15.1.

Procedure

A systematic approach should be followed for all joint injections/aspirations as described in Table 15.2.

Common injection sites and landmarks
Subacromial bursa (Figure 15.1)
Indicated for
- Rotator cuff tendonopathy
- Rotator cuff tears
- Bursitis
- Impingement

Landmarks
1 Palpate the posterior posterolateral edge of the acromion.
2 Insert the needle 1 cm below.
3 Advance the needle aiming slightly upwards under the acromion into the subacromial bursa.
4 Inject the steroid and local anaesthetic whilst slowly retracting the syringe.

Acromioclavicular joint (Figure 15.2)
Indicated for
- Acromioclavicular joint arthritis

Landmarks
1 Palpate the clavicle laterally until a slight depression is felt where it meets the acromion.
2 Inject steroid and local anaesthetic into the joint from a superior anterior (almost perpendicular) approach.

Lateral epicondyle (Figure 15.3a)
Indicated for
- Lateral epicondylitis – tennis elbow

Landmarks
1 With the elbow flexed to 90°, palpate the lateral epicondyle.
2 Inject perpendicular to the skin until the periosteum.
3 Withdraw the needle 1–2 mm and inject slowly.
4 Peppering technique is most beneficial.
5 Withdraw and inject at multiple points over the lateral epicondyle.
6 Elbow joint: aim for the space between an inverted triangle consisting of lateral epicondyle, radial head, and olecranon (Figure 15.3b).

Carpal tunnel (Figure 15.4)
Indicated for
- Carpal tunnel syndrome

Landmarks
1 Identify the palmaris longus tendon by opposing the thumb and little finger with the wrist in neutral.
   a If no tendon is present, identify the midline of the wrist.

ABC of Orthopaedics and Trauma, First Edition. Edited by Kapil Sugand and Chinmay M. Gupte.
© 2018 John Wiley & Sons Ltd. Published 2018 by John Wiley & Sons Ltd.

2 The needle is inserted just proximal to the wrist crease between the tendons of flexor carpi ulnaris and palmaris longus or in the midline of wrist.

3 The needle should be at 30° to the skin and directed towards the ring finger.

  a Advance the needle 1.5–2 cm and aspirate first before injecting.

  b Inject local anaesthetic, initially ensuring there is no resistance and there is no shooting pain.

  c Leave the needle in situ and change the syringe to inject the steroid.

Table 15.1 Complications of joint injections and arthrocentesis

- Infection
- Bleeding
- Pain
- Intravascular injection
- Fat atrophy – particularly with repeated steroid injections
- Tendon damage – avoid injecting directly onto a tendon
- Skin discolouration

Table 15.2 Procedure for joint injection/aspiration

1. Patient should be on the examination table at the correct height with the appropriate joint fully exposed.
2. Ensure the skin over the joint is intact with no active infection.
3. Palpate bony landmarks and identify the correct insertion site.
4. Clean the skin with betadine or chlorhexidine spray.
5. Wear sterile gloves and prepare the needle and syringe using aseptic nontouch technique.
6. Insert the needle into the designated joint and either inject (steroids and local anaesthetic) or aspirate.
   - Local anaesthetic to anaesthetise the skin may be used prior to the injection/aspiration.
7. Dispose of the sharps appropriately.
8. Cover insertion site with a dressing.
9. If fluid is aspirated, make a note of the colour and consistency of the aspirate before sending it to the microbiology lab for further analysis.

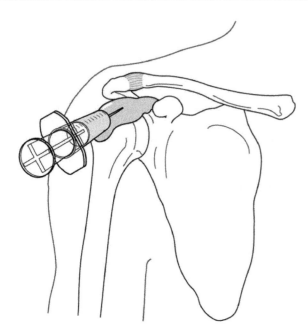

Figure 15.1 Subacromial bursa injection site

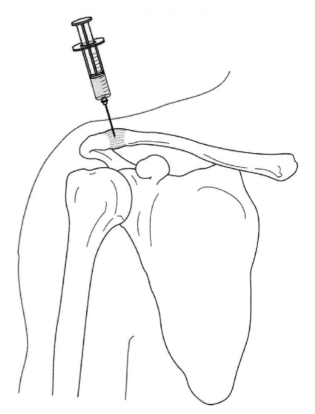

Figure 15.2 Acromioclavicular joint injection site

Wrist (Figure 15.5)

Indicated for
- Septic arthritis

Landmarks

1 Palpate the soft spot 1 cm distal to Lister's tubercle on the dorsum of the wrist, between ECRB and EPL tendons radially, and EDC ulnarly.

2 Insert the needle in a dorsal to volar direction, with a 10° proximal inclination.

3 A give is felt as the joint is entered and aspirate fluid.

Knee joint (Figure 15.6)

Indicated for
- Osteoarthritis
- Septic arthritis
- Crystal arthropathy
- Diagnostic and therapeutic (offloading) reasons

Landmarks

1 Sit the patient on the edge of the examination table with the knee flexed to 90°.

2 Palpate the patella tendon and identify the soft spots either medial or lateral to the tendon (lateral approach is preferred).

3 Advance the needle in either of the soft spots aiming towards the intercondylar notch. The typical dose is 40–80 mg methylprednisolone mixed with 10 mL 1% lignocaine.

Ankle (Figure 15.7)

The safest approach is anterolateral followed by anteromedial approach.

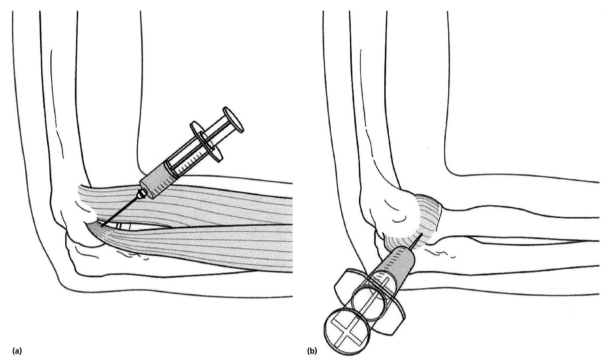

(a)

(b)

Figure 15.3 Elbow injection sites: (a) lateral epicondyle and (b) elbow joint

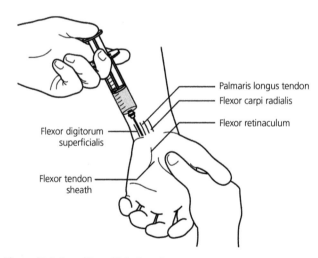

Palmaris longus tendon
Flexor carpi radialis
Flexor retinaculum
Flexor digitorum superficialis
Flexor tendon sheath

Figure 15.4 Carpal tunnel injection site

Indicated for
- Septic arthritis
- Crystal arthropathy

Landmarks
Anterolateral
1 Palpate the distal tip and anterior border of the fibula.
2 Insert the needle approximately 5 mm medial to the anterior fibula, 3 cm proximal to the tip where a soft spot can be felt.
3 Inject in a posteromedial direction and proximal inclination.
4 A give is felt as the joint is entered and aspirate.
Anteromedial
1 Palpate the soft spot just medial to the tibialis anterior tendon and lateral to the medial malleolus, 3 cm proximal to the tip.

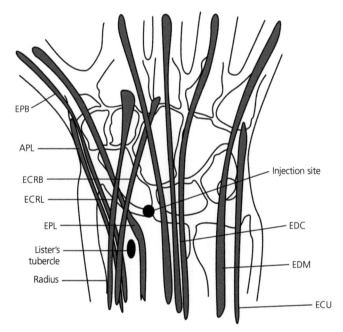

EPB
APL
ECRB
ECRL
EPL
Lister's tubercle
Radius
Injection site
EDC
EDM
ECU

Figure 15.5 Relationship of dorsal wrist tendons to carpus and appropriate site for injection or aspiration of wrist joint: APL, abductor pollicis longus; EPB, extensor pollicis brevis; ECRL, extensor carpi radialis longus; ECRB, extensor carpi radialis brevis; EPL, extensor pollicis longus; EDC, extensor digitorum communis; EIP, extensor indicis proprius; EDM, extensor digiti minim; ECU, extensor carpi ulnaris

2 Insert the needle in a posterolateral direction and proximal inclination.
3 A give is felt as the joint is entered and aspirate.

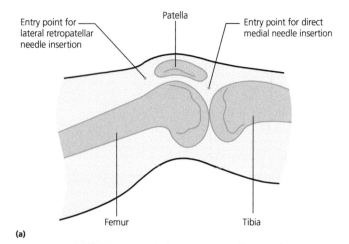

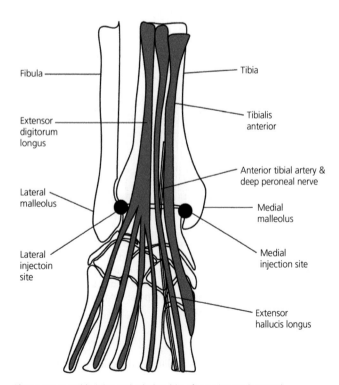

(a)

(b)

Figure 15.6 Knee joint (a) injection entry site and (b) synovial fluid aspiration

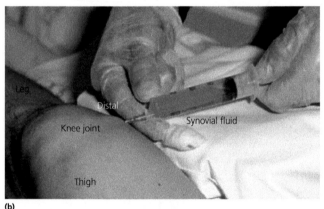

Figure 15.7 Ankle joint and relationship of anterior tendons and anterolateral and anteromedial injection or aspiration sites

Common orthopaedic surgical approaches

Shoulder arthroscopy

Arthroscopy of the shoulder has a number of indications. Accurate examination of the shoulder, together with radiographic imaging such as ultrasound or MRI scans, means diagnostic arthroscopies are rarely performed.

Arthroscopic interventions include:
- Subacromial decompression for impingement
- Biceps tenotomy for chronic tendonitis
- Capsular release for frozen shoulder
- Rotator cuff repairs for acute rotator cuff tears
- Glenoid labrum stabilisation for instability
- Acromioclavicular joint excision for osteoarthritis

The patient should be placed supine in the beach-chair position (sitting up at around 60°). The operative shoulder should be off the table to allow access to the posterior part of the joint. Arm traction can be used in some cases to allow better access to the subacromial space. Although numerous portals have been described, the most common are the posterior viewing portal together with the anterior instrumentation portal. For the posterior portal, palpate the posterolateral tip of the acromion and make a stab incision 2 cm inferior and 1 cm medial (Figure 15.8). The trocar should be directed anteriorly towards the coracoid process and pass between the teres minor and infraspinatus muscles. The anterior portal is made under direct vision from the posterior viewing portal with the aid of a needle. It should be made halfway between the tip of the coracoid process and the anterior edge of the acromion. The trocar is inserted under vision splitting the pectoralis major and deltoid muscle.

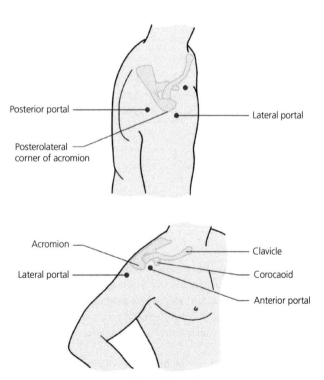

Figure 15.8 Shoulder arthroscopic portal sites

Knee arthroscopy

Knee arthroscopy is one of the most commonly performed orthopaedic procedures. Surgical advances have led to an increased number of indications that were previously performed using open procedures.

Arthroscopic interventions include:
- Meniscal repair or resection
- Anterior or posterior cruciate ligament reconstruction
- Microfracture for osteochondral defects
- Debridement for early osteoarthritic changes
- Removal of loose bodies
- Synovectomy for inflammatory conditions

The patient should be placed supine on the operative table with a thigh tourniquet to minimise bleeding. A leg support should be placed on the side on the table at around the level of the tourniquet. Valgus stress can then be applied against the support giving better access to the medial tibiofemoral compartment.

After prepping and draping the leg, ensure that it is free to flex and extend as these movements will be required to gain access around the joint. The two ports most commonly used are the anterolateral viewing portal and the anteromedial instrumentation portal (Figure 15.9). The anterolateral portal is created first. Flex the knee to 90° and palpate the soft spot between the lateral tibial plateau, the lateral edge of the patella tendon, and the lateral femoral condyle. Make a stab incision through the skin, patella retinacula, and the joint capsule. Insert the trocar with knee flexed, aiming for the intercondylar notch of the femur. Then extend the knee and continue to advance the trocar in to the suprapatella pouch. The anteromedial portal is made in the anteromedial soft spot between medial tibial plateau, medial edge of patella tendon, and medial femoral condyle. The incision is made under direct vision of the medial tibiofemoral compartment through the anterolateral viewing portal. This avoids damage to the medial meniscus or articular cartilage. Occasionally, a superomedial accessory portal is made for water outflow, which can help to give a clearer picture within the joint.

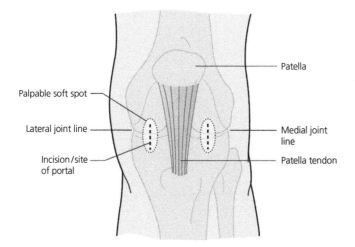

Figure 15.9 Knee arthroscopic portal sites

Labels in figure: Patella; Palpable soft spot; Lateral joint line; Incision/site of portal; Medial joint line; Patella tendon

Approach to hip joint

The anterolateral, direct lateral, and posterior approaches to the hip are the most common for performing hip hemiarthroplasty or total hip replacements. For the anterolateral approach, the patient is best positioned laterally on the operative table with the affected side up. Front and back supports should be used to ensure the pelvis is supported perpendicular to the table.

Palpate the tip of the greater trochanter and the shaft of the femur. Make a 10 cm longitudinal incision centred over the tip of the greater trochanter in line with the femoral shaft. Superficially dissect the skin and subcutaneous fat to expose the fascia lata. Incise the fascia lata in line with the skin incision and apply retractors to hold open the fascia. Excise the trochanteric bursa to expose the attachment of the hip abductors (gluteus medius and gluteus minimus) to the greater trochanter. Deep dissection involves dissection of the anterior two-thirds of the abductors off the greater trochanter. Be sure to leave a cuff of tissue to aid closure. The joint capsule can then be excised or divided to expose the femoral head and neck.

Approach to knee joint

The medial parapatella approach is a common approach used to gain access to the knee joint and provides enough exposure for total knee arthroplasty. The patient should be supine with a side support and a sandbag to support the knee in 90° of flexion. Palpate the midline of the patella and the tibial tubercle. A midline longitudinal incision should be made, starting 6–12 cm proximal to the superior pole of the patella, extended over the midline of the patella ending just on the medial border of the tibial tubercle. Superficial dissection involves dividing the subcutaneous fat and superficial retinaculum to expose the quadriceps tendon, the medial border of the patella, and the medial border of the patella tendon. Deep dissection involves a proximal incision through the midline of the quadriceps tendon, continued distally to the superior pole of the patella. The incision is then curved along the medial border of the patella and then distally along the medial aspect of the patella tendon to the tibial tubercle. Care should be taken to leave a cuff of tissue on the medial patella to aid closure. Flip the patella laterally with the knee extended and flex the knee to 90° to expose the knee joint.

Carpal tunnel decompression

Open carpal tunnel decompression is indicated in patients with carpal tunnel syndrome in which conservative measures such as splinting or steroid injects have failed.

The procedure is usually performed under a local anaesthetic. The technique previously described can be used for the carpal tunnel block. However, only local anaesthetic should be injected and no steroid. Typically, 5 mL of 1% lignocaine mixed with 5 mL of 0.5% bupivacaine is used for infiltration. Alternatively 1:200,000 adrenaline can be mixed with 0.5% bupivacaine so that no tourniquet is required.

After the local anaesthetic block is applied, the patient should be positioned supine with hand on an arm board with appropriate prep and drape. Landmarks should be drawn to ensure a safe incision, avoiding nerves and arteries in the hand (Figure 15.10).

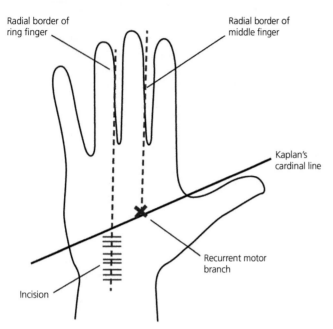

Figure 15.10 Surface anatomy of the palm of the hand and landmarks used for carpel tunnel surgery

- Distal wrist crease – marks the proximal end of incision
- Radial border of the ring finger – marks the direction of the longitudinal incision
- Kaplan's cardinal line – marks the distal end of incision
  - An oblique line is marked from the apex of the inter-digital fold between the thumb and index finger distally towards the ulna side of the palm, passing 4–5 mm distal to the pisiform.

- Danger zones:
  - **Distally**: an incision made distal to this line risks damaging the *superficial palmar arch* arteries.
  - **Radially**: The *recurrent motor branch of the median nerve* is found at the intersection of Kaplan's line with a line drawn along the ulna border of the middle finger.
  - **Proximally**: The *palmar cutaneous branch of the median nerve* usually traverses superficially over the carpal tunnel and originates 5–6 cm proximally to the distal wrist crease.

- The incision is made from the distal wrist crease in line with the radial border of the ring finger distally towards Kaplan's line. Dissect through the skin and longitudinal fibres of the palmar fascia. Use ragnell retractors to sweep away any fat. Expose the transverse fibres of the transverse carpal ligament. Ensure an adequate view of the ligament by readjusting the retractor deeper into the wound. Divide the transverse carpal ligament under direct vision using the ragnell retractor to ensure adequate proximal and distal release. This should be to the fat pad distally and to 1.5 cm of proximal forearm fascia. The median nerve should be visualised. Ensure adequate haemostasis and close the wound with interrupted nylon sutures.

Further reading

Hoppenfeld, S., deBoer, P., and Buckley, R. (2009). *Surgical Exposures in Orthopaedics: The Anatomic Approach*. USA: Lippincott Williams & Wilkins.

CHAPTER 16

Prevention and Postoperative Care

Ahsan Sheeraz

Barts Health NHS Trust, London, UK

OVERVIEW

- Good postoperative care helps to minimise complications such as pressure sores, DVT, pain, and chest and urinary sepsis.
- By undertaking an MDT approach of avoiding falls in elderly patients and carrying out prophylaxis for osteoporosis, we can minimise the chance of patients developing fractures and avoiding unnecessary hospital admissions, surgery and its complications.
- Complications occurring after trauma surgery can be grossly divided into immediate, early, and late complications and also into local or general categories.

Fragility fractures of the hip

Background

The National Hip Fracture Database (NHFD) is a clinically led, web-based quality improvement initiative that is managed by the Royal College of Physicians, all 182 eligible hospitals in England, Wales, and Northern Ireland take part in this by submitting data. The NHFD is now the largest hip fracture database in the world and have devised their own protocol (Figure 16.1).

The Department of Health introduced Best Practice Tariff (BPT) in 2010 (Table 16.1). BPT in simple words is an additional financial reward for a hospital that is achieving all the given criteria in the management of a hip fracture patient. BPT for hip fracture care was one of the first payments by results to be paid on an individual patient basis (currently £1,335 per patient).

The BPT has clearly changed how we manage hip fracture patients over the last few years. There is emphasis on improving overall package of care, by concentrating more on prevention of falls and bone protection to minimise incidence of fractures. In addition, there is a focus on improving postoperative care using enhanced recovery programmes to enhance the patient experience and decrease complications and overall length of stay in hospital.

Falls assessment and prevention

In June 2013, NICE issued guidelines (CG 161) for prevention of falls in elderly patients. They advised to identify elderly patients who had falls in the last year or those elderly patients at risk of falling. These at risk patients then need a multi-factorial falls risk assessment (Table 16.2).

Once such an assessment has been done, these patients should be offered an individualised multifactorial intervention program that should include strength and balance training, vision assessment and referral, and medication review with modification of hazards at home. It is also imperative to involve the patient in this program to gauge their motivation, undergo the balance training and take appropriate bone protection if needed.

Identification and treatment of osteoporosis
Definition

The World Health Organization describes osteoporosis as a "progressive systemic skeletal disease characterised by low bone mass and micro architectural deterioration of bone tissue, with a consequent increase in bone fragility and susceptibility to fracture" (Figure 16.2).

Epidemiology

In the United Kingdom, nearly 200,000 fractures occur each year due to osteoporosis, costing the NHS over £1.73 billion. Approximately one in three women and one in five men will suffer from an osteoporotic fracture in their lifetime. The most common site for these fractures is in the vertebral bodies, hip and distal radius, respectfully. Risk factors are outlined in Table 16.3.

Investigations

Dual-energy X-ray absorptiometry (DEXA) scan applied to the femoral neck to measure its bone mineral density (BMD) is the investigation of choice. In addition to its diagnostic use, this scan provides information on prognosis (i.e. the likelihood of future fractures). Osteopaenia is a milder disease but is on the same spectrum.

ABC of Orthopaedics and Trauma, First Edition. Edited by Kapil Sugand and Chinmay M. Gupte.
© 2018 John Wiley & Sons Ltd. Published 2018 by John Wiley & Sons Ltd.

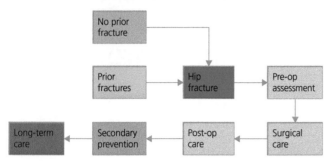

Figure 16.1 Various stages of care in hip fracture surgery (courtesy NHFD)

Table 16.1 Criteria for BPT

The criteria set out for BPT were adopted from the National Institute for Health and Care Excellence (NICE) guidelines, the management of hip fracture in adults (QS16). These include:
1 Surgery within 36 hours of admission
2 Shared care by surgeon and geriatrician
3 Admission using a care protocol agreed by geriatrician, surgeon, and anaesthetist
4 Assessment by geriatrician within 72 hours of admission
5 Pre- and postoperative abbreviated mental test score (AMTS) assessment
6 Geriatrician-led multidisciplinary rehabilitation
7 Secondary prevention of falls
8 Bone health assessment

Table 16.2 Falls risk assessment

1 Assessment of the patient's history of falls along with patient's gait, balance, and mobility
2 Risk of osteoporosis
3 Assessment of visual and cognitive impairment
4 Assessment of medical co-morbidities (e.g. urinary incontinence and cardiovascular causes of falls)
5 Identification of home hazards

Management

Conservative: Supportive measures may be considered before initiating pharmacological treatment for osteoporosis. These include prevention of falls and prolonged immobilisation, as that causes bone loss. Improving the patient's nutritional status by increasing intake of a high-protein diet, along with calcium and vitamin D3–rich foods, has been shown to reduce fracture risk in elderly patients.

Medical: Pharmacological treatment can be initiated (in conjunction with supportive measures). Drug options include bisphosphonates, strontium, hormone replacement therapy, Raloxifene, Teriparatide, and Denosumab. The National Osteoporotic Guideline group have recommended the use of bisphosphonates. These are analogues of inorganic pyrophosphate and inhibit bone resorption.

Alendronate is approved for the prevention and treatment of postmenopausal, glucocorticoid-induced, and male osteoporosis. Bisphosphonates, however, need to be used with care, and patients need to be monitored for rare but serious complications of oesophagitis, mandibular osteonecrosis, and atypical fractures (especially of the femur) that heal poorly. It must be taken on an empty stomach and in an upright position.

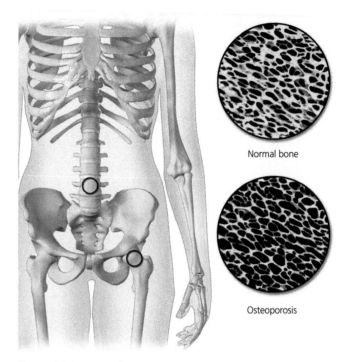

Figure 16.2 Osteoporosis

Table 16.3 Risk factors for fractures independent of age and BMD

Risk factor	Effect
1 BMI (Body mass index)	A low BMI increases risk of hip fractures.
2 History of previous fracture	In osteoporotic area the re-fracture risk nearly doubled.
3 Parental history of hip fracture	Largely independent of BMD.
4 Smoking	In part, effect is dependent on BMD.
5 Steroid use	Other factors are also involved, apart from bone loss.
6 Alcohol use	Intake of 3+ units increases risk of fracture.
7 Rheumatoid arthritis	Risk increases due to multiple factors, including drugs.

Complications in postoperative recovery

It is worth noting that approximately half of all patients suffering a hip fracture can no longer live independently, and one in three will die within a year of the fracture. So it is imperative to work as part of the MDT team to provide optimal postoperative care to prevent complications (see Tables 16.4 and 16.5).

Short-term complications would include the complications associated within the initial 24 hours after surgery; medium-term would include the complications within days to weeks after surgery; and long-term complications would be the ones beyond this period.

The following sections discuss immediate, short-, medium-, and long-term complications.

Table 16.4 Complications of fractures

Time frame	General	Specific
Immediate (<24 hours)	Fat embolus	Neurovascular injury Muscle/tendon injury Haemorrhage/haemarthrosis
Immediate to early *(24 hr < x < 30 days)*	Myocardial infarction Shock Stroke	Compartment syndrome
Early **(<30 days)** ***Early to late*** *(30 days < x > 30 days)*	DVT/PE Infection (UTI, pneumonia)	Poor wound healing and dehiscence Cellulitis and abscess Osteomyelitis Contractures Stiffness
Late **(>30 days)**	Prolonged immobility (stiffness, pressure sores)	Nonunion/malunion Degenerative change/ osteoarthritis Reflex sympathetic dystrophy (i.e. Sudeck's atrophy) – now referred to as chronic regional pain syndrome (CRPS) Avascular necrosis Growth disturbance Disuse osteopaenia/muscle atrophy

Table 16.5 Preventative measures of possible postoperative complications

Postoperative complications	Preventative measures
Anaemia	Monitor haemoglobin, MCV, and clotting function.
Biochemical imbalance	Monitor urea and electrolytes, thyroid function, liver function and bone profile.
Chest infection or atelectasis	• Monitor inflammatory markers (WCC and CRP) and radiographic changes. • Assess cardiorespiratory function by listening to the chest and checking the pulse daily. • Chest physiotherapy and breathing exercises. • Regular nebulisers if wheezy. • Effective analgesia.
Atrial fibrillation and cardiac events	• Check central pulses daily for regular rhythm. • Treat reversible causes like sepsis hypertension and ischaemic heart disease. • Monitor serial troponins and ECGs in chest pain.
Wound infection	Monitor surgical wound, keeping it dry and changing wet dressings.
Urosepsis	• Aseptic urinary catheterisation. • Removal of catheter as soon as mobilising.
Constipation	• Physiotherapy and mobilising • Regular laxatives • Encourage oral hydration
DVT	• Physiotherapy and mobilising • TED stockings and heparin
Delayed recovery	• Enteral nutritional support • Physiotherapy and mobilising • Effective analgesia

Immediate complications

Internal and external haemorrhage

It is well known that fractures can cause significant blood loss. For open fractures after pressure dressings have been applied, the limb should be splinted. It is worth noting that even closed fractures can bleed sufficiently into the compartments before the patient shows signs of hypovolaemic shock, and such patients need to be fluid-resuscitated as per ATLS principles. Patient can lose up to 1–1.5 litres of blood in an isolated closed femur fracture. The use of tranexamic acid, control of clotting function, and pressure dressings can be applied to manage oozing wounds.

Electrolyte imbalance

This can be caused due to the initial tissue damage due to the trauma and later again by the "second hit" from the surgery. Monitor lactate level (an indicator of anaerobic metabolism) and correct electrolyte levels (mainly sodium and potassium).

Nerve injury (also refer to Chapter 22 on peripheral nerve injury)

Nerve injury can result from direct trauma or due to surgery. Nonsurgical closed neurological trauma without vascular compromise does not need urgent surgical exploration unless the nerve is trapped in the fracture fragments (e.g. wrist drop from radial nerve palsy due to distal humeral shaft fractures). Often, patients will develop relatively less serious symptoms like paraesthesias, which can be monitored expectantly. Most will improve in 6 months; for the ones that do not improve, nerve conduction studies and MRI are indicated. If the nerve injury is a result of surgery – for example, a foot drop due to sciatic nerve injury after hip surgery – even this needs to be investigated and patient needs to be returned to the theatre to deal with the likely cause (e.g. haematoma evacuation or severed nerve requiring repair).

Early/medium-term complications

Postoperative infections

Postoperative infections are one of the most challenging complications after surgery. They can be broadly divided into superficial and deep infections.

Diagnosis

Superficial infection is common and pertains to an infected wound or surrounding skin (which appears red, swollen, and may be oozing). Wound swabs can isolate the pathogen and dictate which antibiotic to use. Infections normally manifest 7–10 days postoperatively.

Deep infections, on the other hand, take longer to develop and require longer treatment with antibiotics and surgical washouts. Subtle signs include delayed or nonunion of fracture and persistent pain at fracture site. Most patients present as being systemically unwell (fevers, rigours, sweating, and vomiting). They will have raised inflammatory markers (CRP, ESR, neutrophil count).

The radiological changes often lag behind the clinical picture, and clinicians should not be misled by normal appearance of plain radiographs. MRI scanning helps in diagnosis. Having metalwork in situ presents an additional challenge, as bacteria secretions make it less susceptible to antibiotics. If the fracture has united, then the metalwork would need to be removed and the wound must be thoroughly washed out and debrided, followed by antibiotics to "eradicate" the infection. However, if the fracture has not united, then antibiotics are required merely to suppress infection to allow more time for the bone to heal before the decision to remove the metal can be made.

Prevention

Antibiotic prophylaxis at induction of anaesthesia should be routinely considered to reduce the incidence of postoperative infections. During surgery using aseptic technique, careful soft tissue handling and thorough lavage with warm saline have all been shown to reduce infection risk.

Treatment

If infection has been established, then it is imperative to start treatment with empirical broad-spectrum antibiotics after taking relevant tissue swabs and blood cultures. Once the culture and sensitivities have been identified, empirical antibiotics should be switched to narrow-spectrum antibiotics. Antibiotics are often given intravenously (e.g. PICC line) for 6–12 weeks to fully eradicate the infection. Compliant patients may be suitable for outpatient antibiotic therapy (OPAT) and can be discharged home for the district nurse to administer the antibiotics once or twice a day.

Medical complications (respiratory, urinary, cardiovascular, etc.)

The NHFD has stressed the importance of an ortho-geriatrician being part of the MDT looking after the patient postoperatively in hip fracture surgery. However, the basic principles behind these practices hold for all postoperative patients, which is to be able to prevent and identify potential medical complications before they develop (Table 16.5).

Pressure sores and ulcers
Background

Pressure sores and pressure ulcers are injuries to skin and underlying tissue resulting from prolonged pressure on the skin. Bedsores most often develop on the skin that covers the bony areas of the body, such as the ankles, heels, and sacrum.

Elderly patients who are not very mobile and bed- or wheelchair-bound are susceptible to developing them. Other risk factors include diabetes, steroid use, smoking, poor health and nutritional status, urinary or bowel incontinence and dry skin. Apart from the pain and healing issues, the main risk is infection, especially if the ulcers are deep with exposed tendons or bone (Figure 16.3).

Diagnosis

Diagnosis of pressure sores is clinical and wound swabs are required if infected.

Prevention

This can be achieved by repositioning the patient in bed after every few hours during their inpatient stay. Using supports like gel pads, cushions, and air mattresses to prevent pressure on bony prominences is an important part of the prevention strategy. Applying dressings, keeping wounds clean and dry, as well as keeping patients well nourished with a high-protein diet should be used routinely.

Treatment

If conservative and supportive measures of wound care fail with input from the tissue viability team, then surgical debridement followed by tissue cover (e.g. skin grafts, tissue flaps, synthetic grafts etc.) are required.

Thromboembolic events: Deep vein thrombosis (DVT) and pulmonary embolism (PE)
Background

This is potentially a life-threatening complication, and often presents 3–5 days after surgery (Figure 16.4). DVT often occurs in the calf due to venous stasis, and such a clot may dislodge into the blood stream causing a PE, which can be fatal. Risk factors include immobility, surgery, past history or family history of thromboembolism, oral contraceptive pill, smoking, obesity, pregnancy, or cancer.

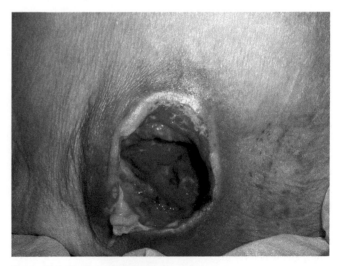

Figure 16.3 Grade 4 pressure sore

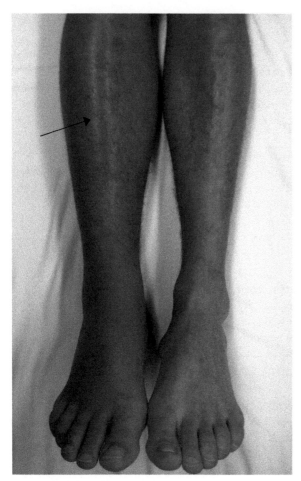

Figure 16.4 Right leg DVT

Prophylaxis

Thromboembolic deterrent (TED) stockings on the ward and pneumatic compression foot pumps (Flowtron) during surgery are routinely used. Pharmacological agents consist of anti-platelets (aspirin) and anti-coagulants (heparin and warfarin) and are chosen to balance the risk of bleeding versus the risk of venous thromboembolism.

Diagnosis

A high index of suspicion should be raised if the patient has calf pain, erythema, or dependent oedema and there is tenderness over the course of the deep veins. However many patients can have all these signs even after routine surgery, so diagnosis may be confirmed by a duplex ultrasound scan. D-dimers will give a falsely positive figure, which can be raised secondary to surgery, so do not measure it postoperatively. PE will classically present with acute shortness of breath and pleuritic chest pain. Signs include sinus tachycardia on the ECG, desaturating on air while being tachypnoeic, and respiratory alkalosis on ABG in the early stages from hyperventilating before decompensating. The gold standard for imaging consists of CT pulmonary angiogram (CTPA).

Treatment

Therapeutic doses of heparin should be started while warfarinising the patient before hospital discharge with follow-up in the anticoagulation clinic.

Compartment syndrome

Compartment syndrome is an orthopaedic emergency as it is limb threatening and can lead to long-term disability if not managed early or appropriately. The problem here is that the osseofascial compartment pressure of a limb exceeds its perfusion/microcirculatory pressure, leading to musculoskeletal (and neural) ischaemia, followed by necrosis, which could lead to limb contracture (i.e. Volkmann contracture). Diagnosis is clinical, and treatment is a fasciotomy of all limb compartments with examination of the musculature. For more information, refer to Chapter 5.

Late/long-term complications

Joint stiffness
Background

This is a common complication and, broadly speaking, happens due to poor surgical treatment and prolonged immobilisation.

Prevention

To avoid stiffness, anatomical intra-articular reduction of fracture is needed. Also avoid splinting of joints and, where possible, start early mobilisation and physiotherapy. The elbow joint and small joints of hands develop stiffness very quickly within a few weeks of immobilisation of casts.

Management

To manage stiffness, physiotherapy is required, and if it fails, then surgery is required to revise the fixation or to break adhesions within the joint.

Delayed union, malunion, and nonunion
Prevention

Definitions related to bone union are outlined in Table 16.6. All three conditions are challenging and can be prevented by good surgical technique, respecting the blood supply to the bone, and minimal soft tissue handling. Apart from surgical factors, certain patient factors (e.g. diabetes, smoking, immunosuppression, and steroidal use) can contribute to these conditions.

Diagnosis

Plain radiography and CT scan can help confirm the diagnosis if there is any doubt.

Table 16.6 Definitions relating to bone union

Delayed union	Union fails to occur in the expected time.
Nonunion	Fracture fails to unite and there are radiological changes, which suggest that this situation will be permanent – can be either atrophic (suboptimal biological environment for healing) or hypertrophic (mechanical instability).
Malunion	A fracture unites in a less-than-anatomical, "malaligned" position.

Treatment

There is no single best treatment option for this condition. Treatment must be tailored individually to the patient, keeping multiple factors in mind, which include managing the patient's risk factors, presence or absence of infection, and the blood supply to the particular bone involved. For instance, nonunion of scaphoid fracture is best managed with revision surgery using bone graft and screw fixation, whereas a nonunion or malunion of a clavicular fracture hardly ever needs treatment, as most patients are asymptomatic and surgical risks outweigh the functional benefits.

Complex regional pain syndrome (CRPS)
Background

Complex regional pain syndrome is a group of conditions associated with increased pain after trauma surgery due to irritation of the local sympathetic nerve supply. The cause of this condition is unknown and the neurology does not fit in with a particular peripheral nerve distribution.

Natural history

While it causes significant disability to the patient, for a majority of patients the condition is self-limiting and improves over 4–12 months.

Treatment

Neuroleptic drugs and sympathetic blockage can be used as adjuncts in patients who fail to improve. Aggressive physiotherapy is often required to prevent restriction of movements.

Avascular necrosis (AVN)
Background

Avascular necrosis is the necrosis of bone due to interference in its blood supply. The most commonly affected bones from this condition are the scaphoid, lunate, head of femur (Figure 16.5), and talus

after fracture due to the retrograde nature of the blood supply to these bones.

Diagnosis

Diagnosis is clinical as the patient presents with persistent pain in the affected area. Radiographic confirmation of diagnosis is late, but a MRI is more sensitive and specific.

Treatment

Treatment is challenging, and most methods are faced with failure. There is a chance that in some conditions revascularisation may take place, but this can take up to 18 months. Once AVN is well established, then it may well lead to secondary osteoarthritis, and at that stage, the options are either excision of the dead bone fragment or joint replacement.

Heterotopic ossification

This was previously known as myositis ossificans. In simple words, this is additional calcification in soft tissues close to a joint after surgery. It leads to restriction of movement and pain due to its mechanical affect. It commonly appears around the elbow and hip joint.

Prophylaxis

Prophylaxis includes radiation therapy or indomethacin for 1–2 weeks.

Treatment

Treatment is in the form of surgical excision of the calcific deposits; however, early surgery almost always leads to recurrence, so it should be carried out 6–12 months after the heterotopic ossification has started. Following surgery, further radiation or indometacin treatment is required to prevent recurrence, which is common.

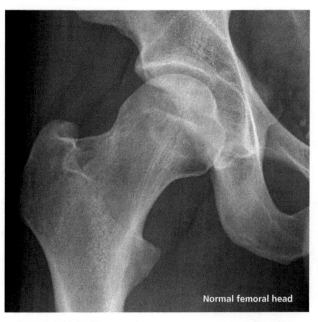 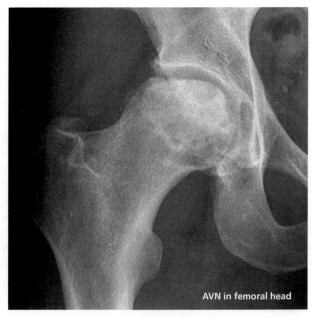

Figure 16.5 Right hip AVN

Metalwork complications including protrusion, irritation, and dislocation of prosthesis
Background
While use of metalwork has revolutionised orthopaedic surgery, it does come with its problems. When used around bones that are easily palpable in the body, like the patella, olecranon, and the ankle, there are often patient complaints of the metalwork being protuberant, easily felt, and irritable to touch. This can be best managed by removal of the metalwork once union has taken place months later.

Common problems
Other problems include broken metalwork, which happens due to loading, and implant fatigue in the case of nonunion. Removal of broken metal can be often challenging and lead to even higher complications, so careful planning, surgical skill, and image guidance are required to retrieve it from the patient.

Metalwork in arthroplasty
Metalwork also presents a different challenge when it is used to replace joints, such as in the case of hip arthroplasty. Patients must follow specific hip precautions to avoid dislocating their joint. Recurrent dislocations are one of the most common causes of revision hip surgery, and all efforts should be made to educate the patient to prevent joint dislocation. This is most likely to occur in the first few weeks after surgery but can happen later as well. There is a shelf life with hip prostheses too, so aseptic loosening after a decade will lead to pain on full weight-bearing and difficulty in standing up from a sitting position.

Surgical approach
A lateral approach to the hip joint can cause the prosthesis to dislocate anteriorly with a leg being short and externally rotated, whereas a posterior approach can dislocate the prosthesis posteriorly with a short internally rotated leg.

Precautions after joint replacement
The surgeon, nurse, and the physiotherapists educate patients; often they are provided with leaflets with written hip precautions to follow. An example is provided in Table 16.7.

Table 16.7 Precautions to protect hip

In order to prevent a dislocation, please follow these instructions:
1 Sit in high armchairs and use a high toilet seat (approx. 24 inches high).
2 Raise your bed to about 24 inches by placing an extra mattress or blocks under its feet.
3 Do not bend the hip more than 90°.
4 Do not cross your knees.
5 When in bed, keep a pillow between your knees.
6 To reach your foot, bring your knee outwards and the foot inwards, so that you see the inner part of your thigh, knee, and leg. If you cannot reach your foot easily, do not force it.
7 If you have to pick up objects from the floor, lean on a piece of furniture.
8 Do the exercises to strengthen the muscles of your hip. Start doing them standing, slowly, gently, a few minutes in the morning and in the evening. The exercises should not hurt. Increase the number of repetitions as tolerated. Once they become easy, you can also do them lying down in bed, which demands a greater effort.

Treatment
In case of a dislocated prosthesis, a full history and examination is required to assess what prosthesis has been implanted and through which approach. Time since surgery and number of times the dislocation has taken place needs to be accounted for. Involvement of sciatic nerve is a key finding, and if involved, patient needs to be taken to the theatre for a reduction of the prosthesis back into joint. This can be either closed or open. If joint dislocation reoccurs, then the patient needs revision surgery.

Further reading

Beaupre, L.A., Jones, C.A, et al. (2005). Best practices for elderly hip fracture patients. A systematic overview of the evidence. *Journal of General Internal Medicine* 20 (11): 1019–1025.

National Hip Fracture Database (NHFD) at www.nhfd.co.uk/2014report

NICE (2013, June). Falls: assessment and prevention of falls in older people.

National Osteoporosis Guidelines Group. (2014, November). *Osteoporosis: Clinical Guideline for Prevention and Treatment*, www.shef.ac.uk/NOGG/ NOGG_Executive_Summary.pdf.

NICE guidelines (CG161), https://www.nice.org.uk/guidance/cg161.

CHAPTER 17

Osteoarthritis

Alexander L. Dodds and Dinesh Nathwani

Imperial College Healthcare NHS Trust, London, UK

OVERVIEW

- Osteoarthritis (OA) refers to a clinical syndrome of joint pain accompanied by varying degrees of functional limitation and reduced quality of life.
- OA is primarily noninflammatory (as opposed to rheumatoid) and involves loss of articular cartilage.
- Radiological findings include **LOSS**: (i) **L**oss of joint space, (ii) **O**steophytes, (iii) **S**ubchondral sclerosis, and (iv) **S**ubchondral cyst formation.
- Treatment involves many modalities, including analgesia, exercise, functional aids, and surgery.
- Surgical options range from realignment osteotomy and replacement of all or part of the joint.

Introduction

Arthritis is one of the most common diseases in the Western world, and its prevalence will increase as the age of the population increases, combined with an increase in obesity. Patient expectations of treatment are also increasing, with a trend towards earlier intervention in the disease process to keep the individual active for as long as possible. The disease therefore has a significant impact on the health care and wider economy.

The most common type of arthritis is OA or degenerative joint disease. It is a chronic, progressive musculoskeletal disorder characterised by gradual loss of articular cartilage, according to the World Health Organisation (WHO). OA refers to a clinical syndrome of joint pain and stiffness accompanied by varying degrees of functional limitation and reduced quality of life. It is the most common disease affecting joints.

Prevalence

Prevalence of OA is high and increases with age, with a systematic review of the literature finding a prevalence of 43% for osteoarthritis of the hand, 24% for OA of the knee, and 11% for OA of the hip.

Due to the high number of cases and chronic nature of the condition, it causes a substantial financial burden on the NHS.

Aetiology

OA is not a single disease but a complex disorder with multiple risk factors, divided into genetic factors, constitutional factors, and local biomechanical factors (Table 17.1).

Genetic risk factors

Genetic risk factors can influence risk factors for OA, such as obesity, skeletal shape, bone mass, and synovitis. Twin studies have shown an apparent genetic influence in the development of OA, and after adjustment the heritability has been calculated at 60% for hip osteoarthritis and 39% for knee OA. There is also evidence that there can be a genetic predisposition to pain sensitivity.

Constitutional risk factors

Trauma is an important risk factor for OA. Incongruity of the articular surface after trauma (both surgical and nonsurgical) is known to lead to an increased rate of OA development. Body habitus also contributes significantly to OA development, particularly in weight-bearing joints, with obesity being identified as a major risk factor. The increase in obesity rates throughout the Western world is likely to significantly increase the burden of OA.

Biomechanical risk factors

Abnormal biomechanics, particularly in the lower limbs, can lead to abnormal wear pattern in joints and OA development. A good example of this is the varus knee, which leads to increased wear of the medial compartment of the knee. Another example is misalignment and poor anatomical reduction due to suboptimal surgical management of a fracture. Thus, it is important when assessing an osteoarthritic joint in an individual to assess the overall alignment of the limb rather than concentrate on just the specific joint.

ABC of Orthopaedics and Trauma, First Edition. Edited by Kapil Sugand and Chinmay M. Gupte.
© 2018 John Wiley & Sons Ltd. Published 2018 by John Wiley & Sons Ltd.

Table 17.1 Nonmodifiable risk factors for development of OA

Age	Gender	Ethnicity	Obesity	Family history

Table 17.2 Important issues to address when taking a history

Pain	Associated symptoms (e.g. stiffness, locking, giving way)	History of trauma	Childhood conditions (e.g. septic arthritis, malalignment)
Other joints affected (inflammatory)	Previous investigations	Treatments tried	Functional disability

History

OA usually affects larger mono-articular joints. Pain is often the major presenting symptom of OA, but other severe debilitating symptoms may also be present. The onset of symptoms is often insidious, and they can worsen over a period of weeks, months, or years. The functional effect of pain on the patient needs to be thoroughly assessed. It can have a detrimental effect on the overall quality of life, causing problems such as inability to sleep, concentrate, and continue with a daily routine. OA in the younger patient can lead to inability to work, and can have a significant economic effect on both the individual and the community as a whole. Due to the high prevalence of the disease, this leads to a significant problem in the Western world. Pain at rest or at night can either indicate severe symptoms due to OA or red flag pathology such as infection or tumour.

Stiffness of joints is another common complaint, with patients having difficulty initiating movement, for example, when moving from a seated position after a prolonged position. Loss of motion of the joint may also be noted, and this may be described by the patient in practical terms, on a spectrum of finding it difficult to use stairs to buttoning one's shirt. Pain and stiffness, often worse in the morning, can occur with OA but may indicate an inflammatory condition such as rheumatoid arthritis.

The history must also focus on contributing factors to the patient's condition (Table 17.2), including previous trauma or surgery to the joint or surrounding area, as well as an overall assessment of the medical and social circumstances. A careful discussion of what the patient hopes to achieve with any form of intervention, in particular surgical, is also essential to meet realistic expectations and rehabilitation goals.

Examination

This must include an overall assessment of the patient's health. Other disease processes may be important if surgery is to be undertaken, such as the presence of systemic disease (e.g. diabetes, cardiorespiratory disease that may affect anaesthesia, or the presence of infection from skin ulcers). Careful neurovascular assessment and range of movement of the limb and their documentation are also crucial pre- and post-operatively.

A thorough examination of the joint itself is essential to ensure that any surgical intervention will bring success. Identification of the exact site of the patient's pain is paramount. Typical findings during the examination will include tenderness on palpation of the joint, swelling in or around the joint, auditory or palpatory crepitus on movement, and loss of function, often seen as a loss of range of movement in the joint. Assessment of the alignment of the whole limb to look for biomechanical problems must be undertaken. The joints proximal and distal to the joint under review should also be carefully assessed, to look for any sources of referred pain (e.g. knee pain stemming from hip pathology).

Investigations

The diagnosis of OA will normally be obvious after the health care practitioner has taken a careful history and examination. Investigations can be used to confirm the diagnosis, but are also a useful adjunct to confirm the degree of severity of joint involvement. Plain film radiographs are the most affordable and accessible form of imaging available (Figure 17.1). Weight-bearing films will be more sensitive in showing osteoarthritic change.

Other imaging modalities may be useful. CT can reveal bony abnormalities in a 3D plane. This is ideal for more complex bony articulations, and is commonly used in guiding foot and ankle surgery. CT scans can also be used to image bony abnormalities such as the cam deformity seen in early hip OA. MRI has also become more widely used in recent years, and is particularly useful in the early stages of the disease process, for example to assess meniscal tears in the knee or labral tears in the hip. Surgical interventions are now targeted at an earlier stage in the disease process, with a trend towards more minimal surgery, may be best planned with MRI.

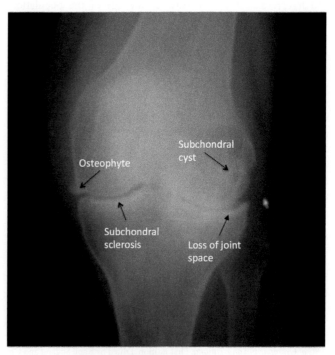

Figure 17.1 Radiological signs of knee OA

Treatment options

Conservative interventions

Treatment options can be thought of as nonsurgical (conservative and medical or pharmacological) or surgical. There is an increasing focus on early and nonsurgical interventions in the primary care setting with the aim of disease prevention and slowing down progression (Table 17.3). Modification of risk factors like weight reduction is one example of this. Simple advice for symptom management may include the use of physiotherapy in some cases, use of analgesia, use of bracing and walking aids, activity modification, intra-articular injections, and psycho-social interventions to make patient expectations of the disease process realistic and manageable.

Medical intervention

Pain relief is often the only interim treatment of OA before surgery becomes the last resort. It is important to titrate analgesia up according to the WHO analgesia ladder to reduce dependency and the side effect profile. The most common painkillers include a combination of oral and topical nonsteroidal anti-inflammatory drugs (NSAIDs) including COX-2 inhibitors, paracetamol, and opioids such as codeine and tramadol.

Minimally invasive interventions

Interventions can also be used with investigations. The use of contrast dye, local anaesthesia, corticosteroid, or hyaluronan injections into the joint via ultrasound or radiography are commonly used, particularly in the foot and ankle surgery. This can be a useful way of identifying local anatomy and the source of the patient's pain.

Arthroscopy

Arthroscopy (Figure 17.2) has been used to the early stages of OA but is now reserved for specific associated pathology that coexists with OA. Specific indications include locking, and giving way in the presence of loose bodies or displaced meniscal tears. It involves inserting a camera into the joint using a mini-surgical approach for both diagnostic and therapeutic indications. In some cases, the procedure is diagnostic, with the aim to assess the severity of the disease process before further interventions are carried out. Arthroscopy can also be used to alter the disease process, with debridement and washout of the diseased joint as a therapeutic intervention. Its main use is in the improvement of mechanical symptoms. However, advances in treatment options mean that reconstruction of structures destroyed as part of the disease process are also possible – for example, the use of allograft menisci in knee joints. Albeit historically used in advanced OA, this practice is diminishing due to lack of evidence and efficacy.

Major surgery

OA is one of the most common indications for surgery, and this has a high cost implication for the NHS. There is an increasing demand

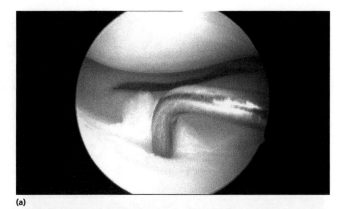
(a)

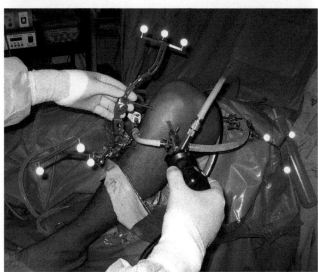
(b)

Figure 17.2 (a) Knee arthroscopy – probe examination showing a tear in the anterior horn of lateral meniscus (b) Knee arthroscopy – external view

with which health care systems are currently struggling with the cost implications of an ageing population to find effective and durable interventions.

Arthroplasty/joint reconstruction

Arthroplasty is one of the most widely performed surgical procedures. Its aim is to either partially or totally replace the native and diseased joint with an artificial joint. The UK National Joint Registry for reports over 80,000 hip and 84,000 knee replacements (Figure 17.3) performed annually, which reflects the success of the operations. However, due to its success, patient expectations have changed, as well as a change in the symptom threshold for the procedure. This has led to a constant attempt at improving modern joint replacements function. Some of these are aimed at improving the life span of the artificial joint, as one of the major concerns with the use of artificial joints in the younger patients is their early failure rate. There has also been a trend towards joint-preserving replacements, such as patella-femoral or medial uni-compartmental knee replacements, particularly if the anterior cruciate ligament is intact. There have been major concerns with the safety of some of the more recent innovations in joint

Table 17.3 Modifiable lifestyle risk factors for the development of OA and conservative management

Education	Physiotherapy	Occupational therapy	Weight loss
Exercise	Orthotics and walking aids	Transcutaneous electrical nerve stimulation (TENS)	Alternative medicine

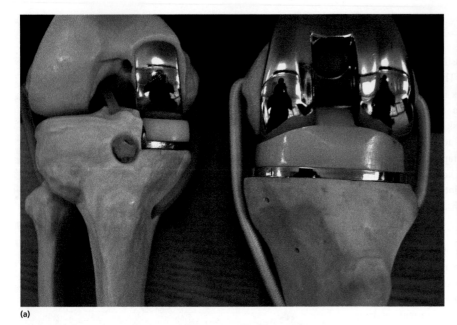

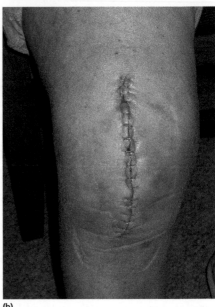

(a) **(b)**

Figure 17.3 (a) Anatomical models showing medial unicondylar (unicompartmental) and total knee replacements (b) Postoperative wound for open knee surgery

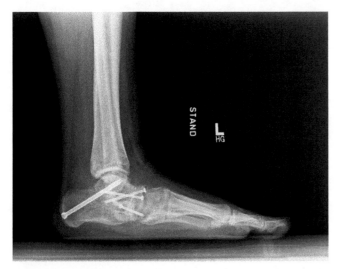

Figure 17.4 Triple arthrodesis – talonavicular, subtalar, and calcaneocuboid joints fused as a last resort

replacement, such as the metal on metal (MOM) hip resurfacings, with wear products leading to systemic adverse reactions and toxicity.

Arthrodesis

Arthrodesis is still a useful surgical procedure in some joints but not in all (e.g. no longer in hips). Arthrodesis of the joint means that the bones around the joint are fused together, so that they are no longer a source of pain, but at the cost of restricting range of movement. In fact, most patients are content to make that compromise to achieve pain relief after years. Yet, a major problem is that it leads to abnormal forces occurring at the joint and the subsequent development of OA. Arthrodesis is commonly used in foot and ankle surgery, where it is used to fuse the lesser toe joints, but may also be used

to fuse larger joints in the hindfoot or midfoot (Figure 17.4). The spine, the shoulder, and the hand are other sites where arthrodesis is still used as a relatively common surgical procedure.

Osteotomy

Osteotomy surgery does not involve direct surgery on the joint, but instead alters the biomechanical axis and forces passing through the joint by surgically breaking and then realigning one of the bones around the joint. A good example of this, which has recently been gaining popularity, is the use of a high tibial osteotomy to realign the biomechanical axis in the varus knee, which is a nonmodifiable risk factor for osteoarthritis (Figure 17.5).

Excision arthroplasty/explantation/Girdlestone procedure

Excision arthroplasty involves surgical removal of the joint, and whilst relieving pain, it also leads to instability at the site of the former joint. It was more commonly used as a treatment for severe OA before more modernised methods of surgical treatments such as arthroplasty were available. In some selected cases, excision arthroplasty is still used in instances like the Girdlestone excision arthroplasty of the hip as a salvage procedure for infection control or revision of failed primary arthroplasty (Figure 17.6).

Future direction

Due to the high incidence and high financial burden placed on the economy by OA, there is a constant drive to improve surgical interventions or to provide novel interventions in the early form of disease treatment. The use of stem cell therapy in the early treatment of OA is one such example. Other new developments in the field of joint replacement surgery include custom-made cutting blocks and computer-assisted orthopaedic surgery (CAOS) using robotic technology (Figure 17.7).

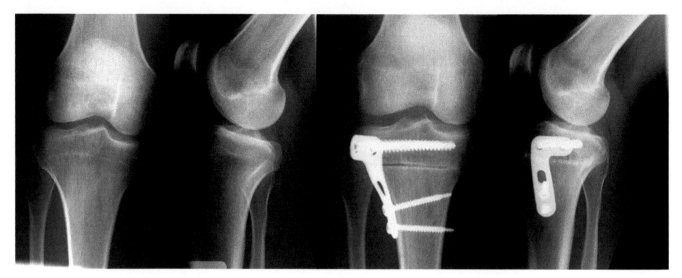

Figure 17.5 High tibial osteotomy

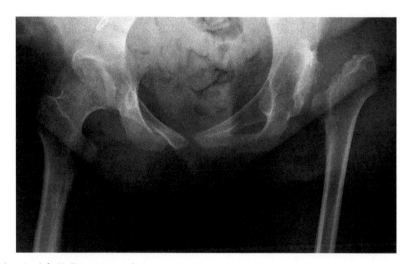

Figure 17.6 Plain radiograph showing left Girdlestone procedure

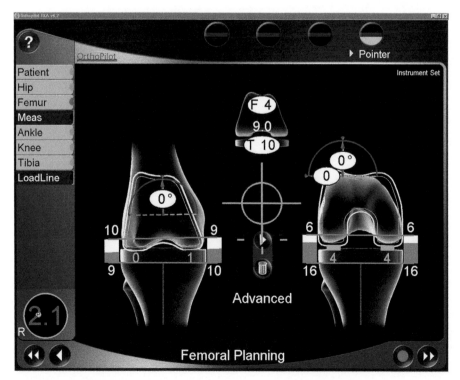

Figure 17.7 Computer-assisted orthopaedic surgery

Further reading

Chen, A., Gupte, C., Akhtar, K., et al. (2012). The global economic cost of osteoarthritis: How the UK compares. *Arthritis*. 698709.

National Institute for Health and Care Excellence, www.nice.org.uk/nicemedia/live/11926/39720/39720.pdf

National Joint Registry, www.njrcentre.org.uk

Pereira, D., Peleteiro, B., Araujo, J., et al. (2011). The effect of osteoarthritis definition on prevalence and incidence estimates: a systematic review. *Osteoarthritis and Cartilage* 19: 1270–1285.

Vales, A.M., and Spector, T.D. (2011). Genetic epidemiology of hip and knee osteoarthritis. *National Review of Rheumatology* 7: 23–32.

World Health Organization, www.archives.who.int/prioritymeds/report/background/osteoarthritis.doc

CHAPTER 18

Inflammatory Diseases

Sanam Kia[1] and Sonya Abraham[2]

[1] Abertawe Bro Morgannwg University, Port Talbot, UK
[2] Imperial College Healthcare NHS Trust, London, UK

OVERVIEW

- Rheumatoid arthritis (RA) is a systemic inflammatory disease characterised by a destructive polyarthritis, most commonly affecting small joints of the hands, feet, and wrist in a symmetrical distribution.

- Only 70–80% of patients will be rheumatoid factor positive; hence, a detailed history and examination is paramount in diagnosis.

- The ultimate goal of therapy is complete disease remission; early referral to a specialist and MDT team is key.

- Early use of disease-modifying anti-rheumatic drugs (DMARDs) and biologics have revolutionised patient care.

- SpAs are classically characterised by: sacroiliitis, inflammatory back pain, and enthesitis, made up of several conditions that often overlap.

- HLA-B27 is not routinely tested. Diagnosis is based on history, examination, and investigations such as MRI.

- Patients with ankylosing spondylitis are typically male (M:F 3:1), less than 40 years of age, and Caucasian, and 20–40% have peripheral joint involvement.

- Inflammatory back pain and limitation of lumbar spine movement are a hallmark of the disease.

- Extra-articular manifestations are categorized by the 6 As.

- Disease management centres on patient education and physiotherapy; pharmacological options include NSAIDs, DMARDs, and biologics.

Rheumatoid arthritis

Background

Rheumatoid arthritis (RA) is an autoimmune disorder of unknown aetiology that primarily affects the synovial membrane of joints, but that may affect other organ systems. The chronic pain and joint dysfunction caused by RA often leads to significant personal disability and has a large health-economic burden.

Incidence and prevalence

There are approximately 400,000 people with RA in the United Kingdom. RA is two to four times more common in women than men. People of all ages can develop RA, but the peak incidence in the United Kingdom is in the seventh decade.

Aetiology

The aetiology of RA is not fully understood. It is thought to be multifactorial, with both genetic and environmental factors playing a role. HLA-DRB1 has been linked with increased risk of RA.

Clinical findings

Signs

RA is characterised by symmetrical polyarthritis. The onset of the disease is often insidious, with morning stiffness, weight loss, and malaise.

Signs of RA include:
- Small joint swelling, especially MCPJs, PIPJs, and wrist. As the disease progresses, more proximal joint may be involved. Erosive changes are seen in Figure 18.1.
- Ulnar deviation and volar subluxation at MCPJs (see Figure 18.2).
- Boutonniere and swan neck deformity (see Figure 18.3).
- Wrist subluxation and prominence of ulnar head (piano key).
- Extensor tendon rupture and muscle wasting.
- Swelling of MTPJs, clawing of toes, and hallux valgus deformity (see Figure 18.4).
- Extra-articular features are outlined in Figure 18.5.

Symptoms

Symptoms of RA may follow a relapsing-remitting pattern, but if disease is poorly controlled, significant irreversible joint damage may occur, resulting in permanent disability. Extra-articular features of RA are a marker of increased disease severity and are more common in patients with high RF levels and in smokers. Extra-articular features are associated with increased overall morbidity and premature mortality.

ABC of Orthopaedics and Trauma, First Edition. Edited by Kapil Sugand and Chinmay M. Gupte.
© 2018 John Wiley & Sons Ltd. Published 2018 by John Wiley & Sons Ltd.

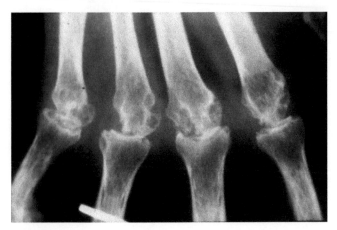

Figure 18.1 Radiograph demonstrating severe erosions affecting the base of MCPs and PIPs

Investigations

No laboratory test results are pathognomonic for RA. Rheumatoid factors (RF) are autoantibodies directed against the Fc portion of immunoglobulin G (IgG). The sensitivity and specificity of RF, depending on the population studied, is 60–70% and 50–90%, respectively. Testing for anticitrullinated peptide/protein antibodies (ACPP) has become common in the evaluation of patients for RA. Anti-CCP antibodies are found in 60–70% of RA patients and are >95% specific for the disease.

FBC is often abnormal in RA, with anaemia and thrombocytosis consistent with chronic inflammation. Checking liver and renal function is essential, as it might influence the choice of medications. Raised urate levels may prompt additional efforts to exclude gout, which can frequently be mistaken for RA.

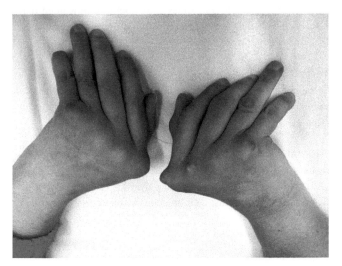

Figure 18.2 Rheumatoid hands: ulnar deviation with rheumatoid nodules

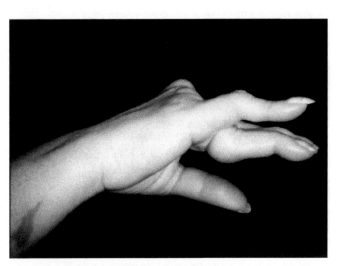

Figure 18.3 Boutonniere deformity of the fifth finger, swan neck deformity of middle and ring finger

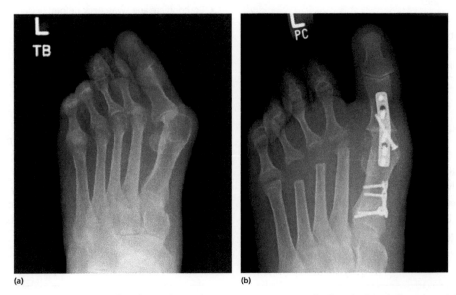

(a)   (b)

Figure 18.4 Radiographs showing (a) subluxation of the first and second MTP. Bones are osteopaenic. There is also a hallux valgus deformity, (b) post-op forefoot arthroplasty 1st MTP joint fusion and basal osteotomy of the 1st metatarsal

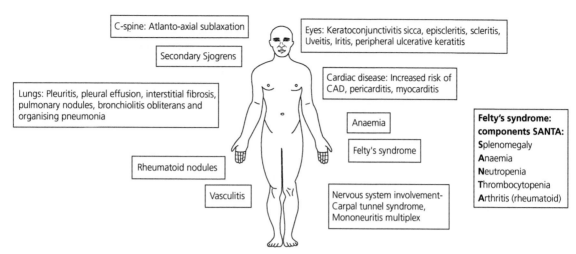

Figure 18.5 Systemic manifestations of RA

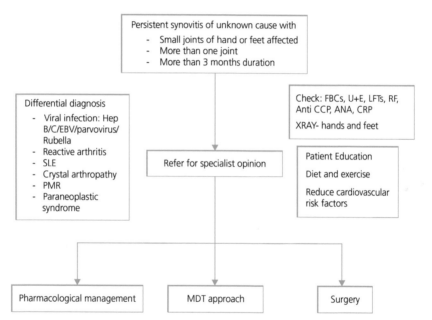

Graph 18.1 Management of rheumatoid arthritis

Diagnosis

Diagnosis of RA requires a careful history and appropriate examination of the patient (Graph 18.1). ACR/EULAR classification criteria (Table 18.1) can be used as guidance in initial diagnosis of the patients.

Management

- *Nonoperative:* A multidisciplinary approach and patient education are crucial to the management of RA and improving patient outcomes. Care is usually led by a consultant rheumatologist, but general practitioners, orthopaedic surgeons, nurse specialists, occupational therapists, physiotherapists, and podiatrists have important roles. Splints and walking aids may also be indicated for continuing daily routines. The therapeutic approach for patients with RA has changed drastically with emphasis on early initiation of disease-modifying antirheumatic drugs (DMARDs; Table 18.2) and, if necessary, with biologics (Table 18.3) to achieve disease remission or low disease activity.

Corticosteroids have a rapid and effective anti-inflammatory effect. They are used to induce remission in conjunction with other DMARDs, followed by rapid tapering to the lowest effective dose due to risk of steroid-induced side effects (osteoporosis, hyperglycaemia, hypertension, skin fragility, peptic ulcer, infections). Response to therapy should be monitored and recorded using composite scoring systems such as Disease Activity Score (DAS)-28.

Nonsteroidal anti-inflammatory drugs (NSAIDs)/COX2 inhibitors can be used for pain control and symptom relief. All oral NSAIDs/COX-2 inhibitors have analgesic effects of a similar magnitude but vary in their potential gastrointestinal, liver, and cardio-renal toxicity.

- *Operative:* Surgical opinion is sought in patients who suffer with persistent pain due to joint damage, deformity, or disability in the form of arthroscopy, arthrodesis, and arthroplasty. Synevectomy may also reduce pain.

Table 18.1 Classification criteria for RA

Classification criteria for RA (The 2010 American college of Rheumatologists [ACR] / European League Against Rheumatism [EULAR] classification criteria).

Score-based algorithm: add score of categories A-D; a score of ≥6/10 is needed for classification of a patient as having definite RA.

Domain	Parameter	Points
A	1 large joint	0
Joint involvement	2-10 large joints	1
	1-3 small joints	2
	4-10 small joint	4
	>10 joints	5
B	Negative RF and negative ACPA	0
Serology	Low positive RF or low positive ACPA	2
	High positive RF or high positive ACPA	3
C	Normal CRP and ESR	0
Acute phase reactants	Abnormal CRP and ESR	1
D	<6 weeks	0
Symptom duration	≥6 weeks	1

Table 18.2 Indications for DMARDs

	Dose	Side effects
Methotrexate	7.5 mg to 25 mg Once weekly	Hepatotoxicity Pulmonary pneumonitis Bone marrow suppression Teratogenic
Sulfasalazine	500 mg daily. Increase by 500 mg weekly to 2 g/daily	Hepatotoxicity Bone marrow suppression
Leflunomide	10 to 20 mg daily	Hepatotoxic GI side effects Pulmonary infiltration/ pneumonitis/reaction Hypertension teratogenic
Hydroxychloroquine	200-400 mg daily	Retinal damage
Azathioprine	1 mg/kg/day- increasing after 4-6 weeks to 2-3 mg/ kg/day	Hepatotoxicity Bone marrow suppression

Complications

Complications of RA such as tendon rupture, nerve compression, and stress fractures may also require surgical intervention. RA is an independent risk factor for cardiovascular disease. Blood pressure and cholesterol monitoring are important in reducing risk of heart attack and stroke. Patients taking DMARDs require influenza and pneumococcal vaccines due to the additional risk posed by immunosuppression.

Seronegative spondyloarthropathies

Introduction

Spondyloarthropathies (SpAs) are a group of inflammatory disorders that includes **PEAR**:
- **P**soriatic arthritis

Table 18.3 Indications for biological agents

	Mode of action	Side effects
Adalimumab	Fully humanised complete anti-TNF monoclonal antibody	Headache, nausea, allergic reaction, serious bacterial infections, Demyelination, worsening of heart failure, reactivation of TB
Etanercept	Recombinant human TNF receptor fusion protein	
Golimumab	Fully humanised anti-TNF monoclonal antibody	
Certolizumab	Pegylated Fab fragment of a fully humanised anti-TNF monoclonal antibody	
Infliximab	Chimeric human –murine anti-TNF monoclonal antibody	
Anakinra	IL-1 receptor antagonist	Injection site reactions, infections, blood dyscrasia
Rituximab	Chimeric monoclonal antibody against CD20 on developing B cells	Infusion reaction, viral infections, Hep B reactivation, progressive multifocal leukoencephalopathy

- **E**nteropathic arthritis
- **A**nkylosing spondylitis (AS)
- **R**eactive/**R**eiter's arthritis

Note that there is also a classification of undifferentiated spondyloarthritis (USpA).

Incidence and prevalence

The estimated prevalence of SpA is 0.5–2% in a Caucasian population with considerable variation worldwide. AS and USpA are the most frequently occurring SpA, and reactive arthritis is much less common.

Aetiology

The aetiology of spondyloarthropathies is complex and may be an interplay between genetic and environmental factors. There is a strong relationship with HLA B27 gene. The HLA B27 gene is positive in 92% of patients with AS, up to 80% with reactive arthritis, and 60% with psoriasis- and IBD-related spondylitis.

Clinical findings

SpAs share the following clinical features (Table 18.4):
- Arthritis of axial skeleton (sacroiliac joints and spine)
- Oligoarthritis of peripheral joints
- Enthesitis (inflammation of tendon insertions)
- Dactylitis (inflammation of a whole digit – *sausage finger*) and digital telescoping in psoriatic arthritis
- Majority are HLA B27 positive and rheumatoid factor negative

A through history is imperative in making an accurate diagnosis in this complex group of patients. Back pain is the predominant complaint in patients suffering from SpAs, and it is important to differentiate between mechanical and inflammatory causes of back pain (Table 18.5).

Table 18.4 Clinical manifestations Of SpA

Musculoskeletal feature – Inflammatory back pain – Peripheral arthritis – Enthesitis – Dactylitis Skin and nails Inflammatory eye disease – Conjunctivitis – Anterior uveitis Gastrointestinal Genitourinary Cardiovascular	Onset before age of 40, insidious onset, pain at night, improve with exercise, worse with rest Asymmetrical, Predominantly affects lower extremities. Can be similar to RA Inflammation around enthesis, relatively specific to SpA. Most common site is the Achilles tendon Swelling of the entire digit. It is not specific for SpA and may be seen in TB, syphilis, sarcoidosis, sickle cell and Gout Psoriasis, keratoderma blenorrhagica, nail disease Anterior Uveitis may be acute, unilateral and the initial presenting feature. Associated with Redness pain and photophobia. Visual impairment is possible if not fully treated. Urgent referral to ophthalmologists is recommended. 10% of patients with Inflammatory bowel disease present with signs and symptoms of SpA. Urethritis, cervicitis Aortic regurgitation, cardiac conduction defect

Table 18.5 Features of inflammatory back pain

- Pain worse with rest
- Improves with activity
- Awakes the patient from sleep
- Morning stiffness that lasts 30 minutes or longer
- Episodes of buttock pain

A more general history will identify systemic symptoms and differentiate between individual SpAs:

- Note onset, pattern, and severity of symptoms.
- Joint swelling – which joints and when?
- Recent infection, one month or less before the onset of arthritis. Any history of urethral or vaginal discharge, or diarrhoea should be included.
- Systemic constitutional features include symptoms such as weight loss and night sweats.
- Past medical history: check for psoriasis, inflammatory bowel disease (IBD), iritis, episodic heel pain.
- Get drug history and sexual history.
- Family history of SpA, psoriasis, and IBD is important.

Initial investigations

At the primary care level, the following investigations should be considered:

- *Haematology*: FBC, ESR, plasma viscosity
- *Biochemistry*: urea and electrolytes, CRP, serum urate, liver function, and bone profile
- *Immunology and tissue typing*: RF, anti-CCP, and autoantibodies (HLA-B27 is not generally useful.)
- *Microbiology*: Urethral or cervical swabs and stool cultures
- *Joint aspiration*: for microscopy, culture and sensitivity, and crystals

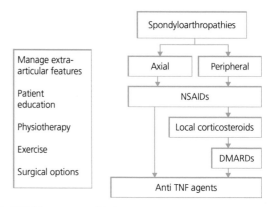

Graph 18.2 Management of SpA

- *Imaging*: a plain antero-posterior (AP) radiograph of the pelvis can be diagnostic of AS if there is evidence of sacroiliitis. Late signs of spinal pathology in AS include 'bamboo spine' to signify spinal fusion. Other imaging modalities such as bone scan and MRI can be useful in confirming the diagnosis in suspected cases.
- Testing for HIV

The clinical manifestations, diagnosis, and classification of the SpA family of disorders in adults will be reviewed in this chapter. Graphs 18.2 and 18.3 show the management algorithm for these patients.

Ankylosing spondylitis

Background

Ankylosing spondylitis (AS) is characterised by the insidious onset of inflammatory lower back pain during late adolescence or early adulthood. AS may involve the whole or part of the spine, with the hallmark being bilateral sacroiliitis. Making the diagnosis is often challenging because there may be few objective signs in early disease.

Diagnosis

Diagnosis is made according to the modified New York criteria.

Clinical parameters

- Lumbar back pain greater than 3 months that improves with exercise but is not relived by rest
- Limited forward and lateral flexion of the lumbar spine
- Limitation of chest expansion relative to normal values correlated for age and sex

Radiological parameters

- Sacroiliitis grade ≥2 bilaterally
- Sacroiliitis grade 3 to 4 unilaterally

A patient is regarded as having a definite diagnosis of AS if he or she fulfils at least one radiological parameter plus at least one clinical parameter.

Examination

The modified Schober test is the standard examination to assess limitation of forward flexion and hyperextension. While standing erect two marks are made on patient's back: 5 cm below and 10 cm

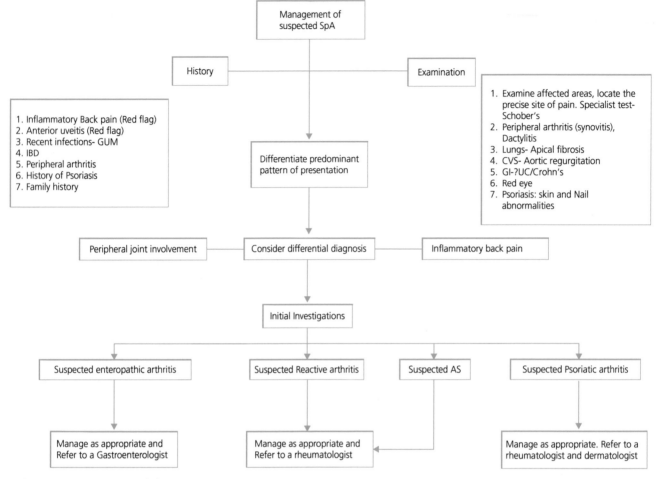

Graph 18.3 Management protocol of SpA

above the sacral dimples. The distance between these marks should increase from 15 cm to 20 cm with forward flexion. Any increase less than 5 cm is considered a restriction.

The characteristic "question mark posture" develops with advance disease due to loss of lumbar lordosis, exaggeration of thoracic kyphosis, and inability to extend the neck. One third of patients with AS also have peripheral mono- or oligo-arthritis.

The Royal National Hospital for Rheumatic Disease (Bath) has produced indices (such as BASFI and BASDAI) for scoring disease activity in patients and can be used to evaluate disease progression and patient's response to therapy.

Management

Graph 18.2 shows the stepwise approach into pharmacological management of AS. Surgery is a last resort for addressing complications that ranges from arthroplasty, spinal fracture fixation, and correction of deformity.

Cardinal rule: A hot swollen joint should be treated as septic arthritis until proven otherwise

Other inflammatory arthritides

Reactive arthritis

Reactive arthritis (ReA) is defined as a form of spondyloarthritis that arises following an infection. Despite the link with infection, cultures of synovial fluid are often sterile and there is no role for antibiotics in treating the arthritis.

Two major clinical features characterise ReA:

1 Preceding infection to the onset of arthritis by 1-4 weeks. Sometimes there is no history of infection, suggesting that subclinical infections or other environmental factors might play a role in the pathogenesis of the disease.

2 Mono- or polyarthritis often involving the lower limb.

ReA has replaced the term Reiter's syndrome, which refers to the triad of:

1 Reactive arthritis
2 Conjunctivitis
3 Urethritis

The bacteria commonly associated with reactive arthritis include:
- *Salmonella* species
- *Shigella* species

- *Yersinia enterocolitica*
- *Campylobacter jejuni*
- *Clostridium difficile*
- *Chlamydia trachomatis*

Most patients achieve complete remission within 6 months. NSAIDs and intra-articular steroid injections are the mainstay symptom control. If synovitis and joint damage persists, DMARDs can be initiated.

Enteropathic arthritis

Enteropathic arthritis (EA) is associated with IBD. Approximately 10–20% of patients with IBD may be affected by joint disease, which may also be the presenting symptom of IBD. The presence of oral ulceration, erythema nodosum, or pyoderma gangrenosum should alert the clinicians to evaluate for the presence of underlying bowel pathology. Other conditions with intestinal involvement and arthritis are outlined in Table 18.6.

There are two main types of EA:

1 Acute peripheral pauciarticular (affecting six or fewer joints) arthritis associated with flares of IBD (type 1 arthropathy), or polyarticular with MCP joints being preferentially involved (type 2 arthropathy).

2 Spondylitis and sacroiliitis: patients generally complain of symptoms of inflammatory back pain. Asymptomatic sacroiliitis is detected by radiography in 4–18% of patients. Involvement of axial skeleton is clinically and radiographically indistinguishable from that of AS.

EA often improves with treatment of gastrointestinal symptoms.

Psoriatic arthritis

Psoriatic arthritis (PsA) is an inflammatory arthritis associated with the skin disease psoriasis. Psoriasis affects 2–3% of the general population, up to 30% of whom develop psoriatic arthritis. The condition affects women and men equally. PsA usually develops within 10 years of onset of psoriasis. In some cases, the onset of psoriasis and arthritis coincide (Figures 18.6 and 18.7).

PsA is classified with the spondyloarthropathies due to presence of spondylitis in up to 40% of patients, HLA-B27 association, and occurrence of extra-articular features common to spondyloarthropathies. There are five clinical patterns among patients with PsA (Table 18.7).

General approach to the management of SpAs

The goal of therapy is to reduce disease progression, manage pain, and improve function. It is achieved through a multidisciplinary approach with physiotherapy, occupational therapy, and pharmacological methods. Patient education is at the heart of management;

Table 18.6 Other conditions with intestinal involvement and arthritis

- Reactive arthritis
- Whipple's disease
- Behcet's disease
- Coeliac disease
- Parasitic infection
- Pseudomembranous colitis
- Intestinal bypass surgery

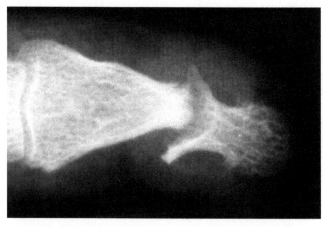

Figure 18.6 "Pencil in cup" deformity is a feature of psoriatic arthritis

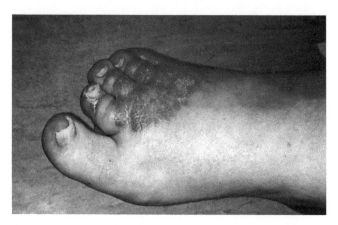

Figure 18.7 Psoriatic arthritis with dactylitis and active psoriasis. There is also nail pitting and onycholysis

Table 18.7 Patterns of joint involvement in psoriatic arthritis

- Distal arthritis: involvement of the distal interphalangeal (DIP) joints
- Asymmetric oligoarthritis: less than five small and/or large joints are affected in an asymmetric distribution
- Symmetric polyarthritis, similar to and, at times, indistinguishable from rheumatoid arthritis (RA)
- Arthritis mutilans: deforming and destructive arthritis
- Spondyloarthritis, including both sacroiliitis and spondylitis

maintaining good posture, preventing flexion contractures, deep breathing exercises, and cessation of smoking all play a role. Treatments options are tailored to patient's wishes and expectations and current manifestations of the disease: severity of symptoms, pain, degree of disability, age, gender, comorbidities, and concomitant drugs. Extra-articular features of spondyloarthropathies should be managed as appropriate with referral to appropriate specialist services (Graph 18.3).

Sacroilitis and spondylitis

Pharmacotherapy includes one or more of the following: NSAIDs, analgesics, DMARDs, and anti-TNF agents. NSAIDs and COX2 selective agents are used for symptomatic relief. Radiographic progression may occur despite the control of symptoms (Graph 18.2).

Peripheral joint disease

Arthritis itself is managed by use of NSAIDs initially. If there is poor response, intra-articular corticosteroids or a trial of oral steroids can be used. In poorly responsive cases, DMARDs (such as methotrexate and azathioprine) and biologic agents are considered. There is some evidence that NSAIDs can induce gastrointestinal flares, hence should be used with caution in patients with irritable bowel disease. If arthritis persists despite the above therapy, TNF-alpha inhibitors (Table 18.3) are recommended.

Further reading

Gladman, D.D. (1998). Clinical aspects of the spondyloarthropathies. *American Journal of Medical Science* 316: v234.

Hakim, A., Clunie, G., and Haq, I. (2011). *Oxford Handbook of Rheumatology*. Oxford University Press, Oxford, UK.

National Institute for Health and Care Excellence. (2010). Psoriatic arthritis – etanercept, infliximab and adalimumab. Technology TA199. www.nice.org.uk/ta199.

National Institute for Health and Care Excellence. (2009, February). Rheumatoid arthritis: the management of rheumatoid arthritis in adults. Clinical guidelines, CG79. www.nice.org.uk/cg79.

National Institute for Health and Care Excellence (NICE). (2008, May). Ankylosing spondylitis- adalimumab, etanercept and infliximab. *Technology appraisals (TA)*143. www.nice.org.uk/guidance/TA143.

Singh, J.A., Furst, D.E., Bharat, A., et al. (2012). Update of the 2008 American College of Rheumatology Recommendations for the Use of Disease-Modifying Antirheumatic Drugs and Biologic Agents in the Treatment of Rheumatoid Arthritis. *Arthritis Care and Research (Hoboken)* 64(5): 625–639.

Vinson, E.N. and Major, N.M. (2003). MR imaging of ankylosing spondylitis. *Seminars in Musculoskeletal Radiology* 7 (2): 103–113.

Zochling, J. (2008). Assessment and treatment of ankylosing spondylitis: current status and future directions. *Current Opinon Rheumatology* 20 (4): 398–403.

CHAPTER 19

Bone and Joint Infections

James Donaldson and Jonathan Miles

Royal National Orthopaedic Hospital, Stanmore, UK

OVERVIEW

- Acute osteomyelitis
  - Usually caused by *Staphylococcus aureus* infection.
  - Most common in children and infants.
  - Treatment is with antibiotics.
- Subacute osteomyelitis
  - More insidious than acute osteomyelitis.
  - Antibiotics and sometimes surgical debridement are needed.
- Chronic osteomyelitis
  - Leads to necrotic bone and often significant soft tissue involvement.
  - Surgery is usually needed but not always successful.
- Septic arthritis
  - Can create an orthopaedic emergency.
- Prosthetic joint infection
  - This is a complex problem.
  - If treated acutely, the implant may be retained.
  - If chronic, the implant will usually need removal and prolonged antibiotic treatment in one or two stages.

General aspects of infection

Infection is a condition in which pathogenic organisms multiply and spread within body tissues.

This usually gives rise to the classical signs of inflammation:
- redness (rubor)
- swelling (tumor)
- heat (calor)
- pain (dolor)
- loss of function (functio laesa)
- fever (pyrexia)

Bone and cartilage is very susceptible to damage from the buildup of pressure characteristically seen in acute infection. The timing of surgery is important. In the acute setting, antibiotics may be all that is needed. If there is pus, it needs to be drained. For chronic infection, the choice between nonsurgical and surgical treatment is more difficult, and each case is decided individually. The principles of treating orthopaedic infections are:
- provide analgesia and supportive measures
- rest the affected body part
- start effective antibiotic treatment after taking microbiology samples
- remove necrotic tissue and bone

Acute osteomyelitis

Osteomyelitis is defined as inflammation of the bone, caused by an infecting organism. It is nearly always seen in children (with the exception of immunocompromised adults).

Aetiology

Infection generally arises from two sources:

1 Haematogenous spread of bacteria is most common. Bacteraemia results in the deposition of bacteria usually in the metaphysis of bone (most commonly around the proximal tibia or distal femur in children and vertebra in adults).

2 Direct inoculation can occur via surgery, trauma, or implant.

Local factors and the host response (extremes of age, malnutrition, immunosuppression, diabetes, etc.) will contribute to the subsequent signs and symptoms. The causal organism can be identified by blood cultures in approximately 50% of patients. Wounds swabs are also important for correct diagnosis. *S. aureus* remains the most common causative organism, but others are prevalent and vary, depending on age (Table 19.1).

Pathology

The predilection for the metaphysis is thought to be due to the relative vascular stasis from hairpin loops in the nutrient artery, which favour bacterial colonisation. In neonates, there is still a connection between the epiphysis and the metaphysis, and infection can settle in the end of the bone. Joint infection (septic arthritis) and growth disturbance can result. In older children, the growth plate acts as a barrier to the spread of infection and acute osteomyelitis is usually confined to the metaphysis (Figure 19.1).

ABC of Orthopaedics and Trauma, First Edition. Edited by Kapil Sugand and Chinmay M. Gupte.

© 2018 John Wiley & Sons Ltd. Published 2018 by John Wiley & Sons Ltd.

Table 19.1 Common orthopaedic infections

Infants (<1 year)	Children (1–16 yrs)	Adults	Special cases
Group B *Streptococcus*	*S. aureus*	*S. aureus*	*Salmonella* (sickle-cell disease)
S. aureus	Group A *Streptococcus*	*Staphylococcus epidermidis*	*Pseudomonas* (intravenous drug users)
Escherichia coli	*Haemophilus influenza*	Gram-negative bacilli	*Neisseria gonorrhoea* (sexually transmitted infections)

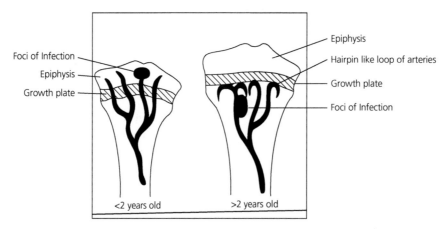

Figure 19.1 Foci of infection in children and in those older

Characteristic patterns of osteomyelitis are:
- Inflammation occurs.
- Suppuration with pus formation occurs by day 2 to 3.
- A rise in intra-osseous pressure causes tissue necrosis and further vascular stasis. Irreparable damage may occur by this stage.
- Dead bone may separate as sequestra.
- Reactive new bone forms at the end of the second week, which slowly thickens, forming an involucrum that encloses the infected tissue and sequestra.
- Resolution and healing is the final stage if the infection is appropriately treated.
- Alternatively, chronic infection may persist.

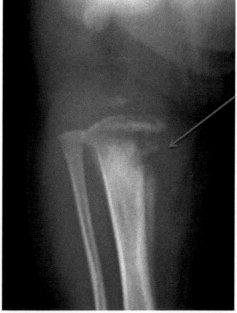

Radiographs of the knee showing destructive changes secondary to infection

Figure 19.2 Destructive changes from osteomyelitis

Clinical features

Pain with localised tenderness as well as fever and malaise are commonplace. The child may be refusing to use that limb and there may be a recent history of infection elsewhere. Local swelling and redness are later signs as the soft tissues become involved. In neonates, the constitutional disturbance may be mild (failure to thrive and irritability).

Investigations

- Blood tests: CRP and ESR are usually raised. It is important to look at uric acid (gout), blood cultures, autoimmunology (e.g. RA, SLE, etc.), and clotting (haemarthrosis).
- Radiographs are often normal initially but changes may include fractures, sclerosis, lytic cavities, or erosions (Figure 19.2).
- Ultrasound may show a subperiosteal collection.
- Bone scan is sensitive but not specific.
- MRI is extremely sensitive and will show periosteal reaction, soft tissue involvement, and bone marrow changes (Figure 19.3).
- Arthrocentesis for synovial fluid analysis: microscopy, Gram-staining, cultures, sensitivity to antibiotics, cytology, and biochemistry.
- Image-guided bone biopsy is often a last resort, since it may have a low yield.

Differential diagnoses

- Cellulitis
- Reactive arthritis
- Flare-up of RA or OA

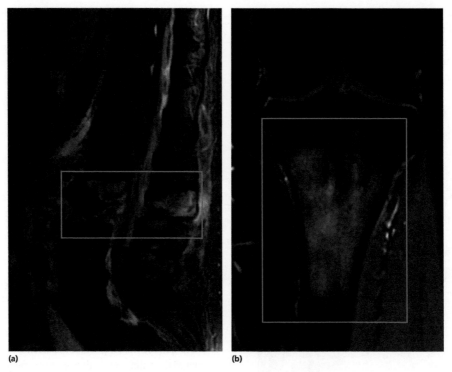

Figure 19.3 MRI images of (a) vertebral osteomyelitis in adult spine, and (b) high signal in the proximal tibia due to infection

- Trauma
- Joint crystalopathy
- Necrotising myositis or fasciitis
- Bone or soft tissue tumour

Treatment
- Supportive treatment includes analgesia, intravenous fluids, and splintage of the limb.
- Antibiotics
  - Commencement of broad-spectrum intravenous antibiotics with recognised anti-*Staphylococcal* and *Streptococcal* activity immediately after culture specimens.
  - Once an organism is identified, the antibiotics can be modified accordingly and converted to oral regimen towards the end of the treatment.
  - Antibiotics are usually required for at least 6 weeks.
  - The earlier the infection is treated, the higher the chance of cure.
- Surgery (either open or arthroscopic) may be required:
  - When significant subperiosteal or soft tissue collections are present and these need to be drained, often repeatedly
  - To debride dead bone
  - To treat recurrent disease or disease that is not responding to antibiotic treatment

Complications of osteomyelitis
- Septicaemia
- Metastatic infection
- Recurrent infection: depends on the site and time to treatment
  - 20% recurrence around the knee
  - 50% in metatarsals
  - early diagnosis 92% cured; late diagnosis 25% cured

- Altered bone growth, deformity, and limb length discrepancy
- Pathological fracture
- Chronic osteomyelitis
- OA
- Subluxation/dislocation

Subacute osteomyelitis

This is more insidious, with fewer symptoms. Pain may be present for some weeks with minimal symptoms. The relative mildness is thought to be due to a less virulent organism or higher innate resistance of the patient. Blood tests may be normal in 50% of cases. The classical radiograph (Figure 19.4) may show a cavity, surrounded by a halo of sclerosis (Brodie's abscess). The most common sites are again the proximal tibia or distal femur (MRI, Figure 19.5).

A benign or malignant bone tumour must be excluded, and often a biopsy is needed to do this. Microbiology is positive in 50% of cases and is almost always *S. aureus*.

Treatment may be nonsurgical with immobilisation and antibiotics. Surgery is indicated if the diagnosis is in doubt or if there is a lack of response radiographically or biochemically to prolonged antibiotic treatment. Overlying abscesses also require incision and drainage supported by antibiotic therapy.

Chronic osteomyelitis

Historically, this often followed acute osteomyelitis. These days, however, it is a more common sequelae to an open fracture or surgery.

Clinical Features

- Systemic features of infection (but not always present)
- Localised pain and discharge
- Thickened and indurated tissues
- Joint contractures and bone deformity

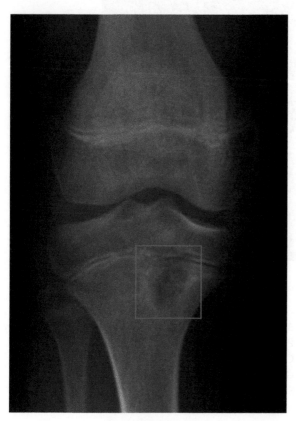

Figure 19.4 Plain radiograph of a Brodie's abscess

The specific symptoms will depend on the physiological condition of the host, the site of involvement, the functional impairment, and the extent of bone necrosis.

Figure 19.6 demonstrate surgical options for infected tibial fracture nonunions.

Imaging

- Radiographs may show:
  - bone resorption
  - periosteal thickening
  - osteoporosis
  - sequestra (infarcted bone) and its surrounding involucrum (periosteal new bone formation; Figure 19.7)
- Bone scan, MRI, CT, and sonograms may be helpful.

Treatment

Chronic osteomyelitis (Figure 19.8) is difficult to treat and antibiotics alone are not sufficient. A specialist bone infection centre should be involved.

- Surgical debridement, excision, and irrigation: Dead bone, infected soft tissue, purulent material, sinus tracks, and foreign material or metalwork all need to be removed.
- Bone loss will need reconstruction: This might include bone graft or limb reconstruction with an external fixator with larger defects (Figure 19.8).
- Soft tissue: May require local tissue flaps or free flaps.
- Antibiotics:
  - Bone cultures and microbiology samples should be taken prior to any antibiotic treatment.
  - Local administration of antibiotic in cement, implants, or via an irrigation system to avoid dead space.

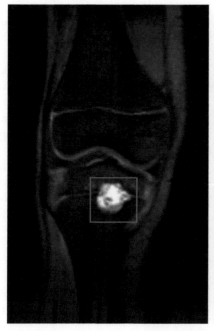
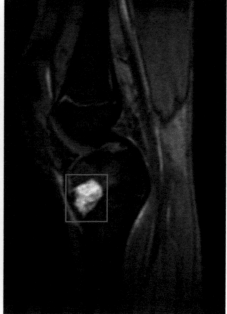

Figure 19.5 The coronal and sagittal views of a Brodie's abscess on MRI

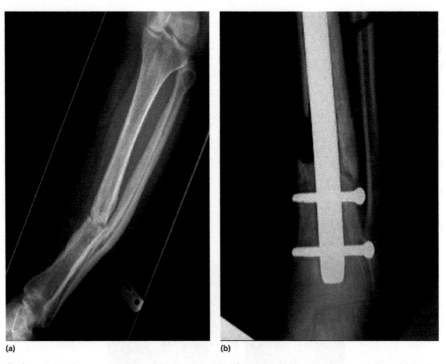

Figure 19.6 Radiographs of infected tibial fracture nonunions (a) without internal fixation and (b) with an intramedullary tibial nail

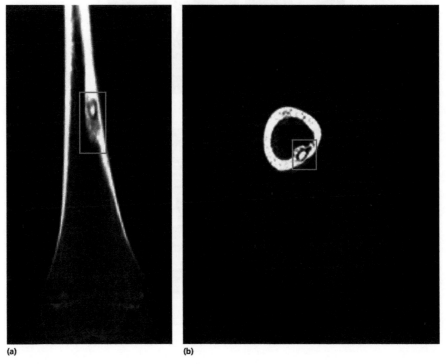

Figure 19.7 A computerised tomography scan show an intracortical sequestrum, (a) coronal and (b) axial image

Prosthetic joint infection

Infection of an orthopaedic prosthesis remains one of the most serious complications of orthopaedic surgery. Its management almost always involves surgical intervention and prolonged antibiotic treatment. Despite sophisticated prevention strategies, infection rates of around 1% persist in elective joint arthroplasty and much higher rates are present following fixation for trauma.

Pathology

Biomaterials and other foreign materials are inanimate materials susceptible to bacterial colonisation. Implants are coated by the body with a layer of protein and platelets, but if bacteria reach the implant first, bacterial adhesion may progress to aggregation that progresses to a structure known as a *biofilm*. Existence within this biofilm represents a survival mechanism by which microbes resist external and internal environmental factors, such as antimicrobial agents and the host's immune system. The most common pathogens include coagulase negative Staphylococcus, *S. aureus* (coagulase positive) and polymicrobial mixture.

Clinical Features
See Table 19.2.

Investigations
No preoperative tests are 100% sensitive and specific. Therefore, a diagnosis can be difficult to make. A careful history is mandatory and may provide crucial clues. Other tests include the following:
- Bloods
- Nuclear imaging: bone scan (will be "hot" for 2 years postsurgery) or labeled white cell scan

- Radiographs (likely to be normal but may show septic loosening in the late stages)
- Microbiology:
  ○ Aspiration (70% sensitive)
  ○ Polymerase chain reaction (high false positive rates)
  ○ Intraoperative samples

Treatment
Surgery (Figure 19.9)
- Extensive and meticulous debridement with retention of the prosthesis:
  ○ For acute (postoperative or haematogenous infection)
  ○ Needs to be done as early as possible (at least within 6 weeks) to prevent biofilm formation
- Revision surgery for chronic infections

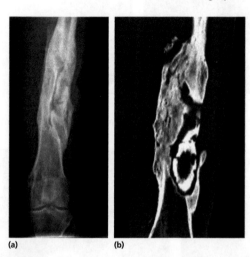

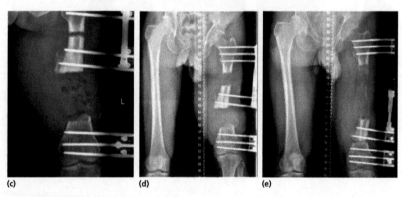

Figure 19.8 Case Study: Distal femoral chronic osteomyelitis. (a) plain radiograph; (b) CT scan; (c) following bone excision; (d) bone more proximal bone being transported; and (e) the bone docking distally with new bone formation following behind

Table 19.2 Clinical features of prosthetic joint infections

Early post-operative	Late chronic	Haematogenous spread
• Immediate post-operative period • The wound may be erythematous, swollen, discharging, and tender. • It may be difficult to differentiate between a superficial or deep infection (deep to fascia). • Implant salvage remains possible at this stage.	• These likely originate at the time of surgery, but a low virulence or inoculum delays the onset of symptoms. • Removal of the device is usually needed to eradicate the infection.	• Sudden, rapid deterioration in the function of an implant. • Usually takes years presenting with symptoms and signs similar to early postoperative infection. • May be triggered by infection elsewhere, such as dental surgery, urosepsis, or remote infection. • Implant salvage is possible if treatment is prompt.

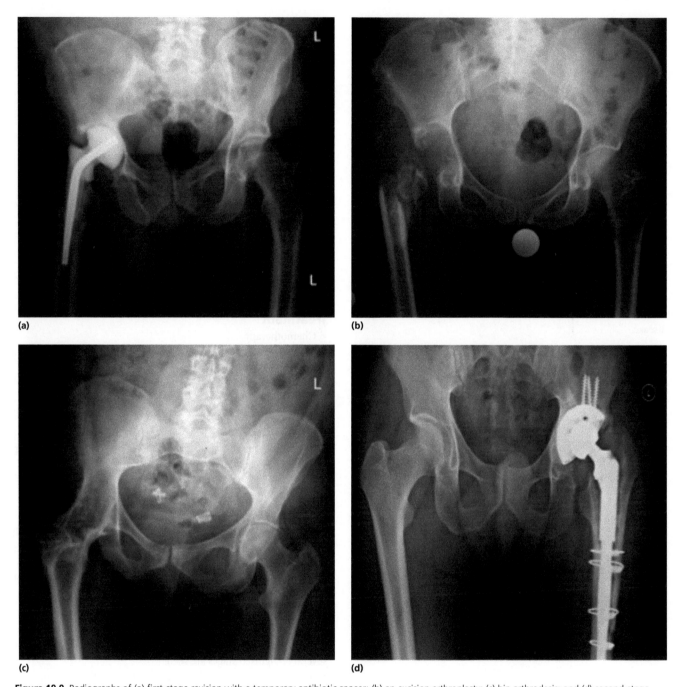

Figure 19.9 Radiographs of (a) first-stage revision with a temporary antibiotic spacer; (b) an excision arthroplasty; (c) hip arthrodesis; and (d) second-stage revision total hip replacement

- One-stage revision requires:
  - Low virulence organisms
  - Good soft tissues
  - No bone loss
  - An identified microorganism and antibiotic sensitivity
- Two-stage revision involves:
  - Success rates are quoted around 85–90%.
  - The first stage involves debridement, removal of the implant, and insertion of a temporary spacer.
  - Revision is followed by antibiotic treatment, often for 6 weeks or longer.
  - The definitive (second-stage) prosthesis is inserted when signs of infection have been eliminated (lack of pain/redness, normal CRP, and ESR)
- Arthrodesis: Largely historical unless the soft tissue envelope is severely compromised.
- Excision arthroplasty (Girdlestone procedure or resection arthroplasty): This is a fairly disabling procedure and is often reserved for the moribund or where the joint is unreconstructable.
- Amputation / disarticulation: This is for recurrent infections with poor bone and soft tissues and when other strategies have failed.

Antibiotics

Antibiotics are required in all cases of revision surgery. The type, mode of delivery, and duration depend on the individual patient, and close liaison with the microbiology department is essential. Where surgery is not appropriate (in those unfit or unwilling to undergo revision procedures), long-term antibiotic suppression is an option. The prosthesis should not be loose. Better results are achieved when the organism and its sensitivities are known. Methods to prevent infections in orthopaedic surgery can be seen in Table 19.3.

Tuberculosis (TB)

Tuberculosis is most common in developing countries with crowding, poor sanitation, and malnutrition. In the developed world, its incidence is on the increase due to an increasingly elderly population, global travel, and immunosuppressive disease states (especially HIV). Only a small number of patients (3–5%) with TB will have osteoarticular involvement, and half of these will have spinal disease.

Pathology

Mycobacterium tuberculosis is an aerobic bacterium that enters the body via the lungs or gastrointestinal tract. It causes a granulomatous reaction, which is associated with tissue necrosis and caseation. The primary focus of infection is usually in the lung and regional lymph nodes. Musculoskeletal involvement is via haematogenous spread. Musculoskeletal disease may begin as a synovitis or osteomyelitis. At this stage, soft tissue swelling is seen with a reduction in movement. Degenerate changes and eventual joint destruction ensue. Healing is often by fibrosing ankylosis.

Clinical Features

Clinical features of TB can be divided into constitutional, pulmonary, and extrapulmonary (e.g. musculoskeletal, Table 19.4).

Investigations

- Plain radiography
  - Soft tissue swelling
  - Peri-articular osteopaenia, erosions

Table 19.3 Preventing infection in orthopaedics

Preoperative	Medical optimisation:
	• Control of blood glucose
	• Cessation of smoking
	• Avoiding surgery with concomitant infection
	• Reducing obesity and vascular insufficiency
	Antiseptic agents and proper bathing
	MRSA decolonisation
Perioperative	Antimicrobial prophylaxis
	Theatre positive pressure ventilation and laminar flow
	Appropriate surgical attire and drapes
	Antibiotic impregnated cement
	Bleeding control
Postoperative	Sterile dressing
	Avoiding disturbing the incision site
	Appropriate hand washing

Table 19.4 Clinical features of extra-pulmonary TB

Constitutional	Musculoskeletal
Low-grade fever	Swelling and stiffness
Night sweats	Restricted movement
Weight loss	Pain
Anorexia	Deformity
Malaise	Sinuses
	Neurological deficit (spine)

- Little or no periosteal reaction
- Spine: bone erosion and collapse around a narrowed or destroyed disc space
- Bloods: raised ESR
- Positive Mantoux test
- Acid fast bacilli (AFB) in synovial fluid
- Tissue biopsy is the most sensitive for AFB

Treatment

- Chemotherapy
  - Specialist anti-tuberculous treatment is essential usually with multiple therapies to limit resistance.
- Surgery is seldom necessary, except:
  - Emergency spinal decompression and stabilisation in cases of impending or actual paraplegia.
  - Joint arthrodesis or arthroplasty once the disease is quiescent. Anti-tuberculous treatment should be given pre- and postoperatively when joint replacement surgery is performed.

Poliomyelitis

Polio is an acute viral disease that affects the anterior horn cells of the spinal cord and brain stem, resulting in asymmetrical lower motor neuron palsy. It is a rare disease in developed countries following widespread vaccination but still persists in 4% globally.

Clinical Features

Only a small proportion of patients exhibit any symptoms but several recognised stages are seen:

- *Acute illness*: fever, headache, flexed joints with pain when they are stretched
- *Flaccid paralysis*: peaks at 2–3 days, may give rise to difficulty in breathing
- *Recovery*: from 10 days to up to 2 years
- *Residual paralysis*: asymmetric weakness may lead to joint deformities
- *Post-polio syndrome*: progressive muscle weakness in both old and new muscle groups due to neural fatigue

Treatment

- Physiotherapy and surgical appliances is the mainstay of treatment
- Surgery, when necessary, is aimed at restoring function with tendon transfers, osteotomies, or joint stabilisations

Table 19.5 Miscellaneous soft tissue infections

Disease	Clinical Features	Organism(s)	Treatment
Cellulitis	• Deep subcutaneous involvement • Often indistinct borders	• Group A *Streptococcus* • *Staphylococcus aureus* occasionally	Antibiotics
Erysipelas	• Superficial, well demarcated • Red, raised, painful plaque	• Group A *Streptococcus* • *Staphylococcus aureus*	Antibiotics
Necrotising fasciitis	• Involves the muscle fascia • Aggressive	• Group A *Streptococcus*	Extensive surgical debridement
Gas gangrene	• Affects muscle • Pain, oedema, and discharge	• *Clostridium perfringens* or *specticum*	Debridement and fasciotomy +/– hyperbaric oxygen
Surgical site infection	• Postoperative wound discharge and erythema	• Varies • *Staphylococcus aureus* • *Staphylococcus epidermidis* • MRSA • Group A *Streptococcus*	Antibiotics +/– wound debridement
Suppurative tenosynovitis	• Swollen and tender, sausage-shaped finger • Flexed position and pain with passive movement	• *Staphylococcus aureus*	Splintage and antibiotics if caught very early; Usually, surgical drainage is required
Paronychia	• Infected paronychial fold along a nail	• *Staphylococcus aureus*	Drainage of pus +/– antibiotics
Bites	• Human or animal	• Multiple	Broad-spectrum antibiotics. Often, wound washout is needed for hand bites (fight bites)
Tetanus	• Neuroparalytic disease from contaminated wounds	• *Clostridium tetani*	Tetanus immunoglobulin if vaccination status unknown

Discitis

Infection limited to the intervertebral disc is rare. In adults, it is usually a result of surgery or haematogenous spread – for instance, in dialysis patients. In children, it is from haematogenous spread. The vertebral end plates are rapidly destroyed and the infection can progress into the vertebral body. Acute back pain, muscle spasm, limitation of movements, and systemic infective features may be seen. Treatment is with prolonged antibiotics. Surgery is seldom indicated except where there is cord compression from abscess formation.

Some more miscellaneous soft tissue infections are outlined in Table 19.5.

Further reading

Bulstrode, C., and Wilson-MacDonald, J. (2011). *Oxford Textbook of Trauma and Orthopaedics*. Oxford: Oxford University Press.

Osmon, D.R., Berbari, E.F., Berendt, A.R., et al. (2013). Diagnosis and management of prosthetic joint infection: clinical practice guidelines by the Infectious Diseases Society of America. *Clinical Infectious Diseases* 56 (1): 1–10.

Rockwood, C. A., Green, D.P., Heckman, J.D., et al. (2001). *Rockwood and Green's Fractures in Adults*. Philadelphia: Lippincott Williams & Wilkins.

Solomon, L., Warwick, D., and Nayagam, S. (2001). *Apley's System of Orthopaedics and Fractures*, 8th ed. New York: London: Hodder Arnold.

Warwick, D., and Nayagam, S. (2010). Apley's System of Orthopaedics and Fractures, 9th ed. Boca Raton, FL: Hodder Arnold.

CHAPTER 20

Metabolic Bone Diseases

Michael Fertleman, Shuli Levy, and Georgina Meredith

Imperial College Healthcare NHS Trust, London, UK

OVERVIEW

- Metabolic bone diseases are an important cause of morbidity, particularly in the elderly.
- One of these diseases, osteoporosis, is the leading cause of fractures in the elderly.
- Vitamin D deficiency and insufficiency are common in the elderly population and contribute to cause of fractures.
- Patient-oriented health goals and specific frailty interventions are essential.
- Gout may present as an inflammatory or septic arthritis.

Background

Metabolic bone disease (MBD) encompasses several different disorders of bone. The most common of these in the United Kingdom is osteoporosis. Worldwide, 200 million people suffer from this disease, making it a significant public health issue. As the population ages, the prevalence of osteoporosis is expected to increase. Other MBDs are vitamin D deficiency or insufficiency (on the spectrum but nonpathological), which are common worldwide. The aim of this chapter is to provide an overview of MBDs, their diagnoses and management, and how to recognise them as early as possible.

Osteoporosis

There are approximately 70,000 hip fractures per year in United Kingdom, with the vast majority being associated with underlying osteoporosis. Approximately 10% of people over the age 65 and up to 25% over age 85 are affected by this MBD. Addressing the prevention of falls as well as early screening for frailty and bone health in the community prior to, and following fracture, all contribute to holistic management.

Osteoporotic bone becomes fragile (due to lack of bone density) and therefore is at a high risk of fracture. Unfortunately, this is a retrospective diagnosis since osteoporosis gives no symptoms until an unexpected or fragility fracture occurs.

Fragility fractures are sustained from low-energy trauma, or from a force that would not usually be expected to cause a fracture. WHO quantifies this as forces equivalent to a fall from standing height or less.

Risk factors

Peak bone mass is reached by the third decade. This is chiefly determined genetically, but modifiable factors such as diet and weight-bearing exercise in earlier life also have a role. Reduced peak bone mass predictably increases the chance of developing osteoporosis in later life. Bone is constantly being remodelled by the resorptive activity of osteoclasts and the re-forming activity of osteoblasts. Under healthy circumstances, these are equally balanced, maintaining normal bone mineral density (BMD). A disruption to this balance leads to osteoporosis, as seen in Figure 20.1.

Aetiology

Osteoporosis is often multifactorial in aetiology, the commonest cause being post-menopausal bone loss, in which lack of oestrogen results in increased osteoclastic activity. As a result, osteoporosis is more common in females (1:2) than males (1:5). Reducing oestrogen levels also contribute to male osteoporosis. Caucasians and Asians are at greater risk, as are those with first-degree relatives with osteoporosis. When associated with ageing or post-menopausal changes, the condition may be termed *primary osteoporosis*. Underlying diseases such as rheumatoid arthritis, glucocorticoid use, and malabsorption, as well as lifestyle choices such as smoking, sedentary lifestyle, and alcohol use, can cause secondary osteoporosis. These all affect bone density in different ways and cumulatively (Table 20.1).

Clinical presentation

Typically, osteoporosis is asymptomatic until a fracture occurs, by which point significant bone loss has already occurred. Common presentations include:

ABC of Orthopaedics and Trauma, First Edition. Edited by Kapil Sugand and Chinmay M. Gupte.
© 2018 John Wiley & Sons Ltd. Published 2018 by John Wiley & Sons Ltd.

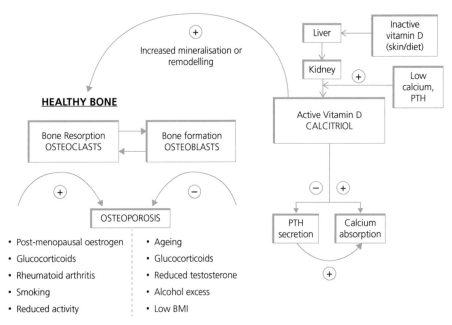

Figure 20.1 Bone metabolism

Table 20.1 Common risk factors for osteoporosis and underlying mechanisms

Risk factor	Effect on bone
Primary Osteoporosis	
Post-menopausal (including premature menopause)	Reduced oestrogen causes increased osteoclastic activity
Ageing, low mobility	Reduced osteoblast activity
Smokers	Impaired osteoblast activity
Secondary Osteoporosis	
Calcium and / or vitamin D deficiency	Increased bone resorption driven by raised PTH to supplement low serum calcium levels
Glucocorticoids and Cushing's	Reduced osteoblast activity, increased osteoclast activity, suppressed calcium absorption
Rheumatoid arthritis	Glucocorticoid use, chronic inflammation causing increased bone resorption
Male hypogonadism	Reduced oestrogen and testosterone levels. Testosterone withdrawal reduces osteoblast activity
Alcohol excess	Reduced osteoblast activity, associated nutritional deficiency (calcium, vitamin D)
Smoking	Upregulation of osteoclast production
Malabsorption	Predominantly due to vitamin D deficiency or insufficiency
Low body mass index (BMI)	Reduced osteoblast activity
Inadequate physical activity	Reduced osteoblast and increased osteoclast activities

Table 20.2 Common osteoporotic fracture sites

- Spinal – particularly lower thoracic and upper lumbar
- Hip – particularly neck of femur fractures in the elderly
- Distal radius:
  - usually Colles' fracture from falling on outstretched hand
  - commonly first presentation of female osteoporosis
- Proximal humerus
- Ribs
- Tibial plateau
- Pelvic fractures (Figure 20.2) – commonly sacral ala, pubic ramus, and ischial ramus

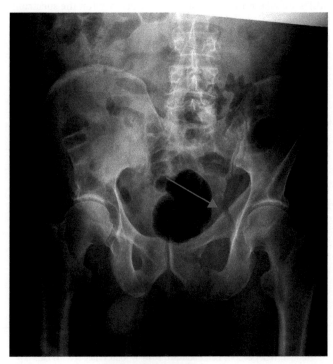

Figure 20.2 Radiograph showing left pubic ramus fracture

- Fragility fracture – a fracture sustained when falling from standing height or less
- Pain – at a new, spontaneous fracture site, or from resultant nerve compression
- Loss of height or progressive kyphosis – due to vertebral fracture

Common fracture sites and types are displayed in Table 20.2.

Spinal/vertebral body fractures

Spinal fractures may present with acute onset of back pain, often spontaneous, with no history of trauma, or after rolling in bed, coughing, or lifting (Figure 20.3). Pain is sharp and localised. Neurological injury is rare unless the fracture is severe, causing nerve root involvement. Two-thirds of vertebral compression fractures are asymptomatic and are diagnosed radiologically. On plain films, there is a loss of height associated with thoracic kyphosis, or lumbar lordosis may occur particularly with multilevel involvement.

Spinal fractures are classified radiologically according to which part of the vertebral body is most affected:
- *Wedge fracture*: anterior compression causing a wedge-shaped deformity. Commonly found in lower thoracic/upper lumbar regions.
- *Biconcave fracture*: central compression.
- *Crush fracture*: posterior compression.

Hip (neck of femur) fractures

Hip fractures are a common presentation of osteoporosis in the elderly, with the vast majority as the result of a fall resulting in a fragility fracture (Figure 20.4). They are associated with significant mortality, long-term morbidity, and loss of function (Table 20.3).

These fractures are classified radiologically according to the fracture site:
- Intracapsular – within the hip joint capsule, requiring hip hemiarthroplasty or total hip replacement
- Extracapsular – distal to the hip joint capsule, requiring dynamic hip screw (DHS), cannulated screws or intramedullary nail

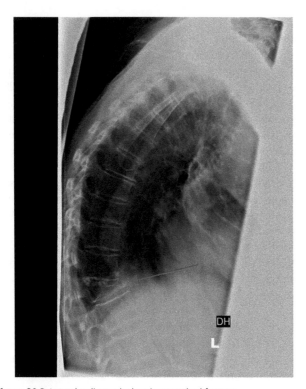

Figure 20.3 Lateral radiograph showing vertebral fracture

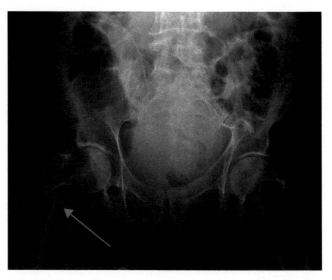

Figure 20.4 Radiograph (AP pelvis) showing a fracture of right extracapsular neck of femur

Table 20.3 Implications of a hip fracture

- Average 21-day inpatient admission.
- 11% readmission rate at 28 days post-discharge.
- Estimated 30-day mortality is 10%.
- Estimated 1-year mortality is 30%.
- 50% of people are permanently disabled to some extent.
- 10–20% of those admitted from home will require institutional care on discharge.

Table 20.4 FRAX tool

- FRAX is the WHO risk assessment tool that is validated to predict a 10-year hip and major osteoporotic fracture probability.
- The algorithm incorporates age, gender, BMI, family history, and key risk factors such as smoking and alcohol to calculate the risk.
- The score can be calculated with or without a formal BMD, thereby allowing treatment decisions without DXA scanning.

Assessment

Assessing osteoporosis is focussed on identifying those at risk of a fracture who meet thresholds for further investigation and treatment. Current NICE guidance recommends that at risk individuals should have a FRAX risk assessment to determine the 10-year predicted fracture risk (Table 20.4).

The following patient groups are considered at risk:
- All women > 65 years; all men > 75 years
- Women < 65 years and men < 75 years with:
  - Previous fragility fracture or family history of fragility fracture
  - Any condition or behaviour that predisposes to secondary osteoporosis (see Table 20.1)

This score can then be used to inform management decisions. The National Osteoporosis Guidelines Group (NOGG) recommends managing patients according to their FRAX score as follows (Figure 20.5):
- Low risk – reassess in 5 years or less; do not initiate treatment.
- Intermediate risk – measure BMD and recalculate FRAX score to determine need for intervention (see Table 20.5).
- High risk – consider treatment without further BMD assessment.

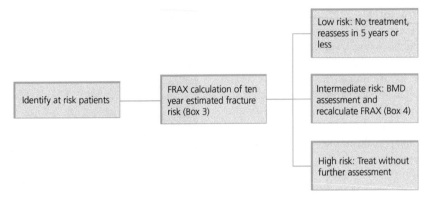

Figure 20.5 Summary of NOGG recommended algorithm for assessment of patients at risk of fracture

Table 20.5 Dual-energy X-ray absorptiometry (DXA) scan

- DXA scans are used to measure BMD, as part of a work-up for osteoporosis.
- The technique uses X-ray absorption by different bones to measure their density.
- Typically, lumbar spine, hip, and proximal femur are evaluated.
- Results are expressed as a T-score or Z-score; the units of measurement are standard deviation from the mean (SD).
  - T-scores compare BMD to that of an adult with peak BMD.
  - Z-scores compare BMD to age and ethnicity matched BMD.
- The WHO stratifies T-score values as follows:
  - 0 to −1 SD = normal BMD
  - −1 to −2.5 SD = osteopaenia
  - −2.5 SD or more = osteoporosis

NOGG additionally recommend that post-menopausal women with a prior fragility fracture should be considered for treatment without the need for further investigation.

Prior to treatment, a few key blood tests may be helpful in eliminating other reversible or contributory causes of osteoporosis. These include calcium, vitamin D, parathyroid hormone (PTH), thyroid function tests (TFT), and consideration of a myeloma screen. However, PTH and myeloma screens are expensive and should only be carried out where clinical history or basic biochemistry suggest further investigations are indicated.

Management of osteoporosis through lifestyle changes

The goal of management for osteoporosis is to minimise the risk of further deterioration in the bone architecture and density. Improving bone health can be achieved by inhibiting or enhancing different elements of the metabolic bone pathway (i.e. osteoclasts and osteoblasts). The guidelines for primary and secondary treatment of osteoporosis in England can be found through NICE.

Before embarking on pharmacological treatment options, it is important to coordinate individual health-oriented goals. Addressing the individual's lifestyle is paramount, and this includes diet and exercise. An exercise prescription that incorporates regular weight-bearing exercise, such as star jumps or hopping, is invaluable and has been shown in post-menopausal women to increase bone mass. "Walking and talking for 20 minutes every day" is a great place to start. Stretching and balance exercises are also recommended, especially outdoors, as this can boost vitamin D levels.

Diet plays a key role in the management of osteoporosis. A balanced diet should incorporate foods high in calcium, such as cheese, fish, vegetables, pulses, beans, and seeds, as well as cereal products and fruit. Minimising alcohol and smoking is also beneficial to bone health.

Management of osteoporosis through pharmacological options

Pharmacological treatment options are determined by an individual's T-score, age, and history of fractures. This is addressed in Figure 20.6.

Calcium and Vitamin D

Daily supplementation with calcium and vitamin D is recommended to all elderly people who live in an institution, as it has been shown to significantly reduce the number of fracture sustained. Any individual who is commenced on other pharmacological treatment for osteoporosis ought to be taking calcium and vitamin D supplements unless it is contraindicated.

Bisphosphonates

Bisphosphonates that promote osteoclast apoptosis to inhibit bone loss are a first-line treatment for osteoporosis. They are routinely used as treatment for secondary prevention for osteoporosis following fragility fracture. Alendronic acid is licensed for use in both men and women and is taken once a week with specific instructions. These include needing to be in an upright position for 30 minutes following ingestion. Compliance with alendronic acid is poor, with up to 80% of patients not being compliant at one year.

If alendronic acid is not tolerated, often due to gastrointestinal side effects, risedronate and etridronate are recommended. Another alternative is the annual intravenous zolendronic acid. A well-recognised side effect is osteonecrosis of the jaw, with advice to seek dental review prior to commencement if indicated.

If taken for more than five years, bisphosphonates are associated with atypical fractures. Their use is contraindicated in patients with renal impairment (eGFR < 30–35 mL/min).

Selective oestrogen receptor modulator (SERM)

Raloxifene is recommended as an alternative treatment to a bisphosphonate in post-menopausal women as a preventative measure for vertebral fractures. It has the serious side effect of tripling the risk

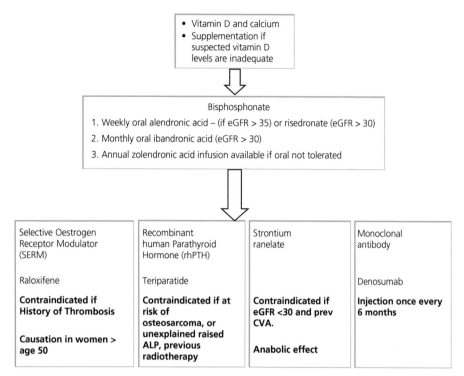

Figure 20.6 Pharmacological treatment of osteoporosis

of venous thrombosis and is therefore contraindicated in any woman who has a past medical history of thrombosis. Caution should therefore be used in starting this medication shortly after a hip fracture. In addition to being an HRT, this medicine has an associated risk with breast cancer. Its usage for osteoporosis prevention in women should be restricted to a specialist bone clinic.

Strontium ranelate

This treatment is also recommended as an alternative in patients intolerant or noncomplaint to bisphosphonates. It has a "dual action," as it increases deposition of new bone by osteoblasts and reduces resorption by osteoclasts. It is contraindicated in patients with an eGFR < 30 mL/min. Its use was severely restricted in 2013 following an association with DVT and increased risk of cerebrovascular and cardiovascular disease, and thus should only be started by a bone clinic.

Recombinant human PTH

Teriparatide is another treatment option if bisphosphonates are not well tolerated in post-menopausal women. It is given as a daily subcutaneous injection for 18 months. Teriparatide versus bisphosphonate therapy as first-line treatment for osteoporosis prevention is currently being reviewed.

Monoclonal antibody

Donosumab inhibits maturation of osteoclasts by inhibiting RANK ligand, a surface receptor on osteoclast precursors. It is administered every 6 months by subcutaneous injections. As with intravenous bisphosphonates, it must not be given in the context of vitamin deficiency or insufficiency.

Vitamin D deficiency

In recent years, the evidence regarding the role of vitamin D in numerous disorders, ranging from cardiovascular disease to cancer, has been growing. However, much of the data in this field remains conflicting. In contrast, the importance of vitamin D in bone health is well established.

The active form of Vitamin D, calcitriol, is derived from sequential hydroxylation of the inactive forms D_2 and D_3 in the liver and kidney (Figure 20.1). Active vitamin D acts directly on bones and on the bowel to increase calcium and phosphate absorption, with an overall action that increases bone mineralisation. Calcium and vitamin D levels are regulated by PTH via complex negative feedback loops. When these mechanisms fail, as in primary hyperparathyroidism, the ensuing metabolic disturbance leads to reduced BMD and osteoporosis.

In the United Kingdom, vitamin D deficiency is common, affecting approximately 15% of all adults, 30% of those over 65, and up to 90% of high-risk groups, including institutionalised and housebound elderly individuals. Most people are asymptomatic, although severe deficiency may cause bone pain and tenderness or result in osteomalacia, in which calcium and phosphate deficiency cause reduced bone mineralisation and bony deformity. Vitamin D deficiency is an important risk factor for osteoporosis, and anti-resorptive treatments for osteoporosis require adequate vitamin D levels to act effectively.

Treatment of deficiency states is with oral colecalciferol according to local guidelines, but occasionally intramuscular preparations may be favoured. Combined calcium and colecalciferol preparations generally do not contain enough vitamin D to raise levels, and should only be used for maintenance.

Paget's disease

Paget's disease, or osteitis deformans, results in bone remodelling and deformity (Figure 20.7). It was first described by Sir James Paget in 1882, and it is characterised by a combination of bone breakdown and formation of new bone.

A classic description of Paget's bone disease is that of either a mosaic or woven appearance under the microscope. There is an increased risk of pathological fractures.

The disease can be divided into three distinct phases:

- *First stage*: involves increased osteoclastic activity and hypervascularity resulting in bone loss (i.e. osteolysis).
- *Second* stage: involves a proliferation of bone through osteoblastic activity and some osteoclastic activity (i.e. mixed phase).
- *Third* stage: an extension of the second with formation of new bone, but this bone can be dense and mineralised.

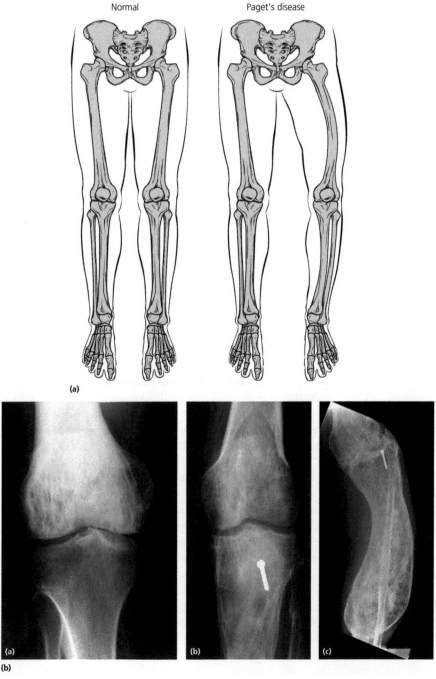

Figure 20.7 Limb deformity with bowing (sabre) tibia

Paget's disease occurs twice as often in men as in women and is uncommon before the age of 40 years. Patients with Paget's disease are often asymptomatic and are diagnosed radiologically or biochemically through a raised ALP. Patients with symptoms report bone pain, joint pain, and occasionally deformities in the pelvis, tibia, and skull. Those in the skull can result in cranial nerve compression such as the facial nerve (CN VIII), causing deafness. A 30% increased risk of osteogenic sarcoma is associated with Paget's disease.

Investigations

Investigations are centralised around imaging, including plain radiography looking for porotic and sclerotic changes and bone scans to look for uptake activity. Biochemical tests can identify raised ALP or calcium.

Management

The primary treatment is with analgesia and bisphosphonates in order to normalise bone formation. Surgery such as arthroplasty or osteotomy is a last resort.

Gout

Presentation

Gout will present in many clinical settings. It is described as an extremely painful, hot, and swollen joint that might mimic flare-up, inflammatory, or septic arthritis. Hence, these sinister differentials need to be ruled out first before confirming gout. The most commonly affected joint is the first MTPJ in nearly half of the cases. Gout is also known as podagra.

Aetiology

Gout is caused by hyperuricaemia (from excess alcohol, dehydration, male gender, genetic influence, or use of diuretics) in which uric acid crystals (i.e. tophi) deposit within joints to cause erosive arthropathy. Deposition in the kidneys may lead to nephropathy and calculi.

Investigations

Appropriate investigations consist of plain radiography looking for erosive changes (usually a late sign), arthrocentesis (e.g. synovial fluid sample from an acutely swollen and hot knee) looking for uric acid crystals, and plasma urate levels in blood testing (beware that the levels may be normal in early acute phase). Other blood tests will also look for high WCC (inflammation), U&E (renal profile), and ESR (chronicity of inflammation). Synovial fluid analysis can identify monosodium urate crystals under polarised light microscopy, which have a needle-like morphology and strong negative birefringence (as opposed to *pseudogout*, where calcium pyrophosphate

dihydrate crystals have a rhomboid shape and weak positive birefringence). Note that pseudogout has different risk factors consisting of hypercalcaemia, hypomagnesaemia, haemochromatosis, and thyroid disease.

Management

Lifestyle changes such as hydration, reduced alcohol intake, exercise, and vitamins can reduce the risk of recurrence, which is generally high. Treatment is usually bed rest and medical intervention with NSAIDs and colchicine in the acute phase, followed by allopurinol (xanthine oxidase inhibitor) for prevention. Using allopurinol in the acute phase may worsen the flare-up. Beware that colchicine and ibuprofen dosaging needs to account for the kidney function, so be careful of their use in renal failure. It is also worth considering prescribing a proton pump inhibitor with NSAIDs in cases more prone to peptic ulceration (side effects).

Renal osteodystrophy

Also known as chronic kidney disease mineral and bone disorder (CKD-MBD), renal osteodystrophy encompasses a range of bone disorders that occur in CKD, resulting from low calcium, high phosphate, poor vitamin D metabolism, and high PTH levels. Low vitamin D levels result in poor intestinal absorption of calcium. In CKD, low calcium and high phosphate levels trigger secondary hyperparathyroidism (thus stimulating PTH), which leads to a high turnover bone state to release calcium. Bone mineralisation may also be inhibited by metabolic acidosis. Less frequently, a low turnover bone state may occur, more commonly in dialysis patients. Both conditions lead to pain, stiffness, and increased fracture risk. Symptoms and signs of hypocalcaemia should also be noted. Treatment is aimed at correcting the driving metabolic disturbance, with dietary modification, vitamin D supplementation, phosphate binding agents, and, at times, parathyroidectomy. Conventional osteoporosis treatment may be considered in certain cases, although it is complicated by renal failure, contraindicating most treatments.

Further reading

Bernabei, R., Martone, A.M., Ortolani, E., et al. (2014). Screening, diagnosis and treatment of osteoporosis: a brief review. *Clinical Cases in Mineral and Bone Metabolism* 11 (3): 201–207.

Kanis, J.A., McCloskey, E.V., Harvey, N.C., et al. (2015). Intervention thresholds and the diagnosis of osteoporosis. *Journal of Bone and Mineral Research* 30 (10): 1747–1753.

Mankin, H.J1, and Mankin, C.J. (2008). Metabolic bone disease: a review and update. *Instructional Course Lectures* 57: 575–593.

Schneider, D., Hofmann, M.T., and Peterson, J.A. (2002). Diagnosis and treatment of Paget's disease of bone. *American Family Physician* 65 (10): 2069–2072.

CHAPTER 21

Bone and Soft Tissue Tumours

Rej Bhumbra

Barts Health Orthopaedic Centre, London, UK

OVERVIEW

- Bone and soft tissue tumours can present in all ages in a variety of ways.
- These conditions are managed in a multidisciplinary setting.
- Unexplained symptoms warrant early radiological assessment and a prompt referral to a supra-regional centre.
- Biopsy of these tumours is performed in the same unit as the surgery.
- Particular malignant tumours may require chemotherapy and/or radiotherapy in their management.

Presentation

Bone and soft tissue tumours present in all ages, with a varying history and different clinical findings, from completely asymptomatic to a pathological fracture. The key initial step is recognition of the possibility that a tumour may exist. NHS England grants patients the right, *"to be seen by a cancer specialist within a maximum of two weeks from GP referral for urgent referrals where cancer is suspected."* There is no definite way to be certain that a tumour is not malignant until examined histologically. Hence, any mass that is removed from a patient must be sent for pathological assessment. Patients present with one or more of the symptoms in Table 21.1.

Epidemiology

In adults, the vast majority of bone tumours are metastatic in origin. The most common primary sites that metastasise to bone are breast, kidney, prostate, thyroid, and lung carcinoma. Primary bone and soft tissue cancers have an annual incidence of approximately 1 and 3 per 100,000 population, respectively. Given the relative rarity of these malignant lesions, multidisciplinary expertise in bone and soft tissue tumours are at the supra-regional level.

Diagnosis

A diagnosis is reached using the triad of:
1 Clinical history and examination
2 Imaging findings
3 Pathological interpretation

Management

In superficial soft tissue lesions that are excised in primary care or at nonspecialist centres, that are less than approximately 3 cm and subsequently turn out to be malignant, a re-resection of the wound bed by a sarcoma service is then performed. With any lesions that are larger than a golf ball, the patient should be referred to a dedicated soft or bone tumour service for primary assessment of their tumour. Inappropriate management of these larger lesions in nonspecialist services jeopardises patient outcome.

Prognosis

Timing and nature of the signs and symptoms are unreliable. Generally, symptoms that do not resolve after 4–6 weeks require imaging unless there is an obvious and proven cause. A low threshold should exist for requesting a plain film on initial presentation. However, the patient may have had a mass for some years, with a new, recent onset of increased growth. This may happen with a lipoma that has undergone malignant transformation into a liposarcoma, or an osteochondroma, the cartilage cap of which has become a chondrosarcoma.

NICE guidelines for referral

See Table 21.2 and the National Institute for Health and Care Excellence (NG12 1.11, June 2015).

Bone tumours

Bone tumours have been traditionally categorised by histological assessment of cell of origin. If a tumour is malignant, it is termed a *sarcoma*. Once malignancy has been confirmed, the lesion is staged locally and the presence of skip lesions are determined with a whole bone MR. Distant staging with a CT chest and assessment of the skeleton is by radioisotope bone scanning. In Ewing sarcoma, certain units use a whole body MR, and for certain soft tissue sarcomas, PET CT is used to facilitate excluding polyfocal sites. However, the mainstay for *initial* radiological assessment of a bone tumour is by plain film radiography. A classification describing the typical radiological matrix type formed is presented in Table 21.3.

ABC of Orthopaedics and Trauma, First Edition. Edited by Kapil Sugand and Chinmay M. Gupte.
© 2018 John Wiley & Sons Ltd. Published 2018 by John Wiley & Sons Ltd.

Osteochondroma

One of the more common benign bone tumours is formed as a result of inappropriate oblique radial outgrowth from the physis growing in continuity with the trabeculae of metaphyseal bone away from the joint (Figure 21.1). This tumour can either be sessile or pedunculated, and either solitary or in association with multiple lesions. Multiple hereditary exostosis (or diaphyseal aclasis) is an autosomal dominant condition, but can occur secondary to spontaneous mutations in 20% of affected patients. Masses are excised if increasing in size, adversely affecting local structures, or if they have a greater than 2 cm cartilage cap in adults. Thicker cartilage caps may mark malignant transformation and warrant excision.

Osteoid osteoma

These lesions cause pain, which is often relieved by NSAIDS secondary to prostaglandin suppression. Fine cut CT identifies a small lucent nidus, surrounded by dense cortical bone (Figure 21.2). The lesions are best managed with radiofrequency ablation if less than 2 cm and if not too superficial or close to critical neurovascular structures or, indeed, the skin. If greater than 2 cm, these lesions are renamed osteoblastomas and usually require surgical curettage.

Osteosarcoma

A malignant osteoid producing tumour that occurs both in children and older adults. These may either be primary or secondary (Pagetoid bone or in sites of previous radiotherapy). It is usually managed with a combination of chemotherapy and surgery. Good prognostic indicators are isolated disease, margin negative resection, and very importantly, a good response (>90% necrosis) to chemotherapy. In younger patients with a good response to chemotherapy and a margin negative resection, the 5-year survival rate is approximately 80%. Systemic relapse is primarily manifested as lung metastases.

Table 21.1 Modes of presentation for bone and soft tissue tumours

- Mass (and mass effect)
- Pain (either relapsing and remitting or nonmechanical in origin)
- Fracture (pathological)
- Reduced function or altered sensation/weakness
- Incidentally on imaging

Ewing sarcoma

Classically presents in the young patient, often in association with systemic disease, with a raised ESR and CRP. The additional radiological features of diaphyseal onion skinning and oedema on MR can complicate the presentation and confuse this with infection.

Table 21.3 Tumour matrix types

Matrix type	Benign	Malignant
Osteoid	Osteochondroma	Osteosarcoma
	Osteoid osteoma	Ewing (reactive periosteal bone deposition)
Cartilage	Enchondroma	Chondrosarcoma
Lytic	Unicameral/aneurysmal bone cyst	Telangectatic osteosarcoma
	Giant cell tumour of bone	
Fibrous	Nonossifying fibroma	Adamantioma
	Fibrous dysplasia	

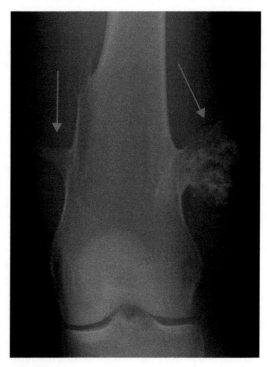

Figure 21.1 Multiple pedunculated osteochondromata in association with diaphyseal aclasia

Table 21.2 NICE guidelines for sarcoma referrals

Soft tissue sarcomas		Bone sarcomas	
Child / young people	Adult	Child / young people	Adult
Very urgent direct access (within 48 hours)	*Urgent direct access (within 2 weeks)*	*Very urgent referral (within 48 hours)*	*Urgent appointment (within 2 weeks)*
1 USS for unexplained growing lump 2 If USS findings suggest soft tissue sarcoma 3 If USS findings uncertain but clinical concern of soft tissue sarcoma persists		• Appointment for specialist assessment if X-ray suggests possibility of bone sarcoma • Assessment for bone sarcoma in those with unexplained bone swelling or pain	• Consider a suspected cancer pathway referral if X-ray suggests possibility of bone sarcoma.

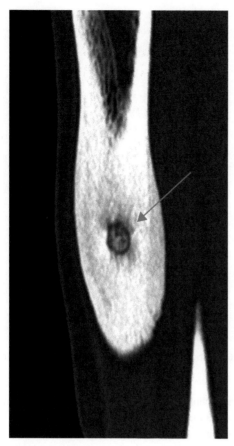

Figure 21.2 Osteoid osteoma (CT)

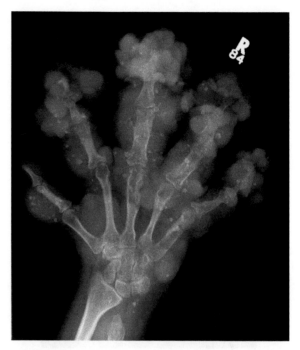

Figure 21.3 Maffucci's syndrome with multiple enchondromata and soft-tissue haemangiomas

A key difference is the presence of what is usually an extensive soft tissue mass found on an MR. This requires chemotherapy and surgery. Pelvic disease can also be managed with additional radiotherapy in order to decrease tumour volume.

Enchondroma

An enchondroma is a benign tumour of cartilage that originates within the medulla of bone. On imaging, the matrix within these lesions appears as spiculated mineralisation. They are often found incidentally in the hand or following pathological fractures. If multiple, the condition is named Ollier's disease or Maffucci's syndrome if found in association with haemangiomas (Figure 21.3). New onset pain, or a rapid increase in size, may be indicative of malignant transformation into chondrosarcoma. Lesions that are large, that are causing endosteal scalloping with cortical breakthrough in association with a soft tissue mass, are highly indicative of malignant transformation (Figure 21.4).

Chondrosarcoma

Usually, these malignant cartilage-producing tumours present in patients older than 40. They represent a spectrum of disease from low grade, which can be managed with curettage, to high grade, which requires a margin negative resection. Importantly, they are currently not sensitive to either chemotherapy or radiotherapy. Recent advances in defining its source genetic mutation may yield a future molecular targeted agent. Currently, the mainstay of

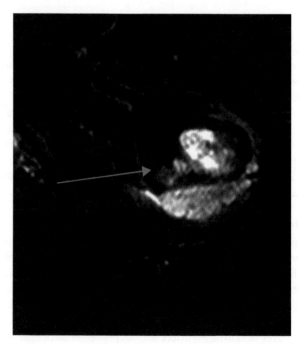

Figure 21.4 MR image demonstrating cortical breakthrough of an aggressive chondroid lesion

treatment is surgery. The most aggressive subtype is de-differentiated chondrosarcoma, in which the classic spiculated mineralisation can be replaced by lytic progression.

Unicameral/aneurysmal bone cyst

These are usually found in the metaphyseal region of the long bones of children. They classically have a small fractured bone fragment that falls to the bottom of the cystic lesion – the *fallen leaf sign*

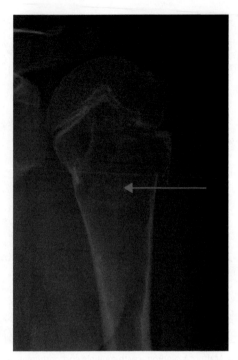

Figure 21.5 Fallen leaf sign in a lytic, pathologically fractured unicameral bone cyst (arrow indicating fallen fragment)

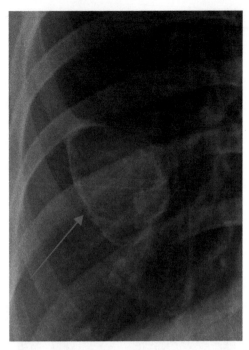

Figure 21.6 Ground-glass appearance of fibrous dysplasia in the rib

(Figure 21.5). These cysts may require intervention if there are ongoing problems with pain and fracture; hence, lesions of the lower limb more commonly require decompression with or without injection of bone marrow aspirate or steroid. In an aneurysmal bone cyst, there are multiple fluid-fluid levels with expansion of the bone around the lesion. Surgical management consists of curettage, breakdown of the loculations and excision of the cystic lining. These procedures are associated with bleeding, especially when performed in the pelvis; hence, preoperative embolisation should be considered. Injection of adjuncts into the individual loculations is a developing area of treatment.

Giant cell tumour of bone

A juxta-articular eccentrically placed lytic lesion with internal septation classically found in patients 30–40 years old. Joint preservation is balanced with the need to completely curette the tumour as well as obtaining postsurgical stability. Although cement is often used to support the bone, long-term aberrant loading of subchondral bone increases the likelihood of subsequent joint replacement. Graft material can be used to fill the defect, but load protection and longer rehabilitation time is required to consolidate bone remodelling. Pelvic and recurrent disease can be problematic, but encouraging results are noted with newer pharmacological treatments, making surgical interventions safer and more effective. Giant cell tumours can (<1%) transform into a malignant form with metastatic potential.

Multiple myeloma

Although strictly a haematological malignancy originating within the bone marrow, it often presents to orthopaedic services with either bone pain or fracture, or radiologically on skeletal screening. Haematological tests will reveal hypercalcaemia, renal failure, anaemia, and high ESR.

Protein electrophoresis, urine Bence-Jones proteins, and bone marrow biopsy are other diagnostic investigations.

Spinal disease and pain are managed with radiotherapy and consideration for either vertebral augmentation using polymethylmethacrylate (PMMA) or surgery with decompression and stabilisation. Long bone disease can be assessed for treatment with either radiotherapy and/or surgery. Surgery includes either skeletal stabilisation or endoprosthetic replacement. Additionally, chemotherapy, steroids, biological therapies, and bone marrow stem cell transplant are the main treatments for myeloma.

Fibrous dysplasia

Abnormal bone and fibrous tissue that replaces normal bone marrow, fibrous dysplasia covers a spectrum of disorders from asymptomatic monostotic disease to florid systemic conditions associated with McCune-Albright. They classically give a "ground glass" appearance on plain film (Figure 21.6) and CT imaging. If found in association with soft tissue myxomas, this condition is termed Mazabraud's disease.

Soft tissue tumours

Soft tissue lesions are more common than bone tumours. Careful history and examination point towards the aggressiveness of the lesion. Masses that are large, deep, rapidly growing, and immobile are concerning. Imaging characteristics on ultrasound can be interpreted with limited capacity, and the imaging modality of choice for these tumours is MRI, which indicates whether the lesion is aggressive, nonaggressive, or marginal (Table 21.4).

Although traditionally classified as cell origin type (Table 21.5), specific genetic markers that are currently used for diagnostic purposes represent a future molecular genetic descriptive system.

Table 21.4 Aggressive appearances include

1 Located deep to fascia
2 >5 cm
3 Lobular contour profile
4 Heterogeneity on T1 and T2 consistent with areas of tissue growth in direct association with necrosis and haemorrhage

Table 21.5 Cell of origin with benign and malignant subtypes

	Benign	Malignant
Fat	Lipoma	Liposarcoma
Vessel	Arterio-venous malformation	Angiosarcoma
Nerve	Schwannoma Neurofibroma	Malignant peripheral nerve sheath tumour
Fibrous	Fibromatosis	Fibrosarcoma
Synovium	Pigmented vilonodular synovitis	

Lipomas

Lipomas are common lesions and can be found in isolation or in multiple sites (Durcum's disease/lipomatosis). Lipomas that contain internal areas of nodularity may be representative of a liposarcomatous de-differentiation.

Liposarcoma

This can be either well or undergo de-differentiation to a more aggressive variety. If myxoid, this cancer is termed myxoid liposarcoma. This tumour type is sensitive to volume reduction in the preoperative radiotherapy setting. Preoperative radiotherapy does, however, increase the chance of wound complications postoperatively.

Arterio-venous malformation (AVM)

AVM can give the patient an aching sensation. The lesions can be and grouped into low- or high-flow lesions. High-flow lesions can be embolised by interventional radiologists, avoiding the need for surgery.

Angiosarcoma

Angiosarcoma are aggressive tumours that can "skip," requiring careful clinical and MR assessment. Prognosis is poor.

Schwannoma

Schwannoma is a benign tumour of the nerve sheath. Tinel's sign can be helpful in obtaining a diagnosis. The lesion is tapped, and distal and proximal pain radiation is produced. MR features are bright on T2, with a target and taper sign (Figure 21.7).

Neurofibroma

Neurofibroma is a fusiform tumour involving the entire circumference of the nerve and not just the Schwann cell.

Fibromatosis

Fibromatosis is found in the hand (Dupuytren's), foot (plantar fibrosis), or the penis (Ledderhose's disease), as well as practically in any other part of the body. Masses are resected if causing local

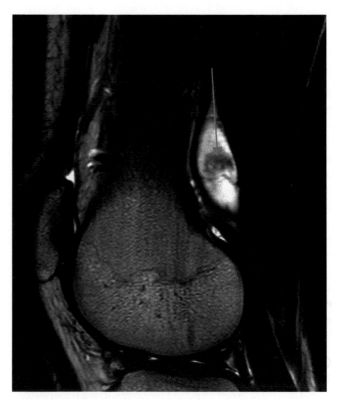

Figure 21.7 Target sign (arrow) and taper sign in a schwannoma (arrow head)

pressure or mass effects, but margin status bears no relation to recurrence. They are better managed pharmacologically or with radiation.

Fibrosarcoma

Fibrosarcoma is a malignant lesion with an infiltrative growth pattern necessitating wide resection margins.

Treatment strategies

These lesions are managed in a multidisciplinary team setting. A collaborative decision on biopsy tract location, input of clinical and medical oncology, resectability, reconstruction, histological interpretation, and subsequent follow-up and rehabilitation is made by a dedicated specialist team. Future molecular targeted therapies may offer hope in improving overall survival once tumoural genetic molecular characteristics are more accurately defined. Earlier diagnosis, combined with biological, morphological, and functional imaging, as well as targeted treatment with improved outcomes, remain long-term aims. Treatment strategy is defined by tumour biology. Malignant lesions are best treated with surgery, with other chemo- or radiotherapeutic agents, depending on the lesion.

Resection margins

A margin-negative resection is the primary surgical aim, with complete removal of the tumour. After this has been achieved, reconstruction of the remaining soft tissues, and if required, bone and neurovascular structures, is performed. A pathological margin classification has both qualitative and quantitative margin data metrics.

1 mm of fascia, periosteum, or adventitia is quantitatively close, but is a "good-quality marginal margin." Marginal resections of an infiltrative tumour growth pattern in muscle, such as a myofibrosarcoma, can raise concerns about the margin quality.

Radiotherapy

If marginal excision (i.e. without a wide margin/cuff of normal tissue) is planned, such as close vascular tumoural contact, then radiotherapy is considered to sterilise the surgical field around the tumour. Radiotherapy can be administered either in the pre- or postoperative context. Although the irradiated volume is smaller in the preoperative setting, the risk of subsequent wound breakdown is twice as likely. The timing of radiotherapy (whether pre- or postoperative) is reflected in the extent of tissue fibrosis, joint stiffness, and oedema secondary to irradiating either just the tumoural site or to completely include the operative and surrounding field.

Modern radiotherapy techniques modulate the intensity (IMRT) and can spare critical healthy structures in relation to conventional two-dimensional beams. Newer radiation techniques are being implemented more widely for other tumour types, such as proton therapy for particular axially located tumours (e.g. chordoma).

Chemotherapy

The use of chemotherapy in the soft tissue sarcoma is variable and should be limited to certain patient subgroups. Its use is more widespread in the United States but less so in Europe, as its role in improving long-term overall survival for the majority of soft tissue sarcomas is poor.

Further reading

Gerrand, C.H., Wunder, J.S., and Kandel, R.A. (2001). Classification of positive margins after resection of soft tissue sarcoma of the limb predicts the risk of local recurrence. *Journal of Bone and Joint Surgery (Br.)* 83 (8): 1149–1155.

Grimer, R.J., and Briggs, T.W. (2010). Earlier diagnosis of bone and soft-tissue tumours. *Journal of Bone and Joint Surgery (Br.)* 92: 1489–1492.

National Cancer Institute. (n.d). SEER stat fact sheets: bone and joint. www.seer.cancer.gov/statfacts/html/bones.html

National Institute for Health and Care Excellence. (2006). Improving outcomes for people with sarcoma. www.guidance.nice.org.uk/csgsarcoma.

National Institute for Health and Care Excellence. (2015, June). Suspected cancer: recognition and referral. NG12 1.11. www.nice.org.uk/guidance/ng12/chapter/1-recommendations-organised-by-site-of-cancer.

O'Sullivan, B., Davis, A.M., Turcotte, R., et al. (2002). Preoperative versus postoperative radiotherapy in soft-tissue sarcoma of the limbs: a randomised trial. *Lancet* 359 (9325): 2235–2241.

Woll, P.J., Reichardt, P., Le Cesne, A., et al. (2012). EORTC Soft Tissue and Bone Sarcoma Group and the NCIC Clinical Trials Group Sarcoma Disease Site Committee. Adjuvant chemotherapy with doxorubicin, ifosfamide, and lenograstim for resected soft-tissue sarcoma (EORTC 62931): A multicentre randomised controlled trial. *Lancet Oncology* 13 (10): 1045–1054.

CHAPTER 22

Peripheral Nerve Injury (PNI)

Rishi Dhir[1], Kapil Sugand[2,3], and Tom Quick[1]

[1] Royal National Orthopaedic Hospital, Stanmore, UK
[2] MSk Lab, Charing Cross Hospital, Imperial College London, London, UK
[3] North West London Rotation, London, UK

OVERVIEW

- There are numerous causes of nerve injury, the most common being diabetes.
- Nerve injuries can be broadly divided into degenerative or conduction block (neurapraxia), and understanding this distinction is important.
- Triple assessment involving a history, examination, and investigations such as imaging or nerve conduction studies help to confirm the diagnosis, localise the lesion, and determine possible prognosis.
- Definitive diagnosis and prognosis may depend on surgical exploration and early recognition, and referral to a peripheral nerve unit is essential.

Structure

The nervous system is composed of three components:
1 The central nervous system: brain, brain stem, and spinal cord
2 The peripheral nervous system: relays information from the periphery to the brain, and vice versa
3 The autonomic nervous system: responsible for sympathetic and parasympathetic function

Anatomy

Peripheral nerves are composed of neural and non-neural tissues. The basic functional unit of a nerve is confusingly also called a nerve or, more correctly, a neurone. The microscopic neurone consists of a cell body (perikaryon), an axon (the elongated functional unit of a neurone), and a terminal structure (e.g. a motor end plate or Golgi sensory organ). The cell body contains a nucleus, cytoplasm (axoplasm), and the various constituents (such as vesicles, axoplasmic reticulum, and microtubules) needed to maintain the physical and physiological function of the axon. Dendrites branch out from the cell body, facilitating communicating with other cell bodies.

Non-neural tissues are present within the nerve such as vascular and connective tissue to nourish and support the axons. There are also glia, which in the peripheral nervous system are called Schwann cells. These glia support the neurone and can either invest a single myelinated neurone or multiple nonmyelinated neurones (Figure 22.1). Schwann cells produce myelin (a fatty sheath that insulates the axon) and allow myelinated neurones to increase their conduction speed. The Schwann cell also has a secretory function to maintain the neurone and is important in redirecting nerve regrowth after injury, via neurotropic chemicals.

Macroscopically neurones are covered in endoneurium, and several neurones group in bundles (fascicles) encased in perineurium. Multiple fascicles form the final nerve trunk (embedded in perineurium).

Nerve injury

Most commonly, nerve injuries present after some history of trauma or injury, but in clinical practice, injuries to nerves can occur by numerous means.

Aetiology

These can be remembered by the mnemonic **DATING ME**.
Diabetes (commonest), **D**rugs
Autoimmune
Traction, **T**rauma
Inflammatory, Iatrogenic, Infection, Ischaemia
Neoplastic
General (systemic)
Motor neuron disease
Electrical/Thermal

There are traditionally numerous classifications of nerve injuries, and these are important in helping to determine prognosis. However, it can be very confusing, as each of these classifications applies to individual axons, not the whole macroscopic nerve. It is

---

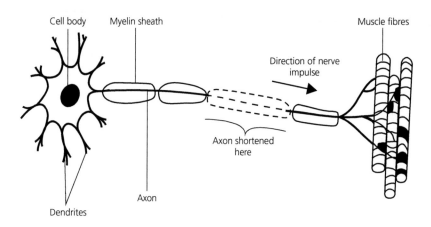

Figure 22.1 Neurone

Table 22.1 PNI classification systems

	Classification system		
Birch & Bonney	Seddon	Sunderland	Pathology
Conduction block (transient)	Neurapraxia	I	Anoxia with recoverable membrane disturbance
Conduction block (prolonged)	Neurapraxia	I	Distortion of myelin sheath
Degenerative (favourable prognosis)	Axonotmesis	II	Axonal disruption; basal lamina, endoneurium, and perineurium intact
Degenerative (unfavourable prognosis)	Axonotmesis	III	Axonal disruption; basal lamina and endoneurium damaged
Degenerative (unfavourable prognosis)	Axonotmesis	IV	Axonal disruption; endoneurium and perineurium damaged; epineurium intact
Degenerative (unfavourable prognosis)	Neurotmesis	V	Loss of continuity of all nerve elements

therefore important to remember that clinically one should bear these classifications in mind but acknowledge that the clinical picture will be a collection of differing injuries to a huge population of many tens, if not hundreds, of thousands of axons. It is this clinical correlate that the Birch, Bonney classification provides, and is thus the most useful in day-to-day practice.

Classifications of nerve injury

See Table 22.1.

Degenerative lesions (axonotmesis and neurotmesis)

These are characterised by axonal loss distal to the injury though a process called *Wallerian degeneration*, where the distal neurone (axon and myelin) is broken down by an acute inflammatory process. The Schwann cells in the distal neurone form "Bands of Bungner," which produce *neurotropic factors* (guiding the "direction of growth" of the regenerating axons). The proximal part of the neurone containing the cell bodies may survive and proliferate (via neurotrophic factors, which stimulate growth) to grow new sprouting axons distally and must reach their appropriate target (via a process called *contact guidance*) before functional recovery occurs.

Recovery is predictable and occurs at a rate of 1 mm/day following a 2-week latent period (*regeneration stagger*) and can be monitored clinically by the (*Hoffman-)Tinel's sign*. The Tinel's sign is elicited after trauma by percussing along the course of the nerve

from distally to proximally. When the percussing finger taps on a regenerating growth cone, the nerve is stimulated and the brain interprets the neuronal signal as originating from the sensory component of the nerve (where a tingling sensation is thus appreciated) e.g. tapping over a regenerating radial nerve will produce tingling over the dorsum of the first webspace of the hand (superficial sensory branch of radial nerve). Therefore, an advancing Tinel's sign is evidence of functional recovery and implies a good prognosis for a degenerative lesion. The advancement of the Tinel's sign (at a rate of 1 mm per day) should be recorded at each clinical visit. After 4 or 6 weeks, the Tinel should have moved an inch or so distally (a minimal distance over which error of measurement of the position of the Tinel to local bony landmarks can be appreciated). If this is the case, the clinical prognosis is good. If the Tinel has not advanced forward, then it is deemed stationary. The axons have not found their path forwards down to the distal stump and the clinical prognosis is poor and intervention is required.

Nondegenerative lesions: Conduction block (aka neurapraxia)

This is known as neurapraxia (*neur-* nerve; *apraxia-* not working) or, more simply put, conduction block (CB). The neuronal structure remains intact but there is loss of physiological function. As there is no Wallerian degeneration, there is not a Hoffman-Tinel's sign at the injury site. This pathology can show a patchy pattern of recovery when the block to conduction has been reversed (e.g. pressure or traction or anoxia). Recovery can take up to 3 months after a single event of CB. Under a persistent conduction block pathology (constrictive scar for example), recovery will never return unless the process is arrested (neurolysis is performed) and from this point, recovery can occur at a point to 3 months from cessation of CB. If persistent CB continues, it may deepen and it can lead to degeneration of the neural elements.

Clinical evaluation

A thorough history, supplemented by a good clinical examination with knowledge of basic plexus and peripheral nerve anatomy gives the majority of information for diagnosis and subsequent management of nerve injuries. In all cases, recognition and subsequent early referral or discussion with a tertiary peripheral nerve injury specialist for definitive assessment and management is mandatory, as delays can adversely affect clinical outcome. With a degenerative nerve injury, "time is muscle," and any delay in reaching an appropriate diagnosis and instituting treatment can reduce final outcome. It is estimated that muscle function degrades at around the rate of 2% per week of delay.[2] Thus, if referral is made a year late in a case where treatment should have been instituted as soon as possible, there is very little chance of gaining any useful motor function – keep this in mind!

History

An adequate history must be taken with relevant questions regarding these issues:

- *Injury mechanism*: closed (more likely to produce stretch or contusion) or open (more likely to involve division) and if cut, the type of blade (clean laceration or serrated/blunt)
- *Time frame* from injury to examination
- *Change in clinical picture* (evidence of recovery? persistence or occurrence of pain?)
- *Any initial intervention* causing change in neurology (e.g. plaster cast)
- *Evidence of ongoing compression* such as pain or worsening neurology
- *Medical comorbidities*

Examination

Clinical assessment of:

- All *modalities* of the nerve (**M**otor, **T**ouch, **S**ympathetic, and **P**ain). Use the mnemonic **M**ight **T**ry **S**omething **P**rofessional.
- *Anatomical location* of the injury (brachial plexus or peripheral nerve).
- *Evidence of a Hoffman-Tinel's sign* indicating the type of nerve injury (degenerative or nondegenerative) and any possible recovery.

Localising the lesion

Nerve injury can occur at the level of the nerve root, plexus (cervical, brachial, lumbosacral), or peripheral nerve. A wide knowledge of anatomy is thus needed.

A typical case encountered in a peripheral nerve injuries unit is a brachial plexus injury. The brachial plexus consists of the anterior rami (branches) of nerve roots C5-T1 (Figure 22.2).

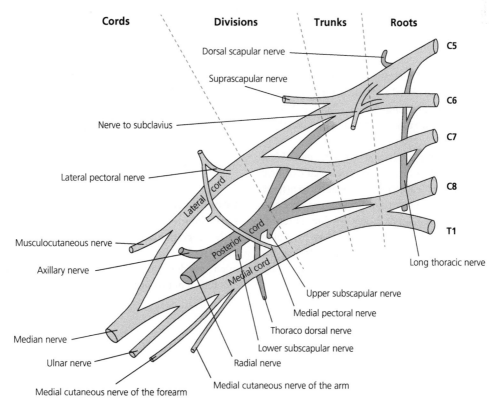

Figure 22.2 Brachial plexus

The different subdivisions can be remembered by this mnemonic:

REAL TEACHERS DRINK COLD BEER

- **Roots** (C5, C6, C7, C8, T1)
- **Trunks** (upper, middle, and lower)   ⎱ Supraclavicular
- **Divisions** (anterior and posterior)   Retroclavicular
- **Cords** (medial, lateral, and posterior)   ⎱ Infraclavicular
- **Branches**

The key question clinically is whether the nerve injury is supraclavicular, infraclavicular, or involves an isolated peripheral nerve.

> The main differentiating nerves to test are:
> - Dorsal scapular (rhomboids): Squeeze shoulder blades together
> - Long thoracic (serratus anterior): Thrust arm forward as if stabbing with a sword
> - Suprascapular (abduction for supraspinatus and external rotation for infraspinatus)
> These three branches come off the supraclavicular plexus. Subclavius also does, but it is difficult to test.

The rest of the nerves can be tested by examining the motor and sensory branches that they supply (Table 22.2).

Investigations

- *Appropriate imaging of the body part,* e.g. plain radiographs (to evaluate underlying fractures), ultrasound, and MRI scans (to exclude a local compressive lesion or associated nerve injuries). Consider compartment pressure assessments and decompression if there is clinical concern.
- Doppler assessment of pulses if clinically concerned – any damaged limb that has a combined neural and vascular injury is likely to present need for surgical interventional, and "pink pulselessness" should not be considered a minor complaint, particularly in children.
- *Neurophysiology: NCS (nerve-conduction studies) and EMG (electromyography)* can be performed to answer a specific clinical question and look at the electrical activity in the nerve to just see what is going on. These can be used to confirm the presence and anatomical location of a nerve injury and any evidence of regeneration. Wallerian degeneration takes several weeks, so doing these tests early on may lead to a false negative. Review the patient regularly and consider referring to these tests at least 3 weeks postinjury after the onset of neurological deficits.

Management

The key decision to make by the peripheral nerve surgeon is whether to operate (explore the nerve) or not. All nonoperative cases should be followed up for evidence of recovery.

Broadly speaking, reasons for urgent exploration would include the following:

- *Known trauma/damage to nerve:* e.g. a penetrating or open injury over the course of a nerve where there is dysfunction of that nerves function mandates exploration of that nerve.
- *Evidence of ongoing compression:* e.g neuropathic pain (suggestive of an ongoing insult to the nerve) or worsening neurologic function (progressive weakness or expanding area of sensory disturbance).
- *No evidence of recovery* despite conservative treatment: e.g. clinically (no advancing Tinel's sign) or neurophysiologically (no evidence of regeneration).

Operative treatment can encompass a variety of techniques ranging from simple nerve exploration (to assess the nerve and confirm the diagnosis, severity of the injury and capacity of the nerve to regenerate) and *neurolysis* (removal of scar tissue from the nerve) to more complex procedures such as nerve repair, nerve grafting, or nerve or tendon transfers (see below).

It often involves a combination of these and depends on several factors, including patient factors, injury factors (type and severity), and surgical factors (expertise of the surgeon).

In reality, definitive treatment will only be decided by the operating surgeon once the nerve has been explored, examined, and tested (neurophysiologically) intraoperatively (Figure 22.3). It is also dependent on the time period postinjury (as in the face of delay, the success rates of direct repair, nerve grafting, and nerve transfers becomes significantly worse, whereas operations such as tendon transfer lose no efficacy and are thus very useful and reliable reconstructive adjuncts).

Common peripheral nerve injuries

In addition to the plexus injuries described earlier, there are numerous peripheral nerve injuries in orthopaedic cases that are too vast to encompass in this text, but some of the typical cases you might meet, their recognition, and management are listed in Table 22.3.

Conclusion

Nerve injuries, either isolated or as sequelae of trauma, require early recognition, adequate clinical assessment, and prompt referral to a tertiary peripheral nerve injuries centre, as these injuries can often have devastating consequences for patient function and quality of life if not recognised or managed urgently.

Table 22.2 Clinical examination of the brachial plexus

Source	Nerve	Root	Motor	Sensory
Roots	Dorsal scapular	C5	Rhomboids	-
Roots	Nerve to subclavius	C5,C6	Subclavius	-
Roots	Long thoracic	C5-C7	Serratus anterior	-
Upper trunk	Suprascapular	C5,C6	Supraspinatus, infraspinatus	-
Lateral cord	Lateral pectoral	C5-C7	Pectoralis major and pectoralis minor (by communicating with medial pectoral nerve)	-
Lateral cord	Musculo-cutaneous	C5-C7	Biceps, brachialis, and coracobrachialis	Lateral forearm (becomes lateral cutaneous nerve of forearm)
Lateral cord	Lateral contribution to median nerve	C5-C7	Pronator teres, flexor carpi radialis	Digital and palmar median sensation (radial 3½ digits)
Posterior cord	Upper subscapular	C5,C6	Upper fibres of subscapularis	-
Posterior cord	Thoracodorsal	C6-C8	Latissimus dorsi	-
Posterior cord	Lower subscapular	C5,C6	Lower subscapularis, teres major	-
Posterior cord	Axillary	C5,C6	Deltoid (anterior and posterior branches) Teres minor (posterior branch)	Posterior branch becomes upper lateral cut, nerve of arm
Posterior cord	Radial	C5-T1	Triceps, supinator, anconeus, brachioradialis, lateral brachialis, and extensor muscles of forearm	Posterior cutaneous nerve of arm and also skin over dorsum of hand (first webspace) by cutaneous branch of radial
Medial cord	Medial pectoral	C8, T1	Pectoralis major and pectoralis minor	-
Medial cord	Medial contribution to median nerve	C8, T1	Flexor digitorum superficialis, palmaris longus (all via median nerve) Flexor pollicis longus, flexor digitorum profundus to second and third digits, and pronator quadratus (via anterior interosseous branch) LOAF muscles (lateral lumbricals 1 and 2, opponens pollicis, abductor pollicis brevis, and flexor pollicis brevis) via recurrent motor branch	-
Medial cord	Medial cutaneous nerve of arm	C8, T1	-	Front and medial skin of the arm
Medial cord	Medial cutaneous nerve of forearm	C8, T1	-	Medial skin of the forearm
Medial cord	Ulnar	C8, T1	Flexor carpi ulnaris, the medial two bellies of flexor digitorum profundus, the intrinsic hand muscles, except the LOAF muscles	Skin of medial 1½ digits

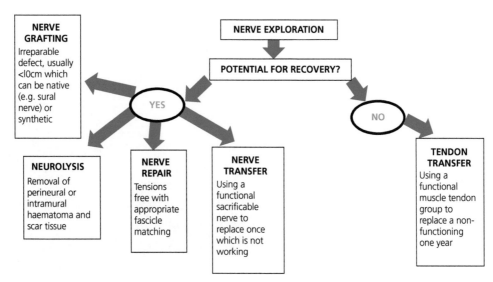

Figure 22.3 PNI surgical options

Table 22.3 Common PNI scenarios

Trauma	Nerve at risk	How to test
Anterior shoulder dislocation	Axillary	• Deltoid (retropulsion of the abducted humerus is the isolated function lost) and sensation over regimental badge (upper lateral part) of shoulder. • Exclude post cord injury by testing subscapularis (upper and lower subscapular nerves) and latissimus dorsi (thoracodorsal nerve) and radial nerve function.
Humeral shaft fracture	Radial	• Test extension of elbow, wrist, fingers, and thumb (wrist drop). • Loss of sensation over dorsum of first webspace. • Exclude post cord injury by testing subscapularis and latissimus dorsi and axillary nerve function. Radial palsy Normal
Paediatric Supracondylar fracture of humerus	Partial median nerve injury (often mistaken as an AIN) Ulnar nerve (at injury or iatrogenic during surgery)	• "Make an OK sign." • Tests flexor pollicis longus (thumb flexion) and flexor digitorum profundus (flexion of DIPJ of index finger). • Check digital and palmar sensation sympathetics and pain. • Check median intrinsics. • "Make a star," "cross your fingers," or "spread your fingers" to check ulnar intrinsics. • Palpate FCU and look for FDP to little finger. • Check digital and palmar sensation sympathetics and pain. • Check ulnar intrinsics.
Perilunate dislocation	Median nerve	Median digital (to radial 3 and a half fingers on palmar side) and palmar sensation sympathetics and pain and motor to LOAF muscles.
Elbow dislocation	Ulnar nerve	Hypothenar wasting, ulnar clawing, and sensory deficit of ulnar 1½ digits.
Posterior hip dislocation / post posterior approach to hip replacement	Sciatic nerve (peroneal division)	• Damage to common peroneal nerve (superficial and deep) can cause foot drop. • Remember to also test tibial (hamstrings/gastroc-soleus) and branches of sciatic sensation sympathetics and pain below the knee (to exclude loss of hip extension and knee flexion).
Knee dislocation/ posterolateral corner injury	Common peroneal nerve	• Foot drop occurs. • Test extension of ankle and toes (tibialis anterior, flexor digitorum longus and flexor hallucis longus (deep branch), and eversion of ankle (peronei) supplied by the superficial branch.

Further reading

Birch, R., Bonney, G., and Wynn Parry, C.B. (1998). *Surgical disorders of the peripheral nerves*. Edinburgh: Churchill Livingstone.

Hing, C., and Birch, R. (2006). Nerve. In: *Basic Orthopaedic Sciences: The Stanmore Guide* (Ed. M. Ramachandran), pp. 95–107. London: Hodder Arnold.

Maggi, S.P., Lowe, J.B., and Mackinnon, S.E. (2003). Pathophysiology of nerve injury. *Clinical Plastic Surgery* 30: 109–126.

CHAPTER 23

Orthopaedic Biomechanics

Hussein Taki[1] and Bernard van Duren[2]

[1] Addenbrooke's Hospital, Cambridge, UK
[2] Yorkshire and Humber Deanery, UK

OVERVIEW

- Basic science and biomechanical concepts are useful in understanding of pathology, diagnosis, and treatment of orthopaedic conditions.
- Trauma and orthopaedic surgeons rely on biomechanical principles in the management of their patients. Examples include:
  - How fractures will displace and therefore how best to fix them
  - What type of implants to use
  - How to configure joint replacements
  - What bearing surfaces to use for joint replacements
  - How best to rehabilitate a patient after surgery

Biomechanics

Biomechanics is a broad term that refers to mechanical principles applied to the structure and function in the human body. Specifically, mechanics is the study of forces and motions produced by their actions. The study of mechanics can be subdivided into (i) statics and (ii) dynamics.

- *Dynamics* is the study of systems in motion. It can be further sub divided into:
  - Kinetics
  - Kinematics
- *Kinetics* examines the forces acting on the body during movement and the motion with respect to time and forces.
- *Kinematics* describes the motion of a body without regard to the forces that produce the motion.
- *Statics* is the study of forces associated with nonmoving or nearly moving systems. It is the branch of mechanics most commonly encountered in day-to-day orthopaedics.

Free body diagram

Creating a free body diagram is an important skill in statics, allowing us to understand the forces going through a joint, otherwise known as the *joint reaction force*. Figure 23.1 represents the forces and moments going through a joint in equilibrium. In order to understand the free body diagram we must first clarify a number of important definitions in biomechanics.

Newton's laws describe the relationship between a body and the forces acting upon it, and its motion in response to those forces.

These three laws of motion form the basis in understanding mechanics.
- **First law:** If there is no net force on an object, it remains at rest or continues to move at a constant velocity.
- **Second law:** The force on an object are equal to its mass multiplied by its acceleration $F = ma$.
- **Third law:** When a first body exerts a force on a second body, the second body simultaneously exerts a force that is equal in magnitude and opposite in direction on the first body.

Other important definitions include:
- **Force:** A force is defined as any cause that tends to alter the state of rest of a body or its state of uniform motion in a straight line. For example, the Système Internationale (SI) unit of force is the Newton. It is defined to be the force that accelerates a mass of one kilogram at the rate of one meter per second^2.
- **Lever:** A lever is a machine consisting of a beam or rigid rod pivoted at a fixed hinge, or fulcrum. A lever is a rigid body capable of rotating on a point on itself, and when a force is applied to it this force is amplified to produce an increased output force. In the body, force is applied by muscles to bones acting as levers, with their fulcrum being joints. An example would be triceps acting on the olecranon of the ulna with the fulcrum being the elbow.
- **Fulcrum:** Fixed pivot point that a lever rotates around.
- **Moment arm/torque:** Perpendicular distance from the fulcrum to the line of action of force acting on the lever.
- **Equilibrium:** A system is in a state of static equilibrium when the resultant of all forces and all moments is equal to zero.
- **Vector:** Most forces have magnitude and direction and can be shown as a vector. A vector is illustrated by a line, the length of which is proportional to the magnitude on a given scale, and an arrow that shows the direction of the force.
- **Vector addition:** The sum of two or more vectors is called the resultant. The resultant of two concurrent vectors is obtained by

---

ABC of Orthopaedics and Trauma, First Edition. Edited by Kapil Sugand and Chinmay M. Gupte.
© 2018 John Wiley & Sons Ltd. Published 2018 by John Wiley & Sons Ltd.

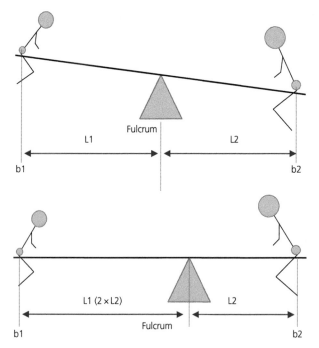

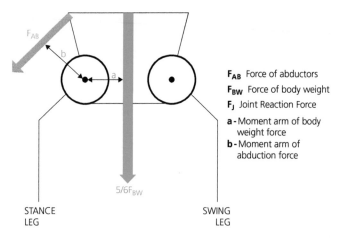

Figure 23.2 Free body diagram of the hip

Figure 23.1 Free-body diagram of two brothers on a seesaw, with b2 being twice the weight of b1, before and after calculation the moment arms to achieve equilibrium

constructing a vector diagram of the two vectors. The vectors to be added are arranged in tip-to-tail fashion. Where three or more vectors are to be added, they can be arranged in the same manner, and this is called a polygon. A line drawn to close the triangle or polygon (from start to finishing point) forms the resultant vector.

To illustrate these basic concepts, consider two brothers are building a seesaw. The older brother (b2) has a weight that is twice that of the younger brother (b1). Their setup is illustrated in Figure 23.1. In order for their seesaw to be balanced (in equilibrium), they would need to place the fulcrum correctly so that the moment arms of the brothers about the fulcrum are equal. Using the free-body diagram of the seesaw beam and given that the moment arm is the distance of the force from the fulcrum, then:

$$F(b1) \times L1 = Fb2 \times L2$$

rearranging this equation we get:

$$L1 / L2 = Fb2 / Fb1$$

The lighter brother would need to be twice the distance from the fulcrum to balance the seesaw with his older brother in Figure 23.1. Building on this simple example, the mechanics of the hip joint can be described, too. A number of assumptions are made, including: (1) the body is in equilibrium, and (2) there is a single-leg stance, (3) the weight of one leg is one-sixth of body weight. During single-leg stance, as is the case during walking, the head of the femur serves as fulcrum; the hip supports the weight of the patient's head, upper extremities, torso, and the contralateral leg. This situation is illustrated in Figure 23.2, where to maintain the pelvis level to the ground, the abductors (gluteus medius and minimus) pull pelvis

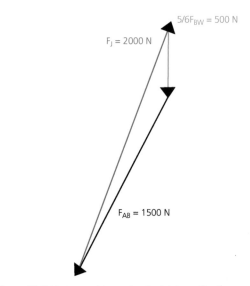

Figure 23.3 Vector used to resolve the joint reaction force

downward toward their attachments on the greater trochanter of the femur lateral to the fulcrum. This is an example of the hip joint to illustrate a free-body diagram:

Figure 23.2 represents the forces going through a hip during a single leg stance.

$$\text{In equilibrium}: F_{AB} \times b = 5/6\, F_{BW} \times a$$

Using the example of a 60 Kg patient, F_{BW} would be 600 N
If $a = 0.15\,\text{m}$ and $b = 0.05\,\text{m}$, then $F_{AB} = 500\,\text{N} \times 0.15\,\text{m} / 0.05\,\text{m} = 1500\,\text{N}$

The joint reaction force can then be calculated by resolving the vector triangle shown in Figure 23.3.

By using a free-body diagram to represent the forces across the hip joint, we can then think about how to change the joint reaction force. Examples would include reducing the body weight to decrease F_{BW}. Other ways include augmenting the abductor moment by adding in additional moments, such as those from using a walking stick in the contralateral hand or carrying a suitcase in the ipsilateral hand. Clinically, this translates into weight loss and walking aids reducing the symptoms of hip pathology by decreasing the joint reaction force. The free-body diagram also explains pathological signs. For example, patients with hip pathology often walk with a Trendelenberg gait, where they move their body over to the affected side, hence lateralising the line of action of F_{BW} and therefore reducing the size of *a* compensating for weakened abductors (often damaged during surgery). This, in turn, reduces F_J.

Deforming Forces

Understanding the forces acting on a joint is especially important in trauma. It allows the surgeon to understand how the fracture will deform and hence allows them to plan which implant and approach to reduction to use (Figure 23.4).

> For example, in subtrochanteric femur fractures, the deforming forces are:
> - **Shortening** – Quadriceps + Hamstrings + Adductors
> - **Proximal fragment**
>   - Flexion – Iliopsoas
>   - External rotation – Iliopsoas + Short external rotators
>   - Abducted – Gluteus medius/minimus
> - **Distal fragment**
>   - Adducted – Adductors (distal half of adductor magnus)

By understanding the deforming forces through the proximal femur, surgeons would plan to reduce a subtrochanteric fracture with traction on the distal fragment and by extending and internally rotating the proximal fragment. This is not always possible to do with a closed reduction, and therefore, the surgeon would be prepared to perform an open reduction *if required*. Another example of commonly encountered deforming forces is in proximal humerus where the humeral shaft is pulled medially by pectoralis major and the proximal fragment abducted by the deltoid.

Biomaterials

Orthopaedic surgeons use several materials in their day-to-day practise. A basic understanding of the principles of material behaviour is paramount to understanding the forces that go through a construct. In many cases, the forces a material can withstand vary according to the direction in which the forces are applied. These materials are named *Anisotropic*. For example, cortical bone is strongest in axial loading or compression but is not as strong under bending forces. Materials that behave identically irrespective of the direction of the force are termed *isotropic*; examples include metals, alloys, and polymers.

Stress and strain are important concepts in understanding how a material responds to an applied force. *Stress* is the force per unit area exerted on a body, causing it to change shape. It is a measure of the internal forces in a body between its particles in reaction to external forces applied on the body. Stress is represented by this equation:

$$\sigma = F\,/\,Ar$$

where: σ = stress, F = applied force, Ar = cross-sectional area

Strain is the *deformation of a solid due to stress*, or more simply, the increase in length divided by original length.

$$\varepsilon = dl\,/\,lo$$

where: ε = strain, dl = change in length, lo = original length

The relationship between stress and strain that a material displays is often represented as a stress–strain curve. The stress–strain curve of a material is unique to it and is found by recording the amount of deformation (strain) at distinct intervals of tensile/compressive loading (stress). Figure 23.5 shows an example stress–strain curve (also known as a force deformation curve).

The section of the curve labelled *a* shows a *linear* relationship between stress and strain where the material deforms when a load

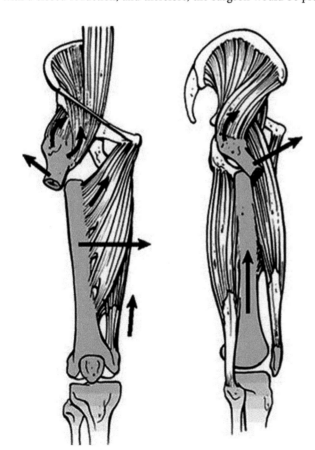

Figure 23.4 Deforming forces on the hip

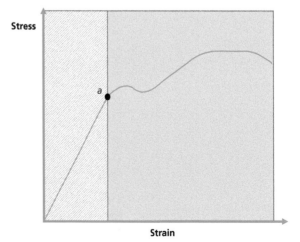

Figure 23.5 Stress strain curve showing the elastic limit *a*. The hatched section represents the elastic region and the shaded section the plastic deformation region

is applied to it and returns to its original shape when the load is removed – this is known as *elastic deformation*. When the force applied to the material deforms it to the extent that it no longer returns to its original dimensions, it is said to have undergone *plastic deformation*. This plastic deformation occurs beyond point in Figure 23.4. Where the relationship between force and deformation during elastic deformation is constant and is termed to be linear, plastic deformation is *nonlinear*.

> Materials are often described by their stress and strain properties. In order to describe a material more completely, Young's Modulus of elasticity is used and is calculated by *Stress/ Strain*. A higher modulus indicates a stiffer (less ability to resist deformation) material (e.g. ceramic > metal like titanium > cortical bone > cement > cancellous bone > tendons/ligaments > cartilage).

Materials that behave identically irrespective of the direction of the force are termed isotropic; examples include metals, alloys, and polymers. The force applied to a material per unit area is termed stress. The change in length of a material divided by the original length gives the strain.

Some materials exhibit time-dependent behaviour, termed *viscoelasticity*. This means the timing of the force being applied will affect the strain. Examples of viscoelastic properties include:

- *Creep:* A material has a constant force applied to it and strain increases with time.
- *Stress relaxation*: A material held in constant strain will require less stress to hold it there with time. An example of this is *hysteresis,* which is the difference between the stress–strain curve during loading and unloading as strain energy is lost as heat or friction.

These principles play an important part in the choice of materials used in the manufacture of implants as well as influencing decisions on what implants to use and how to apply them.

Further reading

Malik, S.S., and Malik, S.S. (2015, June). *Orthopaedic Biomechanics Made Easy* Cambridge University Press.

Online publication date. Print publication year: 2015. Online ISBN: 9781107360563.

Mavrogenis, A.F., Megaloikonomos, P.D., Panagopoulos, G.N., et al. (2017). Biomechanics in orthopaedics. *Journal of Biomedicine* 2: 89–93. doi:10.7150/jbm.19088. Available from http://www.jbiomed.com/v02p0089.htm.

Monk, A.P., Simpson, D.J., Riley, N.D., et al. (2013, September). Biomechanics in orthopaedics: considerations of the lower limb. *Surgery* (Oxford) 31 (9): 445–451.

Orthopaedic Biomechanics Made Easy Sheraz S. Malik and Shahbaz S. Malik.

Cambridge University Press. Online publication date: June 2015. Print publication year: 2015. Online ISBN: 9781107360563.

Surgery (Oxford). Volume 31, Issue 9, September 2013, Pages 445–451. Biomechanics in orthopaedics: considerations of the lower limb. A.P.Monk, D.J.Simpson, Nicholas D. Riley, D.W.Murray, H.S.Gill.

The Surgeon. Volume 2, Issue 3, June 2004, Pages 125–136. Contribution of biomechanics, orthopaedics and rehabilitation: The past, present and future. S.L-Y.WooM.ThomasS.S. ChanSaw.

Woo, S.L-Y., Thomas, M., and ChanSaw, S.S. (2004, June), Contribution of biomechanics, orthopaedics and rehabilitation: The past, present and future. *The Surgeon* 2 (3): 125–136.

CHAPTER 24

Tools of the Trade

Mike Rafferty

North West London Rotation, London, UK

OVERVIEW

- Theatres are designed to decrease infection rates with laminar flow.
- Implants are made of a variety of materials (metals, ceramics, or polymers). Each material has its pros and cons.
- Plates, screws, and K-wires are all used in operative fracture management.
- Fractures and joints can be immobilised using splints, plaster casts, and braces.

Theatre design and considerations

Theatres are sterile environments where protocols are in place to reduce the risk of infection. Outside clothes are changed for scrubs and outside shoes are changed for surgical shoes or clogs to ensure outside contamination is not brought in. Theatres should be entered only through the clean scrub room or the anaesthetic bay and not via the "dirty" or cleaning room.

Laminar flow

Laminar flow theatres aim to reduce the number of infective organisms in the theatre air by generating a continuous flow of bacteria free air. In laminar flow theatres, air is "changed" more than 300 times per hour, compared to standard positive pressure rates of 15–25 air changes per hour. Laminar flow theatres have less than 10 colony-forming units per metre cubed (CFU/m^3) compared to conventional theatres in which there are less than 180 CFU/m^3.

Other methods in reducing infection rates are outlined in Box 24.1.

Different operating tables and setups

Traction tables (Figure 24.1) are designed to aid in the reduction of lower limb fractures by counteracting the deforming forces across the fracture so that fixation can take place. Before using the traction table, care must be taken to ensure that the patient is completely secure on the table. This table can be used for intertrochanteric and subtrochanteric neck of femur fractures for procedures, such as cannulated and dynamic hip screws, and intramedullary femoral nailing. Intraoperative fluoroscopic screening is crucial to ensuring the best reduction possible. Fracture reduction is the cornerstone to successful orthopaedic outcomes, and time should be taken at this crucial step. The modern operating table can be adjusted to accommodate most positions. The majority of shoulder surgery is performed with the patient in the *beach chair* position, as shown in Figure 24.2.

Wrist and hand surgery is performed with the hand on an arm board, which can be connected to the normal table with the patient supine. Tourniquets are used regularly in limb surgery to reduce blood loss. A tourniquet machine maintains a continuous pressure to the tourniquet cuff. The limb must be exsanguinated first to prevent venous pooling in the limb, either through elevation or using a Rhys Davies exsanguinator (a.k.a. the sausage) before deploying the tourniquet. Tourniquet pressures should be set to ~100 mmHg above the patient's systolic blood pressure or 300 mmHg for lower limb and 250 mmHg for upper limb. The time the tourniquet is on for should be closely monitored. The regularly recommended tourniquet time is under *2 hours,* as longer times are associated with ischaemia and postoperative tourniquet pain.

Implant types

Hips

Neck of femur (NOF) fractures make up a large percentage of an orthopaedic surgeon's case load.

Displaced intracapsular fractures

These can be treated with a hemiarthroplasty, which replaces just the femur articulation (Figure 24.3a), or a total hip replacement (Figure 24.3b), which replaces the femur and acetabular articulations and has a liner in between them. The choice depends on patient factors.

ABC of Orthopaedics and Trauma, First Edition. Edited by Kapil Sugand and Chinmay M. Gupte.
© 2018 John Wiley & Sons Ltd. Published 2018 by John Wiley & Sons Ltd.

Box 24.1 **Methods to reduce infection rates in theatre**

- Laminar flow theatre design
- Less people in theatre
- Instruments covered during prolonged inactivity
- Instruments prepared in the sterile room
- Patient warming
- Prophylactic dose of antibiotics prior to implant insertion

Undisplaced intracapsular fractures

These can be treated with cannulated screws or a dynamic hip screw (DHS) (Figures 24.4 a and b).

Extracapsular fractures

These can be fixed with either a DHS or an intramedullary (IM) nail (Figures 24.5a and b). IM nails are usually used for subtrochanteric or unstable intratrochanteric fractures.

Knees

Total knee replacements (TKR) consist of three components, as shown in Figures 24.6a and b:

1 Femoral implant
2 Tibial component
3 Polyethylene insert that goes in between

If there is significant osteoarthritis of the patellofemoral joint, then patella resurfacing may be performed with a polyethylene liner fixed using cement to the back of the patella.

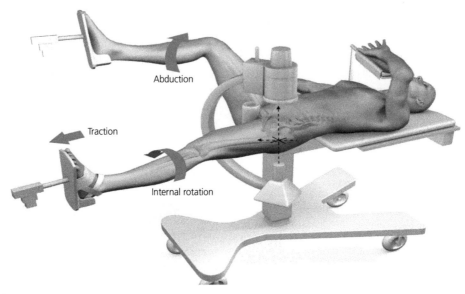

Figure 24.1 Traction table

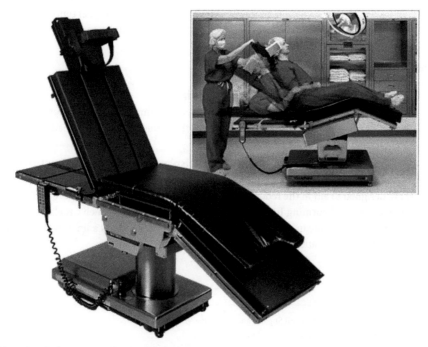

Figure 24.2 Patient should be in beach chair position for shoulder surgery

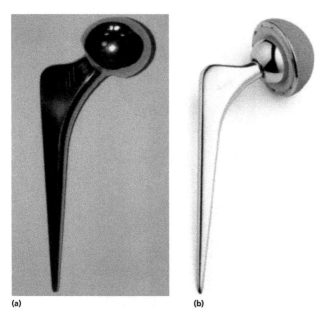

(a)　　　　　　　　(b)

Figure 24.3 (a) Hip hemiarthroplasty implant (b) Total hip replacement implant

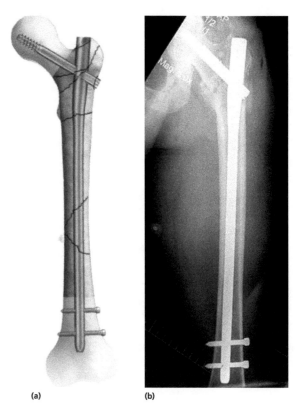

(a)　　　　　　　　(b)

Figure 24.5 (a) Intramedullary femoral nail (b) X-ray of intramedullary nail fixation

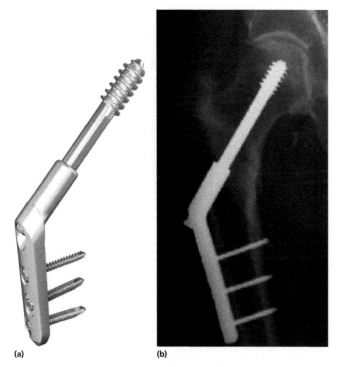

(a)　　　　　　　　(b)

Figure 24.4 (a) Dynamic hip screw (DHS) (b) Radiograph of a dynamic hip screw (DHS)

Shoulders

Shoulder replacements or hemiarthroplasties of the shoulder may be performed electively for severe osteoarthritis; or acutely for comminuted fractures of the shoulder where reconstruction is not technically possible (Figures 24.7a and b).

Implant sciences

Implant design

Ideal materials for implant manufacturing are outlined in Box 24.2 and Table 24.1.

Implant fixation

Total hip replacement (THR) may be cemented or noncemented.

- *Noncemented* implants are designed to allow osseointegration between the implant and the femoral canal. They rely on the patient having good bone stock. The femoral medullary canal is prepared and reamed down so the fit is cortex to cortex.
- *Cemented* implants have similar longevity. They require less reaming of the femoral canal, do not rely on the patient's bone stock to support the implant, and have a lower risk of intraoperative fracture. The use of cement will add 10–15 minutes to the operative time and will increase the rare risk of bone cement implantation syndrome (BCIS).

Cement

History of cement

Cement (Polymethyl methacrylate [PMMA]) was first used in dentistry and has grown in importance especially in joint replacements. In the 1950s, Sir John Charnley popularised cement use in orthopaedics while developing low-friction/torque hip implants that are credited as one of the key developments in the techniques and outcomes seen today.

Cement composition

Cement is resistant to body fluids, has low toxicity and can be moulded before it sets. Most cement comes as two separate components: a polymer powder and a monomer liquid. As the two are mixed, a viscous dough is formed with catalysts such as activators and initiators. The reaction between the two is exothermic, producing heat with a maximum in vivo temperature between 40–47 °C.

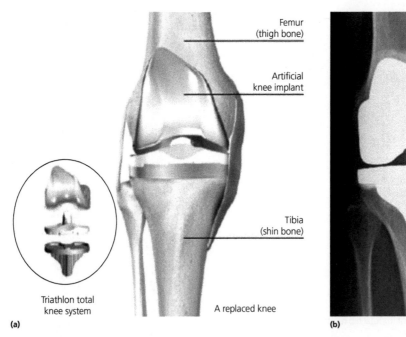

Femur
(thigh bone)

Artificial
knee implant

Tibia
(shin bone)

Triathlon total
knee system

A replaced knee

(a)

(b)

Figure 24.6 (a) Knee replacement implant (b) X-ray of a knee replacement

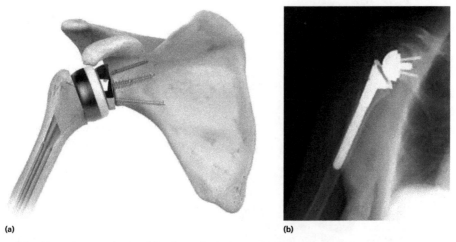

(a)

(b)

Figure 24.7 (a) Reverse total shoulder replacement implant (b) Radiograph of a (reverse total) shoulder replacement

Box 24.2 **Properties of the ideal implant material**

1 Chemically Inert
2 Non-toxic
3 Great strength
4 High fatigue resistance
5 Absolutely corrosion-proof
6 Good wear resistance
7 Inexpensive

A barium additive makes it radio-opaque on imaging and chlorophyll makes it green. Antibiotics are also added in to reduce risk of infected metalwork.

Cement preparation

Cementing is a time-dependent procedure, and care must be taken to ensure that all preparations have been completed and that the implants are ready. The cement timer starts the moment the two components come into contact. The four phases of cementing are shown in Box 24.3.

Bone cement implantation syndrome (BCIS)

Cementing into the femoral canal can cause an increase of up to 500 mmHg of pressure in the femoral canal. This can lead to displacement of fat, bone marrow, and cement, all of which may cause emboli. The residual cement monomer is a vasodilator and may lead to a drop in the patient's blood pressure. Other signs of BCIS are outlined in Box 24.4. The anaesthetist must be informed that the surgeon is about to cement so that the patient can be actively monitored and any changes in the patient's vital signs can be acted on swiftly.

Plates, screws, Kirschner (K-wires)

Plates

Plates must be strong enough not to fatigue or break but flexible enough to encourage bony union (Figure 24.8). A construct that is

Table 24.1 Implant composition

Implant	Composition types	Example	Pros/cons
Metal Alloys	Stainless steel Iron (63%), chromium (18%) nickel (16%), molybdenum (3%), carbon (0.03%)	Plates, screws, external fixators	Pros: • Strong • Ductile • Biocompatible • Relatively cheap Cons: Susceptible to crevis and stress corrosion
	<u>Titanium based</u> Titanium (89%), aluminium (6%), vanadium (4%), others (1%)	Intramedullary nails, plates	Pros: • Corrosion resistant • Biocompatible • Ductile • Fatigue resistant • MRI compatible Cons: Expensive, poor wear characteristics
	Cobalt-Chrome Cobalt 30–60%, chromium 20–30%, small amounts carbon, nickel, and molybdenum	Total knee replacements	Pros: • Corrosion resistant • Biocompatibility • Very strong Cons: Stress shielding and expensive
Ceramics	Alumina (aluminium oxide) Silica (silicon oxide) Hydroxyapatite (HA)	Femoral head, femoral stem HA coating	Pros: • Chemically inert • Best biocompatibility • Strong osteoconductive (HA coated stems) Cons: Brittle, very expensive
Polymers	Ultra-high molecular weight polyethylene (UHMWP)	Liner between articulating surfaces in hip and knee replacements	Pros: Strong, low friction Cons: Eventual wear and can cause debris and aseptic loosening

Box 24.3 **Cementing phases**

1 **Mixing phase**: Lasts up to 1 minute as the powder and liquid are mixed.
2 **Sticky phase:** 2–4 minutes. The cement is too sticky to handle and mould.
3 **Working phase**: 4–6 minutes. The cement is no longer sticky and is viscous enough to prevent blood and fluid from integrating with it reducing it strength.
4 **Hardening phase:** 7–10 minutes. Exothermic reaction as the cement heats.

Box 24.4 **Signs of BCIS**

• Hypoxia
• Hypotension
• Arrhythmias
• Heart failure
• Pulmonary arterial hypertension
• Cardiac arrest

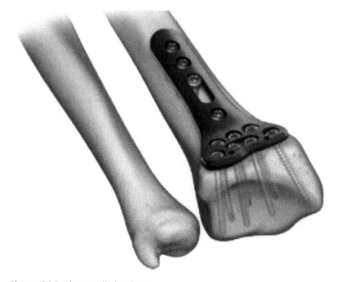

Figure 24.8 Plate applied to bone

too stiff may prevent the union. There are pre-contoured anatomically designed plates for most bones. Preoperative planning is crucial in selecting an implant.

Screws

Screws have different designs, based on their intended use (Figure 24.9).

• *Looking screws* have a thread in the head that will "lock" into the plate's locking holes. Locking into the plate increases the strength of the total construct.
• *Nonlocking screws* simply go though the holes in the plate. Their advantage is that since they do not lock into the plate they can provide compression as each turn of the screw advances the screw head further compressing the plate onto the bone.

Cancellous   Locking   Cortical

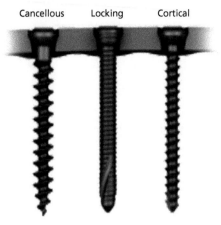

Figure 24.9 Screws with specific purposes

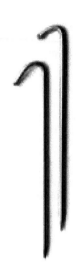

Figure 24.10 Two types of K-wires

Table 24.2 Indications for different types of sutures and clips

Absorbable sutures			
Monocryl		Fine suture that is made of one strand, which makes it suitable for closing skin as it causes less soft tissue reaction and absorbs quickly.	Used for skin closure.
Vicryl		Synthetic. Multiple strands are braided together, making it strong and preventing knots from slipping.	2' Vicryl is thick and used in deep tissues. 2-0 Vicryl is thinner and used in more superficial tissue.
PDS		Synthetic monofilament.	Slower absorption, thick good tensile strength. PDS is used in deeper tissues.
Nonabsorbable sutures			
Ethibond		Braided suture made of polyethylene terephthalate, which optimises its handling. It has to be manually removed.	Good for skin, minimal tissue reaction, sutures must be removed 10-14 days.
Fibrewire		This has a multistranded polyeythelene core and a braided jacket that gives it superior strength and breakage resistance.	Can be used in tendon repairs, Very strong.
Ethilon		A monofilament composed of nylon	Nylon (usually 3-0 or 4-0) is commonly used to close skin.
Other closure devices			
Staples		These have to be removed at 10–14 days, and this can be uncomfortable for the patient.	They are quick to use, which can be desirable in unstable trauma patients, but they rely on the skin edges already being closely opposed.
Dermabond		A cyanoacrylate tissue adhesive that holds wound ends together to allow healing. It also acts as a microbial barrier. Quicker than suturing and results in an equivalent cosmetic appearance.	Used for lacerations or incisions that are small and superficial.

- *Cortical* screws are designed to take hold of cortical bone. They are usually used in a bi-cortical way, meaning the screw thread goes through both the proximal and distal cortex.
- *Cancellous screws* have a deeper thread compared to cortical screws. They are designed to take hold in soft cancellous bone. *Partially threaded cancellous screws* have screw thread at the distal end but not proximally. Passing the threads past the fracture site will mean that there is compression between the screw head and the distal thread with each turn of the screw.

Kirschner wires (K-wires)

K-wires are 1.2–2 mm in diameter and are usually used in a temporary way to hold reductions (Figure 24.10). They are commonly used in wrist fractures and in paediatric fractures. Fractures are reduced and K-wires can be passed via stab incisions using an image intensifier to ensure they are correctly positioned. They are bent at the end and left protruding from the skin. K-wires are usually left in for 4–6 weeks and can be removed in clinic with a set of pliers.

Sutures

The art of suturing can only be perfected with practice. When selecting the suture material, you must ask yourself what you want it to do. Is the suture permanent, or do you want it to absorb with time? What type of tensile strength do you need? The general rule of suturing is to never close structures under tension, meaning that if you need to pull the knot extremely tight and strangle the tissues to close the tissues, then this closure is destined to fail. Instead, sharing the tension by closing in layers from deep to superficial is the preferred method so by the time you come to close the skin, it is already mostly opposed. Their indications are outlined in Table 24.2.

Wound management

Wounds that are grossly contaminated may be left open to allow the infection to drain out. The wound can be packed with either ribbon gauze or antibacterial dressing, which acts as a wick and allows infected tissues to drain. This requires regular wound management and dressing changes and frequent review, potentially in theatre, at 48–72 hours or as the clinical picture dictates.

Vacuum-assisted closure (VAC) devices are being used in greater frequency as their availability increases. Their advantages are outlined in Box 24.5. VAC devices work by siting a foam mesh over the wound and using a clear plastic dressing to achieve a vacuum seal (Figure 24.11). The pump can then be set to various pressure outputs and the fluid is drawn away from the wound and is stored in the canister attached to the pump which can be carried by the patient.

Box 24.5 **Advantages of VAC devices**

- Decrease frequency of dressing changes.
- Patients can be discharged with them and reviewed in clinic.
- Encourage granulation tissue to form and reduce healing times.

Postoperative weight-bearing status

The aim of orthopaedic surgery is to restore the patient to weight-bearing status as soon as safely possible. For lower limb fixation, you must ask yourself if the fixation can support the patient's body weight. For example, ankle fixation will need a time of non–weight-bearing of up to 6 weeks to allow the bone to start to unite. Union is confirmed radiologically and also on examination. The absence of pain is a good indicator of bony union.

Mobility aids

When reviewing a patient's weight-bearing status, think about the individual patient. An elderly patient may find that managing non–weight-bearing status is not possible and the patient might not be able to tolerate crutches; therefore, a frame can be used to keep some of the weight off the lower limb (Table 24.3).

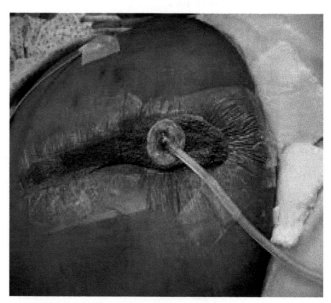

Figure 24.11 Vacuum-assisted closure

Table 24.3 Different types of mobility aids post operatively and their uses

Mobility aid	Picture	Uses
Sticks		A single walking stick may be used to reduce the joint forces after hip and knee surgery. The stick should be held in the hand of the good side (e.g. left hand if your right knee is problematic).
Walking Frames		Elderly patients who cannot tolerate elbow crutches may need a frame. Frames have the benefit of increased stability whilst upright compared to crutches, which require a level of upper body strength.
Crutches		Elbow crutches are less cumbersome than frames and are useful in younger patients. They can be used in patients who are fully or partially non– weight-bearing.

Table 24.4 Types of immobilisation devices for fractures or for postoperative use

	Types	Uses	Advantages/Disadvantages
Casts	**Plaster of Paris**	Fractures	**Pros**: Cheap. Can be moulded to allow three-point fixation to hold fractures in place **Cons**: Heavy, can irate the skin
	Fibreglass		**Pros**: Lighter than plaster and strong **Cons**: Only allows for limited moulding of its position
Splints	**Cricket pad splint**	To keep the leg straight (patella fractures)	**Pros**: Removable and does not irritate skin **Cons**: Bulky, often slips down the leg
	Futura splint	To stabilise the wrist after surgery, or treatment of soft tissue wrist injuries	**Pros**: Comfortable and removable **Cons**: Does not hold the fracture in place
Braces	**Hinge knee brace**	After surgery or injury to control the knee motion	**Pros**: Can set the range of motion and allow early rehabilitation and speed up recovery whilst for restricting movement **Cons**: Bulky, poorly tolerated
	Humeral brace	Used after a humeral shaft fracture	**Pros**: Also applies compression to the fracture "Sarmiento principle" **Cons**: It is initially painful to apply pressure over recent fracture
Air cast boot		After surgery, fractures and soft tissue injuries	**Pros**: More comfortable, absorbs shock, easier to apply and remove than a cast **Cons**: Heavy, bulkier

Immobilisation devices

After an operation, there may be a need to restrict movement of the limb to promote healing and union, which can be done with plaster, splints, or braces (Table 24.4).

Acknowledgement

All images provided in this chapter have been approved for commercial usage by Stryker (Michigan, USA).

References

James, M., Khan, W.S., Nannaparaju, M.R., et al. (2015). Current evidence for the use of laminar flow in reducing infection rates in total joint arthroplasty. *Open Orthopedic Journal* 9: 495–498.

Morykwas, M.J., Faler, B.J., Pearce, D.J., et al. (2001). Effects of varying levels of subatmospheric pressure on the rate of granulation tissue formation in experimental wounds in swine. *Annals of Plastic Surgery* 47 (5): 547–551.

Wheeless, C.R. (2012). Wheeless' Textbook of Orthopaedics. http://www.wheelessonline.com/ortho/extremity_tourniquets. Published 2012. Accessed September 22, 2017.

Index

Page numbers in *italic* refer to figures.
Page numbers in **bold** refer to tables.

ABC of Orthopaedics and Trauma, First Edition. Edited by Kapil Sugand and Chinmay M. Gupte.
© 2018 John Wiley & Sons Ltd. Published 2018 by John Wiley & Sons Ltd.